Kidney Disease
in Primary Care

Kidney Disease in Primary Care

EDITORS

Anil K. Mandal, M.D.
Professor of Medicine
Wright State University
School of Medicine
Chief, Section of Nephrology
Veterans Affairs Medical Center
Dayton, Ohio

N. Stanley Nahman Jr., M.D.
Associate Professor of Medicine
Division of Nephrology
Ohio State University
College of Medicine
Columbus, Ohio

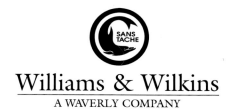

Williams & Wilkins
A WAVERLY COMPANY

BALTIMORE • PHILADELPHIA • LONDON • PARIS • BANGKOK
BUENOS AIRES • HONG KONG • MUNICH • SYDNEY • TOKYO • WROCLAW

EDITOR: Jonathan W. Pine, Jr.
MANAGING EDITOR: Leah Ann Kiehne Hayes
MARKETING MANAGER: Daniell T. Griffin
DEVELOPMENT EDITOR: Karen K. Gulliver
PRODUCTION COORDINATOR: Carol Eckhart
PROJECT EDITOR: Karen M. Ruppert
COVER AND INSIDE DESIGNER: Graphic World, Inc.
TYPESETTER: Graphic World, Inc.
PRINTER AND BINDER: Port City Press, Inc.

Copyright © 1998 Williams & Wilkins

351 West Camden Street
Baltimore, Maryland 21201-2436 USA

Rose Tree Corporate Center
1400 North Providence Road
Building II, Suite 5025
Media, Pennsylvania 19063-2043 USA

Accurate indications, adverse reactions and dosage schedules for drugs are provided in this book, but it is possible that they may change. The reader is urged to review the package information data of the manufacturers of the medications mentioned.

Printed in the United States of America

Library of Congress Cataloging-in-Publication Data
Kidney disease in primary care / editors, Anil K. Mandal, N. Stanley
    Nahman, Jr.
        p.   cm.
    Includes bibliographical references and index.
    ISBN 0-683-30057-1
    1. Kidneys—Diseases.   2. Primary care (Medicine)   I. Mandal,
Anil K.   II. Nahman, N. Stanley.
    [DNLM: 1. Kidney Diseases—diagnosis.   2. Kidney Diseases—
—therapy.   3. Primary Health Care.   4. Managed Care Programs—United
States.   WJ 302 K46 1998]
RC902.K533   1998
616.6′1—dc21
DNLM/DLC
for Library of Congress   97-37957
                                                                    CIP

The publishers have made every effort to trace the copyright holders for borrowed material. If they have inadvertently overlooked any, they will be pleased to make the necessary arrangements at first opportunity.

To purchase additional copies of this book, call our customer service department at **(800) 638-0672** or fax orders to **(800) 447-8438**. For other book services, including chapter reprints and large quantity sales, ask for the Special Sales Department.

Canadian customers should call **(800) 665-1148** or fax **(800) 665-0103**. For all other calls originating outside of the United States, please call **(410) 528-4223** or fax us at **(410) 528-8550**.

Visit Williams & Wilkins on the Internet: http://www.wwilkins.com or contact our customer service department at custserv@wwilkins.com. Williams & Wilkins customer service representatives are available from 8:30 am to 6:00 pm, EST, Monday through Friday, for telephone access.

98 99 00 01 02
1 2 3 4 5 6 7 8 9 10

To my cherished colleagues throughout the world who join
with me in promoting education and research in medicine.

ANIL K. MANDAL

Foreword

With tumultuous changes in the health care delivery system in the United States and the growing reliance of managed care organizations on primary care physicians, it becomes imperative that primary care providers have a systematic approach to clinical problems. The need is particularly acute in nephrology: treatment of end-stage renal disease is supported by the federal government, costing the taxpayers approximately $8 to $10 billion per year for the 200,000 individuals affected. The end-stage renal disease program is growing at a rate of 9 to 10% each year, with no sign of decrease in disease incidence. The major causes for the high mortality rate among patients entering treatment for end-stage renal disease include late referral and inadequate management of problems that fall under the auspices of the primary care physician. The average serum creatinine level at which a patient in the United States is first referred to a nephrologist is greater than 7 mg/dL, suggesting that patient education, vascular access, and preventive aspects of comorbid conditions such as high blood pressure, hyperlipidemia, and anemia are not administered in time to prevent future problems.

Kidney Disease in Primary Care is a book designed to provide primary care physicians with practical approaches to common clinical problems. Interpretation of common radiographic and laboratory techniques are discussed, as are approaches to fluid and electrolyte disturbances. The problem of patients presenting with elevated levels of urea and creatinine is discussed in depth, as are outpatient issues such as the proper approach to proteinuria and management strategies for hypertension, heart failure, edema, diabetes, glomerulonephritis, polycystic kidney disease, kidney stones, and urinary tract infection. In addition, the important issues of patient counseling, proper drug dosing, and nutritional approaches are covered in this very practical book.

Drs. Mandal and Nahman are respected clinicians and teachers who clarify the translation from primary care situations to subspecialty problems for their readers.

WILLIAM M. BENNETT, M.D.

Preface

The health care system is undergoing a revolution. Patient management decisions are being transferred from the specialist to both the primary care physician and allied health care providers. The subspecialty of nephrology has not been spared this swing of the clinical pendulum. Nephrology care is in fact an expanded version of primary care; it is simply directed to patients with renal disease or to patients receiving renal replacement therapy such as dialysis or renal transplantation.

Kidney Disease in Primary Care is designed to guide the primary care provider in the diagnosis and management of some of the more common diseases seen by the nephrologist. Dialysis issues have been left to the domain of the nephrologist; however, issues in transplantation that are relevant to immunosuppressant regimens currently in use are presented.

Because of the inherent complexity of the management issues in nephrology patients, the book has been prepared in a problem-oriented fashion. To serve the purpose of an on-the-spot nephrology consultant, the book combines a basic presentation of relevant pathophysiology followed by practical patient care strategies designed for the primary care provider.

This book will guide the primary care provider in the recognition and assessment of patients with renal problems as diverse as proteinuria, hypertension, and hypokalemia. Clinical features associated with each group of renal diseases are presented, allowing the clinician to synthesize a meaningful framework for diagnostic studies and therapeutic intervention.

The Contents are comprised of **common** nephrology problems the primary care provider may encounter on a daily basis. The reader will be provided with a concise understanding of the problem and appropriate diagnostic and therapeutic options. In addition, indications for nephrology referral are clearly delineated.

ANIL K. MANDAL
N. STANLEY NAHMAN JR.

Acknowledgment

The editors wish to express their deep appreciation for the services rendered by Betty Somers, senior secretary; Sherene Bush, secretary of the Department of Medicine; and all the secretaries of the Word Processing Center at Wright State University School of Medicine. They have all helped immensely in the preparation and completion of this book. The editors would also like to thank Jonathan W. Pine, Executive Editor, and Leah Hayes, Managing Editor, of Williams & Wilkins for their enthusiasm and interest in the preparation of the Nephrology contribution to the growing series of subspecialty textbooks designed for use by primary care providers.

Contributors

Anil Agarwal, M.D.
Assistant Professor of Medicine
Department of Internal Medicine
Division of Nephrology
Ohio State University
College of Medicine
Columbus, Ohio

Amir Alamir, M.D.
Senior Fellow in Nephrology
Department of Internal Medicine
Ohio State University
College of Medicine
Columbus, Ohio

Daniel Bloch, M.D., A.B.F.P.
Assistant Clinical Professor,
Managed Care Director
Department of Family Medicine
Ohio State University
College of Medicine
Columbus, Ohio

Sundeep S. Dhillon, M.D.
Senior Fellow in Nephrology
Department of Internal Medicine
Ohio State University
College of Medicine
Columbus, Ohio

Patrick J. Fahey, M.D.
Associate Professor of Family Medicine
Ohio State University
College of Medicine
Columbus, Ohio

Michael E. Falkenhain, M.D.
Assistant Professor of Medicine
Division of Nephrology
Ohio State University
College of Medicine
Columbus, Ohio

Nabil Farhan, M.D.
Senior Fellow in Nephrology
Department of Internal Medicine
Ohio State University
College of Medicine
Columbus, Ohio

Shelly M. Heidelbaugh, M.D.
Senior Resident in Internal Medicine
Ohio State University
College of Medicine
Columbus, Ohio

Beth A. Holthausen, M.S., R.D., L.D.
Primary Care Dietitian
Nutrition and Food Service
Veterans Affairs Medical Center
Dayton, Ohio

P. George John, M.D., F.R.C.P.
Associate Professor of Family Medicine
Wright State University
School of Medicine
Dayton, Ohio

Neil Katz, M.D.
Assistant Clinical Professor
of Radiological Studies
Wright State University
School of Medicine
Assistant Chief, Nuclear Medicine Service
Veterans Affairs Medical Center
Dayton, Ohio

Julie Beck Kendle, Pharm.D.
Post-Doctoral Fellow
in Infectious Diseases
Ohio State University
College of Pharmacy
Columbus, Ohio

Abdulla Khan, M.D.
Resident in Medicine
Wright State University
School of Medicine
Dayton, Ohio

James L. Knepler, Jr., M.D.
Senior Resident in Internal Medicine
Ohio State University
College of Medicine
Columbus, Ohio

Stephanie E. Ladson-Wofford, M.D.
Assistant Professor of Medicine
Division of Nephrology
Ohio State University
College of Medicine
Columbus, Ohio

John A. Larry, M.D.
Assistant Professor of Clinical Medicine
Division of Cardiology
Ohio State University
College of Medicine
Columbus, Ohio

Anil K. Mandal, M.D.
Professor of Medicine
Wright State University
School of Medicine
Chief, Section of Nephrology
Veterans Affairs Medical Center
Dayton, Ohio

Wanda G. Miller, M.S.N, R.N., C.S., A.N.P.
Adjunct Faculty
Department of Family Medicine
Wright State University
School of Nursing
Veterans Affairs Medical Center
Dayton, Ohio

N. Stanley Nahman, Jr., M.D.
Associate Professor of Medicine
Division of Nephrology
Ohio State University
College of Medicine
Columbus, Ohio

Sucharita Nalagatla, M.D.
Chief Resident in Medicine
Wright State University
School of Medicine
Attending Physician
Veterans Affairs Medical Center
Dayton, Ohio

David E. Neal, M.D.
Assistant Professor of Radiology
Ohio State University
College of Medicine
Columbus, Ohio

Todd E. Pesavento, M.D.
Assistant Clinical Professor of Medicine
Division of Nephrology
Ohio State University
College of Medicine
Columbus, Ohio

Brad H. Rovin, M.D.
Associate Professor of Medicine and Pathology
Division of Nephrology
Ohio State University
College of Medicine
Columbus, Ohio

Shiv K. Seth, Ph.D., R.Ph.
Clinical Assistant Professor of Pharmacy
Ohio State University
College of Pharmacy
Columbus, Ohio

Bruce T. Vandehoff, M.D.
Associate Director
Grant Family Practice Residency
Grant/Riverside Methodist Hospitals
Columbus, Ohio

Kenneth M. Vitellas, M.D.
Clinical Instructor
Department of Radiology
Ohio State University Medical Center
Columbus, Ohio

William A. Wilmer, M.D.
Assistant Professor of Medicine
Division of Nephrology
Ohio State University
College of Medicine
Columbus, Ohio

Gerhard H. Wirnsberger, M.D.
Staff Nephrologist
Department of Internal Medicine
Karl-Franzens University
School of Medicine
Graz, Austria

Contents

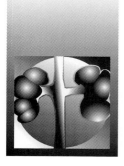

CHAPTER 1

Urinalysis and Assessment of Urinary Electrolytes

Sundeep S. Dhillon
N. Stanley Nahman, Jr.

URINALYSIS

Urinalysis is the most frequently performed clinical laboratory test in the United States. It is a simple but invaluable test in the clinical evaluation of patients with unexplained renal insufficiency, urinary tract symptoms, hypertension, or suspected renal dysfunction. It may help distinguish glomerular from tubulointerstitial disease and thus narrow the differential diagnosis in patients with elevated serum levels of creatinine. Additionally, the urinalysis can be used to monitor disease activity in patients with known renal disease.

Routine urinalysis consists of three parts:

- Evaluation of the physical characteristics of the urine
- Chemical analysis via the dipstick
- Microscopic evaluation of urinary sediment

Sample Collection

Obtaining the Specimen

The urine should be collected in a clean, disposable container that should be sterile if the sample is intended for culture. For routine analysis, at least 15 mL of urine is required from adults. The most common method for obtaining the specimen is the "clean-catch," in which a midstream sample of urine is obtained after appropriate preparation of the external genitalia. The following steps decrease the risk of contamination and allow the specimen to be used for both urine cultures and routine urinalysis:

1. The external genitalia are cleaned with a soap solution.
2. Before voiding, the foreskin is retracted in males and the labia are separated in females.

3. The beginning and end of the urinary stream are not collected; only the midstream flow is collected for analysis or culture.

If urine cultures are not anticipated, extensive external cleansing and the use of a sterile container can be omitted. Bladder catheterization is necessary if a patient has difficulty voiding spontaneously. In females, bladder catheterization may minimize vaginal contamination of the urine, but it is not regularly indicated because of the risk of infection. Suprapubic aspiration of the bladder may be used when infants, children, or adults cannot provide a voluntary specimen.

The first voided sample of the day is the best specimen for analysis. Urine obtained at this time is in its most concentrated and acid form; the relative acidity is conducive to preservation of cellular elements and casts.

Examination of the Specimen

Fresh urine specimens should be examined immediately. Over time, urine stored at room temperature is subject to bacterial overgrowth (which leads to urinary alkalinization) and decomposition of the urinary sediment. Dissociation of cellular elements and casts is further accelerated in dilute or alkaline urine. When assessment of a urine sample is delayed, the authors have stored specimens at 4° C for up to 12 hours.

Chemical analysis of urine is done using a dipstick consisting of multiple test reagents. For analysis, the test areas of the dipstick should be completely immersed in fresh, well-mixed, uncentrifuged urine and then removed immediately. Interpretation of the chemical analysis is based on colorimetric changes of individual test pads.

Microscopic evaluation of urinary sediment should be conducted on the pellet obtained following centrifugation. Approximately 10 to 15 mL of urine is centrifuged at 2000 rpm for 5 minutes. The supernatant is saved for treatment with sulfosalicylic acid (SSA), when indicated. The sediment is aspirated, a drop is placed on a microscope slide, it is covered with a coverslip, and then examined under low (100×) and high (400×) power.

Evaluation of Physical Characteristics of the Urine

See Table 1.1.

Color and Appearance

The color of urine can range from yellow to amber, depending on the concentration. Pale or colorless urine

results from dilution from high fluid intake, diuretic use, or polyuria associated with diabetes mellitus or diabetes insipidus. Common pathologic alterations of urine color include:

- Turbid, creamy appearance from heavy pyuria
- Red to black color from red blood cells or heme pigments
- Yellow–brown or yellow–green color from bilirubin or oxidized bilirubin (biliverdin), respectively

Specific Gravity

The specific gravity of urine is the weight-to-volume ratio of urine compared with the ratio of an identical volume of distilled water at a constant temperature. The ratio indicates the concentration of dissolved material in the urine and, therefore, provides information about renal concentration and dilution. Under appropriate clinical circumstances, the urine-specific gravity can also provide information on the volume status of the patient (the specific gravity tends to be high in dehydrated patients and low in patients with volume-replete states). The physiologic range of urine-specific gravity is from 1.003 to 1.035, with 1.000 used as the standard for distilled water.

Specific gravity is affected by both particle weight and particle number, and the latter is the main variable affecting urine osmolarity. Therefore, when substances with high molecular weights (higher than the molecular weights of normal urine solutes) such as glucose, mannitol, protein, and radiographic contrast media are present in the urine, specific gravity is significantly higher than that expected from the presence of normal urinary solutes. For example, high urinary concentrations of intravenous radiographic contrast media often result in urine-specific gravity beyond the physiologic range (>1.035).

Measuring specific gravity Urine-specific gravity is measured using a urinometer or refractometer. A urinometer is a hydrometer floated in a volume of urine. The relative buoyancy in urine, when compared with water, permits determination of the specific gravity of a given urine sample. A refractometer determines urine-specific gravity by measuring the refractive index (the ratio of the speed of light in air versus a solution). The degree of refraction is proportional to the density of the solution. An advantage of this technique is that the specific gravity can be determined from a single drop of urine.

Recently, reagent strips have been developed to measure specific gravity. These strips contain acid groups, which dissociate in proportion to the ionic

Urinalysis: Diagnostic Implications of Physical Characteristics and Chemical Analysis   TABLE 1.1

Characteristics	Cause	Diagnostic Indication
Color or Appearance		
Pale or colorless	Dilute urine	Polyuria
		Diabetes insipidus
		Diabetes mellitus
Turbid	Pyuria	UTI
Red–black	Hematuria	Upper or lower tract bleeding
Yellow–brown	Bilirubinuria	Hyperbilirubinuria
Yellow–green	Biliverdinuria[a]	Hyperbilirubinuria
Specific Gravity		
Very low	Dilute urine	Water loading
		Compulsive water drinking
		Beer drinking
		Diabetes insipidus
Very high	Concentrated urine or excess osmols	Pre-renal states
		Osmotic diuresis
Very high, nonphysiologic	Presence of exogenous osmols	Presence of glucose
		Presence of mannitol
		Presence of radiographic contrast material
Chemical Analysis (Dipstick)		
Presence of protein	Albuminuria	Glomerulopathy
Presence of glucose	Glucosuria	Diabetes mellitus
		Tubular disorders
Blood	Hemoglobinuria	Hematuria
	Myoglobinuria	Hemolysis
		Rhabdomyolysis
Chemical Analysis (Dipstick and SSA)		
Dip (+), SSA (+)	Albuminuria	Glomerulopathy
Dip (−), SSA (+)	Bence Jones proteinuria	Multiple myeloma

[a] The oxidized form of bilirubin.
UTI, urinary tract infection; SSA, sulfosalicylic acid.

concentration of the urine. A color change indicates the specific gravity of the sample under study.

Chemical Analysis of the Urine via Dipstick

The routine chemical evaluation of the urine utilizes multiple test reagent strips (dipsticks), which are dipped into the sample of interest. A given test strip has eight to nine reagent pads, which allow for qualitative and quantitative measurements of various parameters, including:

- Specific gravity
- Leukocyte esterase
- pH
- Protein (albumin)
- Glucose
- Ketones
- Bilirubin and associated degradation products
- Heme pigments

The reaction times for the development of each parameter range from immediately to 120 seconds. To maintain viability, reagent strips should be stored capped in the original container at room temperature. Exposure to moisture, heat, sunlight, and volatile substances should be avoided.

Urinary pH
Physiologic urinary pH ranges from 4.5 to 7.9. Urinary pH increases after a meal (the postprandial alkaline tide) and decreases with fasting.

Most brands of dipsticks use two indicators, methyl red and bromthymol blue, which provide the color change to identify the exact urinary pH. Litmus paper or nitrazine paper may be used if pH is the only information desired from a given urine sample.

Persistently acid urine   The metabolism of dietary protein generates 50 to 100 mEq per day of fixed acid that must be excreted by the kidney; thus, high protein intake is one cause of persistently acid urine. Other causes include:

- Fever
- Gout
- Severe potassium depletion
- Hyperaldosteronism
- Metabolic acidosis (excluding renal tubular acidosis)
- Ileostomy drainage
- Diarrhea
- Cranberry juice ingestion

Persistently alkaline urine   Conversely, urine pH is persistently alkaline in association with:

- Metabolic alkalosis
- Distal renal tubular acidosis
- Urinary tract infection with urease-producing organisms
- Administration of sodium bicarbonate, sodium or potassium citrate, or acetazolamide

Protein (Albumin)

Proteinuria (albuminuria) is an important marker of renal disease. Normal urinary protein excretion is less than 150 mg/day. Normal urinary protein consists of 60% filtered serum proteins (40% albumin, 15% immunoproteins, and 5% other plasma proteins) and 40% Tamm-Horsfall mucoprotein. Tamm-Horsfall protein is secreted by the cells of the thick ascending limb of the loop of Henle and forms the matrix of tubular casts.

Several transient causes of proteinuria are independent of glomerular disease, including fever, exercise, and upright posture. In contrast, persistent proteinuria is either glomerular or tubulointerstitial in origin. Glomerular proteinuria is often in the nephrotic range (>3 g/day) and consists primarily of albumin. Minor increases in urine albumin excretion (>30 mg/day or 20 μg/min) are termed microalbuminuria. The presence of micro-albuminuria is a strong risk factor for the development of overt nephropathy in both type I

and type II diabetes mellitus and should be aggressively pursued if present.

Methods used to detect proteinuria

DIPSTICK   Proteinuria can be detected via a dipstick. An acid buffer is added to the reagent to maintain a constant pH of 3, which in the absence of urine protein produces a yellow color. False–positive results occur with alkaline urine because increased pH can change the color of the indicator in the absence of protein. Quaternary ammonium compounds and phenazopyridine are also associated with false–positive results, as is gross hematuria.

False–negative results (albumin that remains undetected by this method) are associated with very dilute samples. The reagent test pad for protein is very sensitive for albumin but will not detect Bence Jones proteins (immunoglobulin light chains). The presence of urinary light chains can be detected with SSA. If the dipstick demonstrates negative or trace proteinuria and the patient is at risk for multiple myeloma, the urine should be checked using SSA or the heat test.

SULFOSALICYLIC ACID   Proteinuria can also be detected by an acid protein precipitant. The most commonly used agent is a 20% solution of SSA. SSA will detect all proteins, including Bence Jones proteins, glycoproteins, globulins, and albumin. Bence Jones proteins are immunoglobulin light chains that are present in the urine of patients with plasma cell disorders such as multiple myeloma, plasma cell leukemia, and plasmacytoma. The presence of Bence Jones proteinuria is suggested by a positive SSA result in conjunction with a dipstick test that is negative for albumin. Quantitation of proteinuria using SSA is based on the degree of turbidity following the addition of 8 drops of SSA to 10 mL urine. False–positive results may occur if tolbutamide, large doses of penicillin, sulfonamides, or radiographic contrast media are present in the urine. False–negative results can be caused by a highly alkaline or dilute urine.

HEAT (PUTNAM) TEST   Proteinuria can be detected by heat precipitation of Bence Jones proteins. Five milli-liters of urine is centrifuged in a 15-mL test tube, and supernatant is pipetted out in another 15-mL test tube. One milliliter of 2M acetate buffer (pH 4.9) is added to the supernatant, and the test tube is kept in an incubation bath at 56° C for 15 minutes. A precipitate will form if Bence Jones proteins are present in the urine. By increasing the bath temperature to 100° C for 3 minutes, the precipitate will dissolve and the urine will be clear again. By reducing the bath temperature to

37° C, precipitate will reappear if Bence Jones proteins are present in the urine.

Glucose

Glucosuria is detected by color change resulting from the oxidation of glucose by glucose oxidase. The glucose oxidase test is specific for glucose and does not detect other carbohydrates, such as fructose and lactose. False–negative results occur in patients with high urinary concentrations of vitamin C, which inhibits the enzymatic reaction and, thus, the color change. Glucosuria reflects pathologic levels of urinary glucose and results from conditions in which the renal threshold for glucose is exceeded (e.g., diabetes mellitus) and from tubular disorders of glucose reabsorption (e.g., renal glucosuria).

Blood Pigment

The test reagent for occult blood uses the peroxidase-like activity of hemoglobin and myoglobin. In most reagent strips, the indicator that is oxidized is tetramethylbenzidine. This method to detect hemoglobinuria and myoglobinuria is able to identify intact red blood cells because the cells lyse on the test pad, thus freeing the hemoglobin. Because of the lack of specificity of this test, a diagnosis of hemoglobinuria or myoglobinuria is often made when the dipstick is positive for blood and there is an associated absence of intact red blood cells on microscopic examination. The sensitivity of the test for true hematuria is quite good: five intact red blood cells per microliter is the lower threshold. False–negative results may occur in the presence of elevated urinary levels of ascorbic acid. Pigmented antiseptic solutions (povidone–iodine) may give false–positive results.

Leukocyte Esterase and Nitrite

The presence of pyuria and bacteriuria is determined through the use of reagent strips that detect leukocytes by reacting with leukocyte esterase. Leukocyte esterase generates an indoxyl, which reacts with a diazo salt on the reagent pad to produce a purple color in 60 to 120 seconds.

Gram–negative bacteriuria may be detected by the enzymatic conversion of nitrate to nitrite. Nitrites are produced by Gram–negative bacteria and react with either *p*-arsanilic acid or sulfanilamide, causing a color change on the reagent strip. Detection of nitrites to diagnose urinary tract infection has several important limitations. False–positive results can occur if urine is left standing at room temperature (allowing organisms

to produce nitrite). False–negatives results can occur as a result of:

- The presence of bacteria that do not form nitrite
- Inadequate time for bacteria to generate nitrite
- Enzymatic conversion of nitrite to nitrogen

Despite these limitations, use of the leukocyte esterase and nitrite tests together result in a sensitivity of 85% and a specificity of 65% for Gram-negative urinary tract infection associated with greater than 10 colony-forming units per milliliter.

Microscopic Evaluation of Urinary Sediment

Preparation of urinary sediment for microscopic evaluation should be conducted in the standard fashion discussed at the beginning of this chapter to produce comparable results. Initially, the slide should be examined on low power to scan for the presence of casts, and since placement of the coverslip tends to push casts to the periphery of the slide, scanning the edges may be more rewarding. High power is then used to identify cells and types of casts.

Cellular Elements of Urinary Sediment
See Table 1.2.

Erythrocytes Red blood cells are not normally found in the urine. When present, they appear as pale, smooth, biconcave disks (Fig. 1.1A). Red cells may lyse in alkaline or severely hypotonic urine, and the membranes become colorless and empty. In hypertonic urine, the cells will shrink and crenate, with the resulting spiky appearance. Red cells are smaller than leukocytes and epithelial cells but are larger than fungi; yeast cells can be distinguished from red cells by their ovoid shape, evidence of budding or pseudohyphae, and the presence of a doubly refractile border.

DIAGNOSTIC IMPLICATIONS OF ERYTHROCYTES Hematuria indicates glomerular or lower urinary tract bleeding. The microscopic morphology of red blood cells can help localize the site of bleeding. Acanthocytes are dysmorphic red blood cells associated with glomerular bleeding (Fig. 1.1B); greater than 5% acanthocyturia in a urine sample is over 90% specific for glomerular hematuria. However, the most specific sign of glomerular bleeding is the presence of a red blood cell cast (discussed below). The presumed cause of the morphologic change in cell shape is passage through rents in the glomerular capillary basement membrane.

Acanthocytes may be doughnut-shaped or spherical but microcytic, or they may demonstrate membrane blebs (Mickey Mouse ears).

Leukocytes   Normal urine does not contain leukocytes; when they do appear in the urine, they are spherical and larger in size than red blood cells. This size difference is similar to that seen between leukocytes and red cells on a Wright stain of peripheral blood. When present, leukocytes can be distinguished from other cells by the presence of cytoplasmic granules or lobulated nuclei.

DIAGNOSTIC IMPLICATIONS OF LEUKOCYTES Pyuria implies inflammation from infectious or noninfectious sources. Most urinary leukocytes are neutrophils; however, eosinophiluria may occur in a high percentage of patients with drug-induced allergic interstitial nephritis. Hansel's stain (methylene blue, eosin y, and methanol) can be used to identify eosinophils. Additional clinical signs of allergic interstitial nephritis include fever, skin rash, and peripheral blood eosinophilia.

Epithelial cells   Epithelial cells may appear in the urine and generally consist of tubular epithelia (Fig. 1.1A), transitional epithelia from the ureters or bladder, or squamous epithelia from the vaginal vault. Tubular epithelial cells are slightly larger than leukocytes and exhibit distinct, laterally placed nuclei. Transitional epithelial cells are rounded with small tail-like projections and may be slightly larger than tubular epithelial cells. Squamous epithelial cells are large, irregularly shaped cells with nuclei that approximate the size of leukocytes.

DIAGNOSTIC IMPLICATIONS OF EPITHELIAL CELLS Large numbers of renal tubular epithelial cells suggest tubular damage, as is associated with acute tubular necrosis. The presence of transitional epithelial cells is of no specific pathologic significance, and large numbers of squamous epithelial cells indicate vaginal contamination of the sample.

Casts in Urinary Sediment

Casts are formed in the distal tubule and collecting ducts of the nephron. Tamm-Horsfall protein, secreted

---

TABLE 1.2   Diagnostic Implications of Cells and Casts Found in the Urinary Sediment

Element in Sediment	Cause	Diagnostic Indication
Cells		
Erythrocytes: normal morphology	Bleeding at any level of the urinary tract	Renal or urologic disease
Erythrocytes: acanthocytes	Glomerular bleeding	Glomerulopathy
Leukocytes: polymorphonuclear leukocytes	Inflammation at any level of the urinary tract	Infection Noninfectious inflammation
Leukocytes: eosinophils	Allergic interstitial nephritis	Drug-induced allergy
Epithelial cells: tubular	Slough from renal tubule	Generalized damage to nephron
Epithelial cells: squamous	Typically vaginal contamination of sample	Vaginal contamination of sample
Casts		
Hyaline	Tamm-Horsfall protein	Normal finding Decreased renal perfusion
Red cell	Glomerular bleeding	Glomerulopathy Glomerulonephritis
Leukocyte	Renal parenchymal inflammation	Pyelonephritis Interstitial nephritis Acute glomerulonephritis
Granular	Hyaline cast with granular matrix	Tubular damage
Granular: densely pigmented "muddy brown"	Sloughed tubular cells	Acute tubular necrosis
Granular: waxy appearance	Degenerated granular cast	May indicate tubular damage
Broad	Slow urine flow in dilated collecting ducts	Chronic renal failure

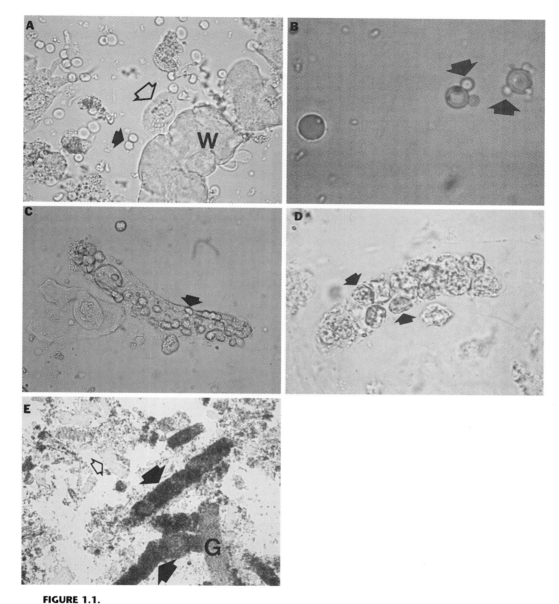

FIGURE 1.1.

Examples of elements found in unstained samples of urinary sediment. **A.** Erythrocytes *(solid arrow)* of normal morphology. A waxy cast *(W)* and tubular epithelial cell *(open arrow)* are also present (800×). **B.** Acanthocytes as seen in patients with glomerular bleeding. Note character-istic blebs *(arrows)* in the cell membrane. A normal-appearing red cell is seen at *left* (1600×). **C.** Red cell cast from a patient with glomerulonephritis. The erythrocytes are well preserved in the matrix of the cast. The *arrow* indicates an intact erythrocyte (800×). **D.** Leukocyte cast in a patient with interstitial nephritis. There are several leukocytes (two of which are indicated by the *arrows* in this particular cast) (1000×). **E.** Numerous casts: granular cast *(G)*, densely pigmented granular (muddy brown) casts *(solid arrows),* and hyaline cast *(open arrow)* (200×).

in the thick ascending limb of the loop of Henle and in the distal tubule, is thought to form the matrix of casts. They are cylindrical in shape (molded in the form of the tubule) with parallel sides and rounded ends. Cast formation is promoted by urinary stasis, an acid pH, increased osmolarity, and proteinuria.

Casts should be distinguished from random collections of cellular debris and mucous strands; the former generally lack a distinct border, and the latter often exhibit irregular, tapered ends.

Identification of specific types of casts helps to narrow the differential diagnosis in patients with renal dysfunction and may be considered a "poor man's renal biopsy."

Hyaline casts Hyaline casts consist of Tamm-Horsfall protein and have no evidence of granularity and cellular elements. For these reasons, hyaline casts are transparent and colorless and can be easily missed. Scanning the sediment with decreased light intensity may help distinguish hyaline casts from the background.

DIAGNOSTIC IMPLICATIONS OF HYALINE CASTS A few hyaline casts can be seen in normal urine, and their numbers can increase after exercise or in clinical conditions associated with decreased renal perfusion, such as congestive heart failure and dehydration.

Red blood cell casts Red cell casts contain distinct erythrocytes (Fig. 1.1C) and may have orange–brown pigmentation. A degenerating red cell cast may show portions of red cells with a pigmented, granular matrix.

DIAGNOSTIC IMPLICATIONS OF RED BLOOD CELL CASTS Mixed red cell–white cell casts, as well as white cell casts, may be present in patients with acute glomerulonephritis. Proteinuria is also present. There is less evidence of inflammation (fewer white cell casts), and the sediment is dominated by granular casts and acanthocytes in patients with chronic forms of glomerulonephritis and in patients with healed glomerular lesions. Patients with acute renal failure who have red cell casts in the urine may have acute glomerulonephritis, and renal biopsy should be strongly considered.

Leukocyte casts Leukocyte casts can be identified by the presence of nucleated or granular polymorphonuclear leukocytes in the cast matrix (Fig. 1.1D). The leukocytes should be contained within the border of the cast; cells that protrude beyond the border of a cast may not be fused with the matrix and likely represent free-floating cells "stuck" to the cast. Ambiguities can be clarified by gently tapping the edge of the coverslip with the tip of a pen or pencil while watching for the cell to

be dislodged. Under these conditions, free-floating cells frequently dissociate from the cast, whereas leukocytes truly engulfed in the matrix do not separate.

DIAGNOSTIC IMPLICATIONS OF LEUKOCYTE CASTS Leukocyte casts are associated with all forms of renal inflammation, including infectious conditions such as acute pyelonephritis, and noninfectious conditions such as acute and chronic interstitial nephritis, glomerulonephritis, and vasculitis.

Granular casts Granular casts are identified by the granular matrix within the borders of the cast and by the lack of distinct cellular elements (Fig. 1.1E). The granular matrix may range from very fine to extremely coarse. Degenerated granular casts may develop a homogenous appearance, with a matrix that has the consistency of paraffin (a waxy cast; Fig. 1.1, A and E).

DIAGNOSTIC IMPLICATIONS OF GRANULAR CASTS The presence of granular casts indicates generalized damage to the tubules. Granular casts may be colorless or stain yellow or orange if other pigments are present in the urine (e.g., in the case of bilirubinuria). In the absence of chromogens, granular casts that are

Summary of Diagnosis

- A dipstick negative for protein in a patient with anemia or renal failure should raise the suspicion of Bence Jones proteins (light chain immunoglobulin).
- A dipstick positive for leukocyte esterase and nitrite in a patient with dysuria is evidence of a urinary tract infection and indicates the need for treatment.
- Normal or near normal urinalysis in a patient with acute renal failure is associated with pre-renal failure.
- Microscopic hematuria without proteinuria is more suggestive of bleeding from the urinary tract (the pelvis, ureter, or bladder) than from glomerular or tubular sources.
- Abnormally shaped red blood cells (acanthocytes) on microscopy accompanied by 2+ to 4+ proteinuria suggest glomerular disease.
- Many eosinophils on urinalysis in a patient with impaired renal function are a strong indication of drug-induced acute interstitial nephritis, warranting review and discontinuation of the suspected medication.

densely pigmented (dark brown or black; called "muddy brown") represent degenerated cellular debris from sloughed tubular epithelia. These casts are associated with the diagnosis of acute tubular necrosis (Fig. 1.1E). A true muddy brown cast remains opaque under high power with maximal light intensity.

Broad casts As the name suggests, broad casts have a larger diameter than other casts and likely originate from dilated collecting ducts.

DIAGNOSTIC IMPLICATIONS OF BROAD CASTS Broad casts are associated with chronic renal disease and are suggested to result from slow urine flow through di-

lated collecting ducts. A careful urinalysis, including microscopic evaluation of urinary sediment, should facilitate a presumptive diagnosis in a patient with proteinuria, impaired renal function, or both. Diagnostic considerations based on the urinalysis are presented in Table 1.3.

ASSESSMENT OF URINARY ELECTROLYTES

The evaluation of urinary electrolytes via the random spot test (Table 1.4) based on a single voided sample of urine, with volumes as small as 1 to 2 mL, provides information concerning renal tubular concentrating

Diagnostic Considerations Based on the Urinalysis   TABLE 1.3

Pattern of Disease	Characteristic Features on Urinalysis	Additional Urinary and Clinical Findings
Glomerular Disease		
Glomerulopathy	Proteinuria	Acanthocytes
		Red cell casts
Acute glomerulonephritis	Red cell casts	Acanthocytes
	Proteinuria	Leukocyte casts
Tubulointerstitial Disease		
Pyelonephritis	Pyuria	
	Leukocyte casts	
	Positive urine cultures	
Interstitial nephritis	Pyuria	
	Leukocyte casts	
	Sterile urine	
Allergic interstitial nephritis	Eosinophiluria	Peripheral blood eosinophilia
	Pyuria	Skin rash
	Leukocyte casts	Fever
	Sterile urine	
Acute tubular necrosis	Muddy brown casts	Granular casts
	Epithelial casts	Tubular epithelial cells
Multiple myeloma	Proteinuria negative by dip but positive by SSA	Light chains on urinary immunoelectrophoresis
	Positive heat test	
Vascular Disease		
Renal artery stenosis	Typically benign urine	Leukocyte casts
		Granular casts may occur with prolonged ischemia
Atheroembolic disease	Typically benign urine	Occasional granular or muddy brown casts if acute tubular necrosis or cortical necrosis supervenes
HUS/TTP	Typically benign urine	Acute renal failure and systemic manifestations predominate
Small vessel vasculitis	Red cell casts	Systemic evidence of vasculitis
	Proteinuria	

HUS/TTP, hemolytic uremic syndrome/thrombotic thrombocytopenic purpura; SSA, sulfosalicylic acid.

TABLE 1.4	Diagnostic Utility of Spot Urinary Electrolytes
Urinary Electrolytes	**Diagnostic Indication**
Spot Test Urine Sodium Level	
< 10 mEq/L	Volume depletion
	Prerenal causes of renal hypoperfusion
> 40 mEq/L	Acute tubular necrosis
	Adrenal insufficiency
	Diuretic use (acute)
	Osmotic diuresis
10–40 mEq/L	Consider measuring FE_{Na}; < 1% suggests prerenal causes of acute renal failure
Spot Test Urine Chloride Level	
< 15 mEq/L	Extrarenal chloride losses
	Vomiting
	Diuretic use (chronic)
	Chloride-responsive metabolic alkalosis
> 15 mEq/L	Renal chloride losses
	Diuretic use (acute)
	Bartter's or Gitelman's syndrome
	Primary hyperaldosteronism (chloride-resistant metabolic alkalosis)
Urinary Anion Gap with an Associated Hyperchloremic Metabolic Acidosis	
> 0	Renal bicarbonate wasting
	Renal tubular acidosis
	Administration of a carbonic anhydrase inhibitor
< 0	Extrarenal losses of bicarbonate
	Diarrhea
	Pancreatic fistula or drainage

$$FE_{Na} = \frac{(U_{Na}) \times (P_{creat}) \times 100\%}{((P_{Na}) \times (U_{creat}))} \text{ ; Urinary anion gap} = (U_{Na} + U_{k}) - U_{cl}.$$

ability, volume status, and the origin of some forms of metabolic alkalosis. In addition, measurement of urinary sodium, chloride, and potassium concentrations allows calculation of the urinary anion gap, which may help identify the source of bicarbonate wasting in patients with a hyperchloremic (non-anion gap) metabolic acidosis.

Urinary Sodium Levels

In patients with oliguric acute renal failure, a urine sodium level less than 10 mEq/L determined by a random spot test indicates hypoperfusion of a generally intact nephron and confirms that there is pre-renal failure, caused by at least one of numerous possibilities. Urine sodium levels greater than 40 mEq/L indicate a loss of proximal tubular concentrating ability and are consistent with physical damage to the tubules, as seen in acute tubular necrosis. Urine sodium levels greater

than 40 mEq/L may also be present in volume-replete patients, in patients with adrenal insufficiency, and in those with histories of recent diuretic use, glucosuria, and advanced renal insufficiency.

Ambiguous Urinary Sodium Levels

Ambiguous urinary sodium levels in the range of 10 to 40 mEq/L may be further assessed by calculating the fractional excretion of sodium (FE_{Na}). The FE_{Na} is the ratio of sodium clearance to creatinine clearance and corrects for changes in glomerular filtration, which may alter sodium reabsorption:

$$FE_{Na} = \frac{((U_{Na})(V))/(P_{Na})}{(((U_{creat})(V))/(P_{creat}))} \times 100\%$$

In this equation, U_{Na} and P_{Na} represent the urinary and plasma sodium concentrations, respectively, and

U_{creat} and P_{creat} represent urinary and plasma creatinine levels, respectively. V represents volume and is the same in both expressions; therefore, it can be canceled from the equation. Because volume is not necessary for the calculation, the FE_{Na} can be derived from random spot test urine samples. After canceling V and rearranging, the FE_{Na} expression reads:

$$FE_{Na} = \frac{(U_{Na}) \times (P_{creat})}{((P_{Na}) \times (U_{creat}))} \times 100\%$$

Values for FE_{Na} less than 1% indicate pre-renal azotemia and greater than 1% suggest structural tubular damage, as is seen in acute tubular necrosis.

Urinary Chloride Levels

A random spot test to determine the urinary chloride level can help identify the cause of metabolic alkalosis. Urinary chloride losses from indiscriminant diuretic use, Bartter's syndrome, and Gitelman's syndrome may result in metabolic alkalosis. Prolonged vomiting, with gastric hydrogen and chloride losses, may also trigger metabolic alkalosis. Chloride levels determined by spot test may help distinguish between gastrointestinal and renal chloride wasting states in this situation. Spot test urine chloride levels less than 15 mEq/L suggest a gastrointestinal source for chloride losses, whereas urine chloride levels greater than 15 mEq/L indicate renal chloride wasting states. Urine chloride levels less than or equal to 15 mEq/L also suggest severe volume depletion and are associated with long-term diuretic use.

Urinary Anion Gap

The urinary anion gap is a useful tool for differentiating between urinary and gastrointestinal losses of bicarbonate in patients with a hyperchloremic metabolic acidosis. The urinary anion gap is the difference between the sum of urine sodium and potassium concentrations and the urine chloride concentration:

$$\text{Urinary anion gap} = (U_{Na} + U_K) - U_{Cl}$$

The calculation utilizes a spot test urine sample. The normal urinary anion gap is zero, or slightly negative. The U_{Cl} is an indirect reflection of urinary ammonium excretion, which eliminates acid in the urine.

In patients with hyperchloremic metabolic acidosis, an increase in the urinary anion gap reflects decreased ammonium excretion (and hence a decrease in U_{Cl}) and is indicative of renal bicarbonate wasting. Conversely, a decrease in the urinary anion gap results from increased ammonium excretion, with an increase in U_{Cl}. This is seen with gastrointestinal losses of bicarbonate (caused by, for example, diarrhea or external drainage of the pancreas).

KEY POINTS

- The first voided sample of the day (morning sample on awakening) is the specimen of choice for analysis.

- A fresh urine specimen should be examined immediately. In case of delay, the specimen may be refrigerated at 4° C for up to 12 hours.

- Dipstick is adequate to detect for proteinuria, hematuria, and urinary infection in office practice. Dipstick is negative for Bence Jones proteins.

- Dipstick is sensitive for true hematuria, with five red blood cells per microliter.

- Dipstick test is a good method to test for leukocyte esterase and nitrite.

- Microscopy of red blood cells can help determine whether hematuria is of glomerular or extraglomerular origin.

- Most urinary leukocytes are neutrophils; however, eosinophiluria may occur in drug-induced acute interstitial nephritis.

REFERRAL

The goal of referral is to identify treatable diseases and reversible causes of renal failure.

- **Renal parenchymal disease.** Nephrology referral should be considered when any aspect of the urinalysis suggests renal parenchymal disease. Indicators of renal parenchymal disease include proteinuria, hematuria, or both, and elevated serum creatinine levels.
- **Isolated hematuria.** Urologic evaluation is indicated for patients with isolated hematuria (i.e., hematuria without proteinuria).
- **Abnormal anatomy.** Urologic evaluation is indicated for patients with abnormal anatomy recognized during the course of radiologic evaluation (intravenous pyelography (IVP), computed tomography (CT), or ultrasound).

SUGGESTED READINGS

Fogazzi GB, Ponticelli C. Microscopic hematuria diagnosis and management. Nephron 1996:125–134.

Geyer SJ. Urinalysis and urinary sediment in patients with renal disease. Clin Lab Med 1993;13(1):13–20.

Graff L. A Handbook of Routine Urinalysis. Philadelphia: Lippincott, 1983.

Kohler H, Wandel E, Brunck B. Acanthocyturia—a characteristic marker for glomerular bleeding. Kidney Int 1991; 40:115–120.

Yager HM, Harrington JT. Urinalysis and urine electrolytes. In: Jacobson HR, Striker GE, Klahr S, eds. The Principles and Practice of Nephrology. 2nd ed. St. Louis: Mosby, 1995:90–100.

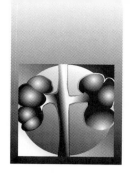

CHAPTER 2

Radiologic Studies of Common Renal Diseases

David E. Neal
Kenneth M. Vitellas

OVERVIEW OF IMAGING STUDIES

Genitourinary tract radiology is an exciting but sometimes confusing area because of the many imaging studies available. There is no best method for imaging the kidneys and urinary tract; the various modalities need to be evaluated for efficient, timely, and cost-effective workup. The availability of local expertise has a profound impact on the type of study ordered. For example, some radiologists have a great interest in ultrasound, whereas others prefer to solve problems primarily through the use of computed tomography (CT). Before ordering an imaging test, it is important to determine if the information to be acquired is really necessary for effective patient care. Also, the importance of providing adequate history on the radiology request cannot be overemphasized. This information is invaluable in tailoring the study to answer the clinical questions most effectively.

Excretory Urography

Despite the popularity of radiologic studies such as CT, ultrasound, and magnetic resonance imaging (MRI), excretory urography (also called intravenous pyelography or IVP) remains a very useful tool for overall evaluation of the urinary tract. Unlike many other tests, urography provides information about both anatomy and function of the kidneys.

Indications

Common indications for excretory urography include:

- The initial workup of hematuria
- Flank pain or suspected ureteral stone
- Certain cases of recent trauma

Contraindications

Contraindications may include:

- History of allergy to contrast media
- Impaired renal function
- Early pregnancy

Preparing a Patient for Urography

Many radiologists prefer that the patient undergoing urography have the colon cleaned before the test to reduce gas and colonic fecal material. Usually, an oral laxative is taken 12 to 18 hours before the study and a rectal suppository is inserted the morning of the test. This practice can probably be eliminated because it is uncomfortable for the patient and improves image quality minimally, if at all. The patient should refrain from eating solid foods at least 3 hours before the study in case vomiting occurs from the contrast injection, but dehydration should be avoided.

Performing Urography

Excretory urography requires constant monitoring and tailoring while being performed. The procedure is as follows:

1. A preliminary film is taken before injection of the contrast agent to detect renal calculi before they are obscured by contrast material collecting in the kidneys. Other conditions, such as barium retained in the colon from a prior gastrointestinal tract study, can be detected and, if necessary, the study can be postponed.
2. Approximately 30 seconds after injection of contrast media, the kidneys begin to appear radiographically. An image is taken at this point, and the size, shape, and position of the kidneys are evaluated. The normal size of the kidneys

varies, but a rough rule of thumb is that the length of the kidney should equal approximately 3.5 vertebral bodies, including the disc spaces. The inferior pole of the kidneys lies lateral to the superior pole; therefore, the axis of each kidney follows the course of the ipsilateral psoas muscle.

3. In most cases, tomograms, which are coronal slices through the kidney, are obtained for more accurate evaluation of the renal outlines and for detection of a renal mass.
4. Images of the abdomen, including the kidneys, ureters, and bladder, are then obtained at 10 and 15 minutes (Fig. 2.1). These films provide a great deal of information, including the presence or absence of ureteral obstruction, ureteral deviation, collecting system filling defects, and bladder abnormalities.
5. If no abnormalities are detected, a final image is obtained after the patient voids. This postvoid film allows detection of postvoid residual volume and is useful for evaluating the bladder mucosa. The distal ureters, which are often obscured by a full bladder, also can be assessed.
6. If evidence of ureteral obstruction is demonstrated on the 10- or 15-minute images, additional delayed images are needed to determine the location and, hopefully, the cause of the obstruction.

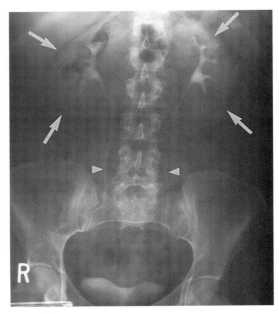

FIGURE 2.1.
Normal excretory urogram (15-minute film). Note the normal kidneys *(arrows)*, ureters *(arrowheads)*, and bladder.

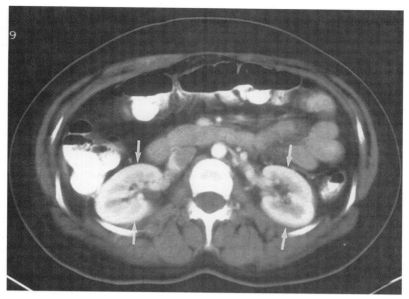

FIGURE 2.2.
Normal contrast-enhanced CT of the kidneys *(arrows)*.

Computed Tomography (CT)

CT has made a dramatic contribution to uroradiology. Unlike conventional radiographs, which display structures in a single plane, CT records internal body structures in predetermined slices. The x-ray tube (which is firing the x-rays) moves around the body in a circle (analogous to a ring on a finger) as the camera records images. The result is many views of the body from many different perspectives. Using a sophisticated mathematical program, the computer reconstructs a cross-sectional image based on the data acquired from these views.

Indications

Most patients have their kidneys imaged as part of a routine abdominal CT scan done for problems unrelated to the urinary tract (Fig. 2.2). Incidental renal pathology is occasionally detected, some of which requires additional workup.

Common indications for CT of the urinary tract include:

- Evaluation of an abnormality (e.g., possible renal mass) demonstrated on excretory urography or ultrasound. The patient with a mass suspected to be renal cell carcinoma on ultrasound can undergo CT for confirmation of the mass and preoperative staging.
- To rule out a neoplasm in a patient with persistent hematuria despite negative findings on urography and cystoscopy

- To exclude a renal or perirenal abscess in a patient with pyelonephritis that is not responding to therapy
- In some centers, use of noncontrast CT to initially assess the presence of urinary tract calculi, which completely replaces use of excretory urography
- To depict traumatic injuries of the kidneys, renal vasculature, and surrounding structures much better than urography, although impact on patient outcome is controversial

CT angiography is a developing field that is proving useful in evaluation of renal artery stenosis (RAS).

Contraindications

Relative contraindications to CT with contrast media are similar to those of urography:

- Impaired renal function
- Allergy to contrast material
- Early pregnancy

Performing Renal CT

If a renal CT scan is requested, the kidneys are usually imaged in thinner sections than are normal in routine abdominal CT. This increases the quality of the images and allows characterization of smaller abnormalities. The procedure is as follows:

1. Initially, the kidneys should be scanned **before** injection of intravenous contrast media.

2. The kidneys then are rescanned **after** intravenous administration of the contrast agent.

The noncontrast images are helpful in detecting renal calculi that are otherwise obscured by the contrast material collecting in the kidneys (stones and intravenous contrast are both bright on CT). Additionally, the images of lesions that are indeterminate precontrast can be compared with the postcontrast images to detect lesion enhancement, which is an important sign of neoplasms.

Ultrasound
Efficacy
Ultrasound is a cornerstone in diagnosing many renal abnormalities. However, the contribution of ultrasound to a diagnosis is extremely dependent on operator skill and experience.

The basic principle behind ultrasound is the visualization of structures by recording sound waves. The ultrasound transducer—the part of the machine placed on the patient during an examination—contains a crystal that vibrates when exposed to an electric current. This vibration produces sound waves that travel into the body, deflect off structures, and return to the body surface where they are detected by the transducer. Some structures, such as renal stones, reflect sound readily and will thus appear bright on the image. Other substances, such as fluid, reflect sound poorly and will appear dark. The computer determines how deep a structure is by the time it takes for the sound wave to make a round trip into the body and back to the transducer.

Advantages   The advantages of using ultrasound are:

- The lack of radiation
- No need for intravenous contrast media
- Relatively low cost
- Ability to conduct the procedure at bedside
- Capability of imaging in any plane

Disadvantages   The disadvantages of using ultrasound include:

- Marked dependence on operator skill
- Inability to image structures deep to bowel gas (such as the ureters)
- Images from obese patients are generally degraded

Ultrasound is the safest method of examining the kidneys in a patient who cannot receive an intravenous contrast agent. Specific examples include ruling out obstruction as the cause of acute renal failure or excluding a renal mass in a patient allergic to contrast material. If an indeterminate mass is detected on an excretory urogram or a CT scan, ultrasound can often determine if it is a simple cyst or a more worrisome solid mass.

Reading the Ultrasound Image
Bright structures on ultrasound are called hyperechoic; darker structures are referred to as hypoechoic. The normal appearance of the kidneys on ultrasound is shown in (Fig. 2.3). The central hyperechoic portion of the kidney is the renal sinus, consisting of fat, blood vessels, and the collecting system. The more hypoechoic renal cortex is the peripheral band of tissue surrounding the renal sinus. The small, focal, dark structures near the junction of the cortex and the renal sinus are the renal pyramids, which should not be mistaken for lesions. The renal cortex should generally be equally or less echogenic (bright) than the adjacent liver. The ureters are difficult to see with ultrasound because they are small structures and are often obscured by bowel gas. The conspicuity of the ureters increases as they become dilated. Occasionally, a calculus will be seen within a dilated ureter, but urography remains the preferred test for evaluating stone disease in the setting of normal renal function.

A gross evaluation of the bladder can be accomplished with ultrasound, including the following:

- Bladder volume
- Presence of postvoid residual volume
- Overall assessment of the bladder wall
- Large bladder masses and bladder wall thickening; however, other tests, such as cystoscopy, are much more accurate at excluding smaller lesions

Doppler Imaging
The renal arteries and veins can be assessed with Doppler imaging, which can produce both sound waves and color images of the blood vessels. Much research in the use of Doppler imaging is being conducted, and new applications are constantly emerging. Currently Doppler imaging is useful for the following:

- Evaluating the renal veins for thrombosis
- Aiding in the diagnosis of inflammatory and neoplastic renal lesions
- Assessing the vascular integrity of renal transplants

The utility of Doppler imaging in the assessment of RAS remains controversial but has generally been disappointing.

Magnetic Resonance Imaging
Efficacy
The role of MRI in the evaluation of the urinary tract is evolving.

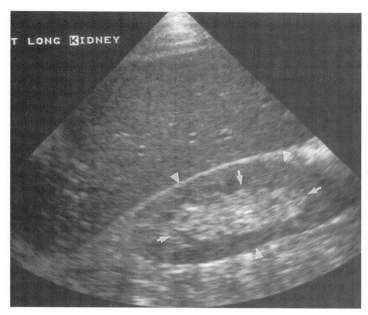

FIGURE 2.3.
Normal ultrasound of the right kidney. The renal sinus *(arrows)* and renal cortex *(arrowheads)* are demonstrated.

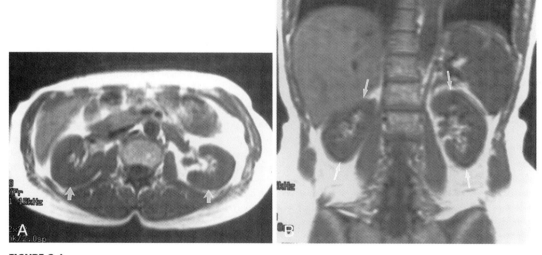

FIGURE 2.4.
Normal axial **(A)** and coronal **(B)** MRI of the kidneys *(arrows)*.

Advantages   This relatively newer modality has the advantages of:

- Imaging in any plane (i.e., axial, sagittal, coronal, etc.) (Fig. 2.4)
- Lack of ionizing radiation
- Excellent depiction of vascular structures without

the requirement for iodinated intravenous contrast material

Disadvantages   The main disadvantages include:

- High cost
- Lengthy examination time

- Difficulty or inability to image claustrophobic patients (sedation with oral diazepam can often help)

MRI is capable of detecting small renal masses and distinguishing cysts from solid tumors. However, these tasks are generally accomplished more easily and less expensively with ultrasound or CT. MRI is the method of choice for evaluating renal lesions suspected to be malignant in patients who have poor renal function or who are allergic to iodinated intravenous contrast material. The majority of allergic patients can safely receive intravenous gadolinium, a contrast agent used for MRI.

Another use for MRI includes staging renal cell carcinoma, particularly if the renal veins and inferior vena cava are not seen adequately on CT. MRI is also showing great promise in the diagnosis of RAS in patients with renovascular hypertension. MRI research is progressing rapidly, and many more applications to renal imaging will likely emerge in the near future.

Cystography

Indications
Cystography (Fig. 2.5) is indicated to:

- Detect vesicoureteral reflux
- Assess abnormalities in patients with neurogenic bladder
- Rule out bladder rupture in a trauma setting

Contraindications
Contraindications for cystography include:

- An uncooperative patient
- A frail patient

Performing Cystography
Cystography is usually done in a fluoroscopic room, which enables the radiologist to visualize the ureters and bladder in real time. The examination is tailored to meet the specific clinical indication. The general procedure is as follows:

1. The urethra is catheterized, and contrast material is injected into the bladder under fluoroscopic visualization.
2. In cases of possible reflux, the bladder is filled until the patient is certain that he or she can void.
3. The catheter is then removed, and the ureters are examined for evidence of reflux during voiding.
4. To rule out bladder rupture, the full bladder is imaged in multiple projections.

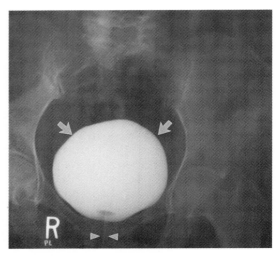

FIGURE 2.5.
Normal bladder *(arrows)* demonstrated on a cystogram. Note Foley catheter *(arrowheads)* in place.

Extravasation of contrast media or a small fistula may not be apparent until the voiding study is obtained.

Urethrography

Urethrography is done to exclude urethral injury following trauma and to assess for a urethral stricture in patients with voiding difficulties.

Indications
Less common indications include:

- Incontinence evaluation
- Suspected urethral tumor
- Urethral fistula

Contraindications
Contraindications include:

- An uncooperative patient
- A frail patient

Performing Urethrography
The procedure for urethrography is as follows:

1. The urethra can be imaged by inserting a small catheter and injecting contrast media while directly visualizing the study with fluoroscopy.
2. When the urethra is completely opacified, multiple images are obtained. At this point, some contrast material will have entered the bladder.
3. The patient is then instructed to void, and the urethra (particularly the posterior urethra) can be

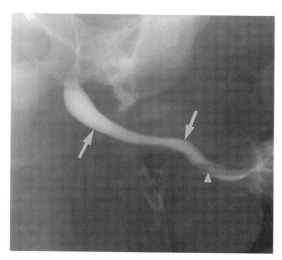

FIGURE 2.6.
Urethrogram demonstrating a normal urethra *(arrows)*. Note catheter tip in distal urethra *(arrowhead)*.

re-imaged. Attempting to examine the urethra on excretory urography is suboptimal.
4. If urethral pathology is suspected, dedicated urethrography should be done.

A normal urethrogram is shown in Figure 2.6.

Angiography

Efficacy

Angiography is an invasive technique used to evaluate the renal arteries and veins. Advancements in noninvasive imaging modalities such as MRI, CT, and ultrasound have eliminated the need for angiography in many cases.

Indications

Angiography remains important in:

- The diagnosis of RAS
- The evaluation of suspected renal arterial injury
- Occasionally, delineation of the vascularity of large renal tumors and arterial malformations before surgery or interventional therapy

Contraindications

Contraindications include:

- Allergy to contrast media
- Renal insufficiency

Performing Angiography

Angiography is the best available method for evaluating the renal arteries; however, the technique is costly and

carries some risk. Although the complications are generally rare, they include hematoma at the puncture site, arterial damage, infection, and a reaction to the contrast material.

The technique is as follows:

1. A catheter should be placed in the femoral artery and then guided into the renal artery using fluoroscopic control.
2. Contrast material is then injected, and multiple images are obtained.

Contrast Material and Complications

Injection of contrast media is necessary for doing excretory urography and cystourethrography and dramatically improves the quality of CT images. Unfortunately, many side effects and potential complications are associated with these agents, as there are with excretory urography and scintiscan. The most serious complication is an allergic response. Allergic reactions can range from mild skin itching or hives to life-threatening cardiorespiratory arrest. It is difficult to predict who will have an allergic response. **Patients who have had a previous contrast reaction are clearly more prone to a second reaction and should only be given contrast media with great caution,** and if the previous reaction was severe, reexamination is generally contraindicated. Those patients with extensive allergy lists (e.g., many drugs or foods) and patients with asthma also are more likely to react to the contrast agent.

Assessing the Risks

Before administering an intravenous contrast agent to a patient with one of the risk factors, other modalities such as ultrasound or MRI should be considered. If these will not answer the clinical question, the indication for the contrast examination should be reviewed. If the benefit of the examination in terms of improving patient outcome outweighs the risk of a contrast reaction, the study can be done using newer (low osmolarity, or nonionic) contrast agents after administering a pretreatment regimen. A 50-mg oral dose of prednisone given 13, 7, and 1 hour before the study, along with 50 mg of diphenhydramine with the last dose of prednisone, has been shown to have a protective effect.

Risks for Patients with Renal Insufficiency

Patients with preexisting renal insufficiency may be at increased risk for further kidney damage if administered an intravenous contrast agent. If the serum creatinine measurement is not available, many radiology departments will proceed with a contrast examination if the patient has no history of renal disease. Therefore, it is important to alert the radiologist ahead of time if there is evidence of renal insufficiency. If renal dysfunction exists, ultrasound or MRI should be used when possible. If a contrast study is required, the risk of nephrotoxicity may be reduced by hydrating the patient and by using smaller doses of the agent.

Summary of Diagnosis

- Excretory urography (IVP) remains a very useful tool for an overall evaluation of the urinary tract. Unlike other radiologic studies such as ultrasound, CT, and MRI, urography provides information about the anatomy and function of the kidneys.
- A CT scan of the kidneys is often necessary for further evaluation of an abnormality (i.e., a possible mass) revealed on an excretory urogram or on ultrasound.
- CT is also the best test for excluding a renal or perirenal abscess in a patient with pyelonephritis who is not responding to therapy.
- CT can identify traumatic injuries to the kidneys, renal vessels, and surrounding structures much better than urography or other modalities.
- Ultrasound is the safest method of kidney examination in a patient with a previous history of allergy to contrast material or at risk (of, for example, renal failure) from its use.
- In cases of suspected lower urinary tract obstruction, ultrasound is the most effective noninvasive method of investigation.
- MRI is the method of choice for evaluating renal mass lesions suspected of being malignant or renal vascular lesions, such as RAS, in patients who have poor renal function or histories of allergy to contrast material.
- Cystography is used on patients with recurrent urinary tract infections in whom there is a high suspicion of vesicoureteral reflux, and to rule out bladder rupture in a trauma setting.
- Angiography remains important in the diagnosis of RAS and in the evaluation of suspected renal arterial injury.

IMAGING EVALUATION OF RENAL DISEASES

Renal Failure

The general approach to the patient with a first-time diagnosis of renal failure is focused on determining if the cause is pre-renal, primarily renal, or post-renal. Pre-renal failure can be determined clinically; however, ultrasound is the method of choice for differentiating primary renal from post-renal causes. CT and excretory urography can also aid in diagnosing post-renal obstruction, but their use is limited by the relative contraindication of administering an intravenous contrast agent to the patient with renal failure.

Post-renal failure can be caused by obstruction of the urinary tract anywhere along its course. Obstruction usually has to be bilateral to cause significant azotemia or decreased urine output. Specific causes of post-renal failure include:

- Bladder outlet obstruction (e.g., caused by prostatic hypertrophy or tumor, neurogenic bladder, bladder tumor, malfunctioning Foley catheter, etc.)
- Bilateral ureteral obstruction from a mass or retroperitoneal fibrosis

When obstruction occurs, the renal collecting system upstream from the blockage will dilate (Fig. 2.7). Once urinary tract dilatation is identified, the sonographer should search for the underlying cause.

False–Negative and False–Positive Ultrasound Findings

Ultrasound can detect dilatation of the urinary tract, but some circumstances are associated with a false–

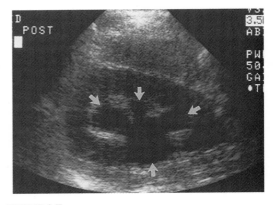

FIGURE 2.7.
Renal ultrasound demonstrating a dilated, obstructed renal collecting system (arrows).

negative result. If the obstruction is recent, dilatation may be absent or minimal. Additionally, if acute renal failure is superimposed on chronic obstruction, urine production may cease and the collecting system will not dilate. Conversely, dilatation of the urinary tract is not always caused by obstruction. Urine reflux from the bladder into the ureter and renal collecting system can produce an image on ultrasound nearly identical to that of obstruction. Other causes of false–positive results include:

- Postobstructive atrophy
- Congenital megacalyces
- Pregnancy
- Parapelvic cysts

Equivocal Results

If no dilatation is present, the cause of the azotemia may be intrinsic to the kidneys (medical renal disease). Chronic renal failure usually can be distinguished from acute renal failure by the history and physical examination, before radiologic tests are undertaken. In equivocal cases, imaging (particularly ultrasound) can determine the chronicity of the renal dysfunction and can, therefore, provide prognostic information. Acutely failing kidneys are usually large, with smooth borders. The echogenicity (brightness on ultrasound images) is usually normal. Small, atrophic kidneys indicate that the renal failure is chronic, especially if the echogenicity is increased (Fig. 2.8). Differentiating among the causes of chronic renal failure is generally not possible since most chronic diseases are associated with a shrunken echogenic kidney as visualized by ultrasound.

Stone Disease

Urinary calculi are a common problem encountered by the primary care provider. Patients experiencing renal colic typically present with hematuria and acute flank pain, which may radiate to the lower abdomen, groin, testes, or labia. However, some patients do not have pain and may present with hematuria only. Radiologic tests can determine if the patient's symptoms are caused by urinary stones, determine the presence and degree of urinary tract obstruction, and help determine the likelihood that a stone will pass spontaneously without the need for intervention.

Excretory Urography

Excretory urography is the test most frequently done for the initial evaluation of stone disease. Approximately 85% of urinary calculi are calcified and therefore can be detected on the preliminary (scout) radiograph (Fig. 2.9). There are, however, many calcified structures that may overlie the urinary tract and mimic urolithiasis. These include:

- Phleboliths (which often have lucent centers)
- Calcified lymph nodes
- Lateral margin of the vertebral body transverse process
- Gallstones
- Costochondral calcifications

Appearance of Calcifications in Radiographs

If calcifications are seen overlying the kidneys on the preliminary radiograph, additional views, such as

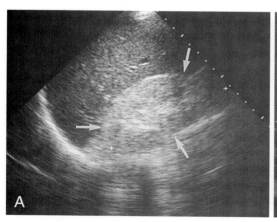
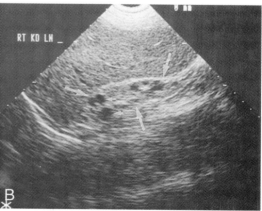

FIGURE 2.8.
A. Renal ultrasound shows an echogenic (bright) kidney (*arrows*) secondary to renal disease.
B. Ultrasound of a small, echogenic kidney (*large arrows*) consistent with chronic renal failure. Note the acquired renal cysts from dialysis (*small arrows*).

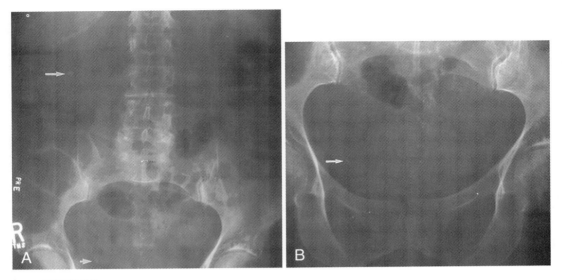

FIGURE 2.9.
A. Preliminary radiograph for an excretory urogram shows a renal stone *(large arrow)* and distal ureteral stone *(small arrow).* **B.** Limited view of the pelvis better demonstrates the ureteral stone *(arrow).*

oblique projections and tomograms, are obtained to determine their exact location. On oblique images, renal calculi move posteriorly with the kidney, whereas gallstones and costochondral calcifications move anteriorly. At least 15% of urinary stones will not be visible on plain radiographs because of many factors:

- Stones may be radiolucent (such as uric acid and cystine stones)
- Stones may be too small to see definitely
- Stones may be obscured by superimposed bowel gas and bony structures

After administration of the contrast agent, the acutely obstructed kidney initially appears fainter than the opposite, normal kidney. As time progresses, the affected kidney becomes denser and the dilated collecting system begins to opacify. This dilatation transforms the normally sharp, cupped calyces into blunt, clublike structures (Fig. 2.10). When delayed imaging is used and images are taken from different positions (upright, prone), the ureter can usually be opacified to the point of obstruction, often displayed as a standing column of contrast. At this point the stone may not be visible because it is surrounded by contrast material of similar density. Careful review of the preliminary film, with attention to the expected location of the obstruction, usually reveals the calculus. Once the stone is confirmed, it can be measured to predict the chance

of passage. The majority (90%) of stones less than 4 millimeters in diameter are likely to pass spontaneously, compared with 50% of stones 5 to 7 millimeters in diameter. Stones measuring greater than 8 millimeters are unlikely to be passed into the bladder.

CT Scan for Radiolucent Defects
If a radiolucent defect is causing the obstruction, it could be:

- A radiolucent stone
- A blood clot
- Sloughed papilla
- A neoplasm

CT can help to differentiate a stone from other possible causes of obstruction. A stone on a CT scan will usually appear quite dense (bright), despite its lucent appearance on the plain radiograph. Occasionally the entire ureter will be dilated (to the level of the bladder) with no calculus visible. In such a case, a stone may have recently passed into the bladder, producing edema and partial obstruction at the ureterovesical junction.

Ultrasound for Evaluation of Acute Renal Colic
Some authors advocate ultrasound as the initial test for evaluation of acute renal colic. Although it is true that ultrasound can detect urolithiasis as well as urinary

tract dilatation, it does have limitations. For example, an acute obstruction (such as occurs with a calculus) may not dilate the collecting system, and the result via ultrasound would be false–normal. Also, the midureters are commonly obscured by bowel gas, making detection of ureteral calculi difficult. However, because it does not involve radiation, ultrasound is useful in evaluating the pregnant patient with suspected renal colic.

CT Without Intravenous Contrast Media

A CT scan of the urinary tract without the use of intravenous contrast media is an alternative to excretory urography, particularly in patients who have had a previous allergic reaction to contrast media. This technique can be useful because it:

- Demonstrates calculi
- Determines the presence of collecting system dilatation
- Detects nonurologic causes of pain
- Is quicker and less labor intensive than excretory urography

In fact, some centers have replaced excretory urography with noncontrast CT for the initial evaluation of patients with suspected renal colic.

Renal Masses

Most renal masses are detected on radiologic studies done for nonurologic reasons. Further imaging is often needed to determine whether the incidentally detected mass is malignant. The usual approach is to first determine if the mass is cystic or solid. Solid masses may represent a renal cell carcinoma and are usually removed, either by complete or, in some cases, partial nephrectomy. Conversely, masses that strictly fulfill the criteria for a benign simple cyst can be safely left alone. Unfortunately, many lesions fall in between these two categories and are classified as indeterminate lesions.

Excretory urographic findings of a renal mass may include:

- A focal bulge of the renal outline
- Displacement of the collecting system
- Enlargement of the entire kidney

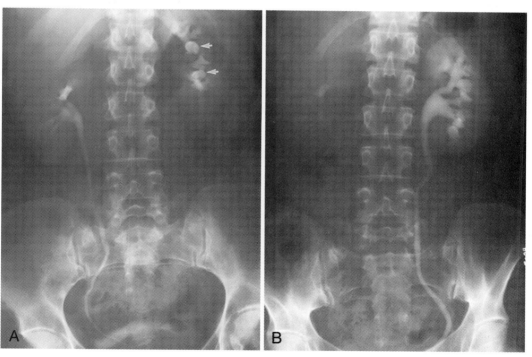

FIGURE 2.10.

Left ureterovesical junction obstruction. Fifteen-minute film from excretory urography demonstrating a normal right collecting system and ureter. The left calyces are dilated *(arrows)* **(A).** Thirty-minute film shows dilated left ureter and intrarenal collecting system **(B).**

Use of CT and Ultrasound to Determine the Nature of Renal Masses

Once a mass is detected on excretory urography, CT or ultrasound is usually needed to confirm its cystic or solid nature. The following findings on the urogram suggest a cyst:

- Smooth borders
- Sharp interface with normal parenchyma
- Relatively low density

An ultrasound is then used for confirmation (Fig. 2.11). To meet the criteria for a simple cyst on ultrasound, the lesion must have:

- No internal echoes (be completely black)
- Well-defined smooth walls
- Good, thorough enhancement (structures behind the cyst will be bright)

Findings on the urogram that suggest a solid mass include:

- Lobular contour
- Density equal to or greater than that of normal kidney parenchyma
- Calcification

CT is the preferred next step because it can confirm that the mass is solid and help determine stage at the same time (Figs. 2.12 and 2.13). Frequently, a mass thought to be solid on the urogram turns out to be a cyst once the CT scans are reviewed. The CT criteria for a simple cyst include:

- A round, well-defined lesion with an imperceptible wall
- Internal density near that of water

Indeterminate Lesions

Lesions that do not meet the ultrasound or CT criteria for a simple cyst or solid mass are called indeterminate. For example, these lesions may have thick septations, calcifications, wall irregularity, internal echoes on ultrasound, or higher density than water on CT. These lesions are best evaluated by a combination of ultrasound and CT. They usually turn out to be simple cysts that have undergone hemorrhage or have been infected in the past. However, the more noncystic features a lesion has, the more likely it is to be malignant.

Management of Indeterminate Lesions

The management of indeterminate lesions (detected on ultrasound or CT) is complex, but, in general, they can

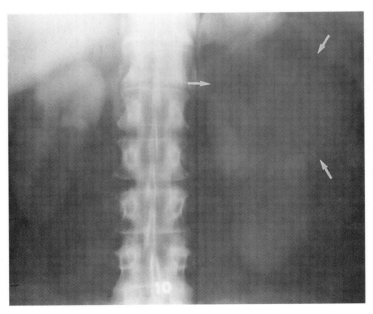

FIGURE 2.11.

Left renal mass. Tomogram from excretory urography demonstrates a large, well-defined left renal mass *(arrows)*. Ultrasound (which showed the mass to be a simple cyst) should be the next imaging step.

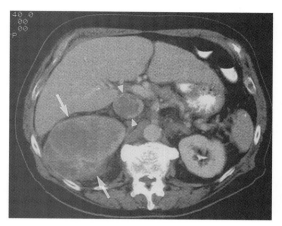

FIGURE 2.12.

Right renal cell carcinoma. CT demonstrates a large, solid, heterogeneous mass replacing most of the right kidney *(arrows)*. Also note the tumor extension into the inferior vena cava *(arrowheads)* and normal left kidney.

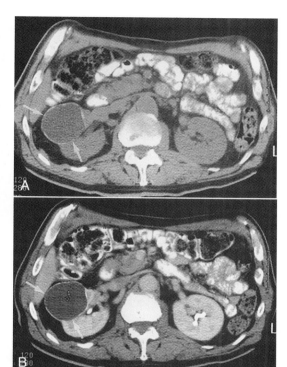

FIGURE 2.14.

CT workup of an indeterminate renal cystic lesion. **A.** CT before administration of intravenous contrast media shows a cystic lesion *(arrows)* with a calcified wall (therefore this is an indeterminate lesion). **B.** After administration of intravenous contrast media, the lesion *(arrows)* does not enhance, indicating that it is a benign cyst.

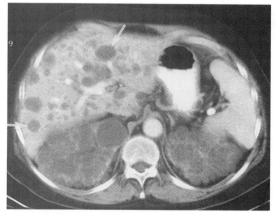

FIGURE 2.13.

Polycystic kidney disease. The excretory urogram (not shown) demonstrated multiple indeterminate renal masses. CT shows multiple bilateral renal cysts. Also note the multiple associated hepatic cysts *(arrows)*.

be followed, imaged further, or surgically removed. Lesions with minimal noncystic features can be followed (i.e., for 3 months, 6 months, and 1 year) to ensure that they are not changing or growing. More complicated cystic lesions, including those with nodular walls, thick irregular septa, or any solid components, should be treated surgically. Indeterminate lesions on ultrasound can be further evaluated with CT by imaging the kid-

neys before and then after the administration of intravenous contrast media (Fig. 2.14). Contrast enhancement (an increase in density following administration of the contrast agent) is an important sign of malignancy. MRI with gadolinium can be substituted for CT in patients with renal failure or allergy to contrast agents.

Renal Lesions Smaller Than 1.5 Centimeters

A particularly challenging situation arises when very small (< 1.5 cm) renal lesions are discovered incidentally. The radiologist will often report these as too small to characterize further. Statistically, a majority of these lesions are cysts. Those that turn out to be tiny solid neoplasms usually have a slow growth rate. What to do about these lesions is controversial and not based on any solid data. In general, management should be based on clinical factors, such as advanced age and the presence of underlying disease. Patients who are non-surgical candidates (i.e., with an underlying heart or lung disease or other life-threatening illness) should not undergo further workup of small renal lesions. It can also be argued that older patients (75 years or older) are unlikely to benefit from extensive evaluation because they are more likely to die of other causes before a small renal lesion grows to a life-threatening size. Younger, healthier patients should undergo ultrasound and dedicated thin-section renal CT to characterize a small lesion further. If the lesion cannot be categorized further, a follow-up examination (CT or ultrasound) in 6 months and then yearly is recommended to confirm stability.

Percutaneous Needle Biopsy of Renal Masses

Percutaneous needle biopsy of a renal mass is generally not done because of its low diagnostic yield, small but real risk of hemorrhage, and the controversial notion that tumor seeding along the needle track may occur. However, needle biopsy and aspiration of a renal mass can be done in nonsurgical candidates in whom a pathologic diagnosis is needed for management, when there is a question of a primary renal neoplasm versus a solitary metastatic lesion, or when an infected lesion is suspected.

Hematuria

Patients presenting with hematuria may have a urinary tract calculus, infection, or neoplasm (anywhere along the urinary tract). These patients are best studied with excretory urography (including tomography). This test provides an overall evaluation of the kidneys, collecting systems, and ureters but is insensitive in detecting small renal and bladder masses. Therefore, in addition to urography, patients usually undergo cystoscopy for further evaluation of the bladder. If these tests are negative and the hematuria persists, the kidneys are examined by CT scanning.

Once a solid renal mass is discovered (Fig. 2.15), a specific diagnosis usually cannot be made radiographically except in the case of an angiomyolipoma, which has specific radiographic features (Fig. 2.16). This benign tumor consists of fat, smooth muscle, and vascular tissue. On ultrasound, it is typically a very echogenic (bright) lesion. If such a lesion is discovered sonographically, CT should be done to confirm the presence of intralesional fat, which is virtually pathognomonic for an angiomyolipoma.

Urinary Tract Infection

Infections that involve the lower urinary tract usually respond rapidly to antibiotics without the need for diagnostic imaging. Likewise, most cases of pyelonephritis are uncomplicated and, with appropriate therapy, will resolve promptly with no adverse renal effects. However, imaging is indicated when a patient is suspected of having complicated pyelonephritis including:

- Poor response to therapy
- A high risk for complications (e.g., immunosuppressed or diabetic individuals)
- The presence of underlying obstruction, stones, or recurrent pyelonephritis

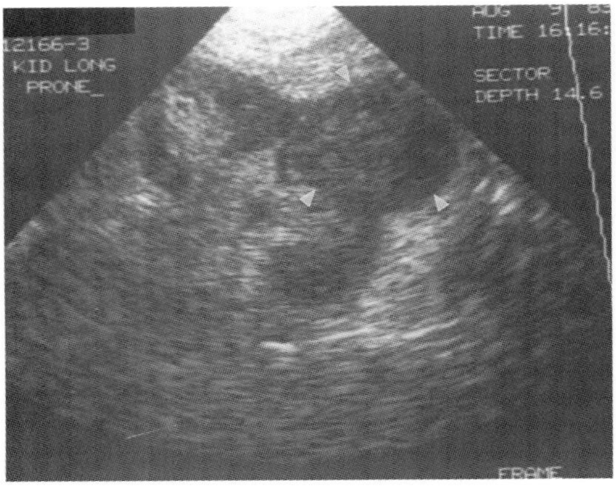

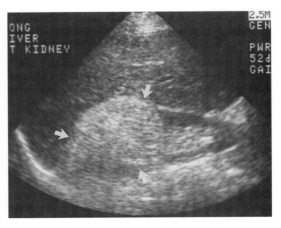

FIGURE 2.15.
Renal cell carcinoma. Renal ultrasound demonstrates a solid mass (arrowheads) projecting from the renal cortex.

FIGURE 2.16.
Renal angiomyolipoma. Ultrasound shows an echogenic mass (arrows) in the superior pole of the right kidney, proven to contain fat on a CT scan.

The optimal imaging strategy is based on the acuteness, complexity, and severity of the patient's clinical condition.

Pyelonephritis in Patients with Diabetes or an Altered Immune Status

Pyelonephritis associated with diabetes or altered immune status can progress to:

- Focal bacterial nephritis, which is a severe form of focal infection often producing a mass effect (Fig. 2.17)
- Renal abscess
- Perirenal abscess
- Emphysematous pyelonephritis (a gas-forming renal infection)

Contrast-enhanced CT is the best way overall to evaluate disease extent, and it plays a major role in guiding therapy. Ultrasound can be done in those patients with renal dysfunction but is less sensitive in detecting perirenal extension of the inflammatory process.

Pyelonephritis in Patients with Other Conditions

Patients with acute pyelonephritis and a history of stones, patients with recurrent pyelonephritis, or males with their first documented renal infection can be imaged initially with excretory urography. Ultrasound is an alternative study, particularly in patients unable to receive an intravenous contrast agent or when pyonephrosis is suspected.

At least half of acute, uncomplicated cases of pyelonephritis will not demonstrate significant findings on conventional imaging studies. In the remaining cases, the urogram or CT scan may show:

- An enlarged smooth kidney
- Decreased renal density
- Delayed opacification of the collecting system

Sonographic findings include renal enlargement and decreased echogenicity.

Imaging Masses Caused by Pyelonephritis

A renal abscess is formed by severe pyelonephritis that produces parenchymal necrosis and liquefaction. The urographic findings include a unifocal mass, which may efface a portion of the collecting system. On ultrasound, abscesses appear as complex hypoechoic masses containing internal debris. CT, the imaging modality of choice, typically reveals a low-density cystic mass with thick, enhancing walls. The small, isolated abscess may resolve with antibiotics, but drainage is usually required for larger lesions or when peri-nephric spread has occurred. If intervention becomes necessary, percutaneous placement of a drainage catheter with CT guidance is curative in up to two-thirds of patients.

Pyonephrosis

Pyonephrosis is the presence of infected material within an obstructed renal collecting system (Fig. 2.18). **Because of the risk of urosepsis and potential death, pyonephrosis is one of the few urologic emergencies.** Ultrasound can reliably differentiate pyonephrosis from hydronephrosis by demonstrating echogenic debris within the dilated collecting system. Once the diagnosis is established, relief of obstruction by

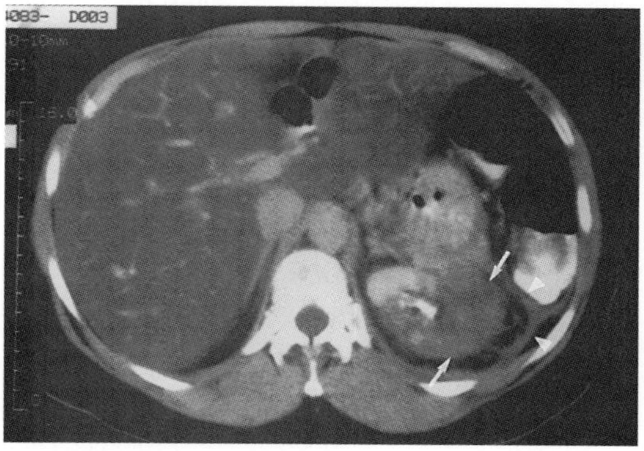

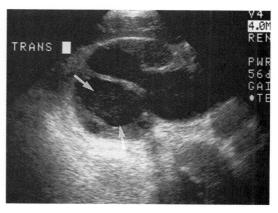

FIGURE 2.17.
Focal bacterial pyelonephritis. A low-density, ill-defined infectious process involving the left kidney *(arrows)*, with extension into the perinephric space and thickening of Gerotas fascia *(arrowheads)*.

FIGURE 2.18.
Pyonephrosis. Ultrasound demonstrates echogenic, infected material in a dilated, obstructed renal collecting system *(arrows)*.

percutaneous nephrostomy and treatment with appropriate antibiotics are indicated.

Emphysematous Pyelonephritis

Emphysematous pyelonephritis is a severe infection associated with infiltration of gas throughout the renal parenchyma. The condition should be suspected in diabetic patients with the following symptoms:

- Flank pain
- Fever
- Nausea
- Vomiting

Although intrarenal gas can be shown on plain films and ultrasound, the extent of involvement and choice of therapy should be determined with the aid of CT. Some patients can be effectively treated with antibiotics and percutaneous drainage, but most patients will require a nephrectomy.

Trauma

Indications for Imaging

The indications and imaging sequences for the radiologic evaluation of renal injury are somewhat controversial. In general, imaging should be obtained in patients with the following signs and symptoms:

- Gross hematuria
- Microscopic hematuria with signs of hemodynamic instability
- Penetrating injury
- Suspected multiorgan trauma

Classification of Blunt Renal Trauma

In the setting of blunt trauma, renal injuries are classified as minor, intermediate, and major. Most injuries (75 to 85%) are minor and are managed conservatively. Injuries classified as minor include:

- Renal contusions
- Small subcapsular or perirenal hematomas
- Small superficial lacerations
- Subsegmental infarcts

Intermediate injuries may or may not require surgical intervention. Intermediate injuries include the following:

- Deep corticomedullary lacerations
- Segmental infarcts

Major injuries require surgery. Major injuries include:

- Multiple renal lacerations
- Injury to the renal vascular pedicle
- Avulsion of the ureteropelvic junction

Plain Film Imaging

All patients with significant abdominal injury should be evaluated with plain films of the abdomen. Fractures can provide important information on location and severity of trauma. In addition, the presence of pneumoperitoneum may necessitate immediate surgery. Although informative, plain films are usually not sufficiently sensitive to direct management, and other imaging modalities are generally necessary.

Excretory Urography

Excretory urography is a good screening tool if blunt trauma is thought to be isolated to the renal area. If the examination is normal and the patient is hemodynamically stable, significant injury is unlikely.

CT

If urography is abnormal or equivocal, further evaluation with CT is required. Furthermore, CT should be the first imaging study (Figs. 2.19 and 2.20) if:

- The trauma is severe
- Multiorgan injury is suspected
- The patient is hemodynamically unstable
- The injury is penetrating

Angiography

CT is extremely accurate at diagnosing the entire spectrum of renal (and abdominal) injuries, including renal vascular trauma. Angiography, once the mainstay of renal trauma evaluation, has largely been replaced by

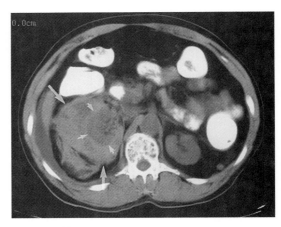

FIGURE 2.19.
Renal hematoma following a percutaneous kidney biopsy. CT scan shows a large hematoma *(large arrows)* involving the right kidney *(small arrows),* with extension into the perinephric and pararenal spaces.

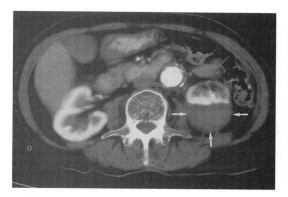

FIGURE 2.20.

Subcapsular hematoma. CT demonstrates a left subcapsular hemorrhage *(arrows)*.

CT for this purpose. Angiography remains indicated in
cases of suspected posttraumatic arteriovenous fistula
or pseudoaneurysm. Angiography can directly aid the
diagnosis of traumatic renal hemorrhage and guide
therapy via transcatheter embolization, thus obviating
the need for surgery.

Ultrasound

The role of ultrasound is limited in the acutely trau-
matized patient, largely because of technical factors.
Difficulty with patient positioning, skin wounds, dress-
ings, tubing, bowel gas, and broken ribs are just some
of the obstacles encountered in obtaining access for
diagnostic imaging. However, ultrasound can be used
to follow injuries that have been characterized by CT,
such as renal and perirenal hematomas.

Imaging for Ureteral and Bladder Injuries

Ureteral injury, usually secondary to penetrating
trauma, can be diagnosed with excretory urography in a
stable patient with good renal function. However, considering the common association with other injuries
(lacerations of the small bowel, liver, and spleen), surgical exploration is frequently done immediately. Some
surgeons prefer to assess the degree of injury with a CT
scan before making management decisions. Ureteral obstruction secondary to posttraumatic strictures can be
relieved with interventional techniques, such as percutaneous nephrostomy and antegrade ureteral stenting.

Bladder and urethral injury can be caused by
blunt, iatrogenic, or penetrating trauma. Retrograde
cystography is the modality of choice for evaluating
bladder injury but generally should not be done until
after a retrograde urethrography has excluded a ure-

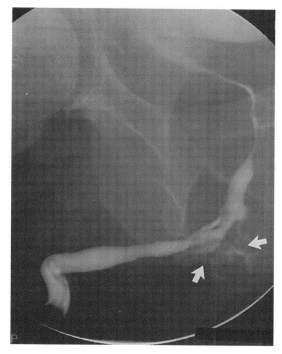

FIGURE 2.21.

Urethral rupture. Urethrogram demonstrates contrast
extravasating from the ruptured urethra *(arrows)*.

thral injury (Fig. 2.21). CT or excretory urography
cannot be substituted for conventional cystography
because of lack of sensitivity in detecting bladder
rupture. Urethral injury may give rise to urethral
stricture (Fig. 2.22).

Renal Artery Stenosis

Essential and secondary hypertension affect approximately 60 million Americans and is associated with
significant morbidity and mortality. RAS, the major
cause of secondary hypertension, is important to diagnose because it is potentially correctable. Many radiologic tests have been advocated for screening hypertensive patients suspected of having RAS, but their
accuracy and utility vary greatly.

Selecting an Imaging Modality

Available imaging modalities include conventional
arteriography, captopril renography, duplex Doppler
ultrasound, CT angiography, and MR angiography.
The different modalities are discussed below. Excretory
urography (i.e., hypertensive urography) is no longer
used as a screening test because of its low sensitivity.

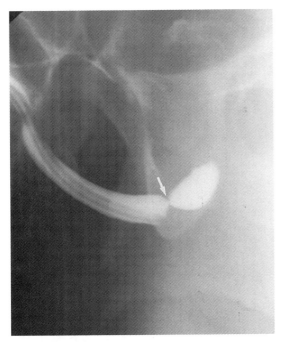

FIGURE 2.22.
Posttraumatic urethral stricture. Urethrogram shows a focal narrowing *(arrow)* of the urethra that developed following trauma.

The most effective imaging strategy is based on many factors, including:

- The likelihood that RAS is present
- The patient's renal function
- The expertise and preference of the involved imagers

Conventional Arteriography

Conventional arteriography, traditionally considered the gold standard for RAS evaluation, should be the initial test when the index of suspicion is high and renal function is normal (Fig. 2.23). Angiography provides the best anatomic detail of the renal arteries and serves as a guide for treatment with balloon angioplasty. However, angiography cannot be used as a screening test for all patients, especially if the index of suspicion is low, because of its invasiveness and relatively high cost.

Captopril Renography

If the index of suspicion is high and angiography is contraindicated (e.g., because of allergy to contrast media, poor renal function, etc.), captopril renography is an acceptable alternative.

Doppler Ultrasound

Many investigators have recommended Doppler ultrasound as a screening test because it is relatively inexpensive, does not involve radiation, and can be used safely in patients with renal failure. The velocity of flowing blood within the main renal arteries and the appearance of the intrarenal arterial sound waves are the important items to consider. As blood flows through a significant stenosis (generally considered to be 50% or greater), its velocity increases. For example, a main renal artery velocity greater than 100 cm/sec or a renal artery:aortic velocity ratio greater than 3.5 is considered diagnostic of a hemodynamically significant stenosis. Theoretically, a significant stenosis of the main renal artery will produce a change in the appearance of the intrarenal Doppler sound wave, including dampening of the Doppler tracing and loss of the early systolic peaks.

Problems associated with ultrasound include difficulty in visualizing the entire main renal arteries (especially in obese patients or in the presence of bowel gas) and the long examination times required. Additionally, the accuracy of ultrasound is highly variable, and many recent investigators have been unable to duplicate the high accuracies initially reported in the literature. At this time, ultrasound cannot be recommended for screening except in those centers that have proven its utility. These institutions typically have dedicated technologists and physicians highly skilled in the performance and interpretation of these examinations.

CT Angiography

CT angiography is a relatively new technique for the detection of RAS. When done well (dedicated imaging protocols using sophisticated software), CT angiography is capable of depicting the main renal arteries with excellent anatomic detail. As with any new technique, sensitivities and specificities vary, but most results have been encouraging. One major disadvantage of CT angiography is the need for intravenous contrast media. However, in the patient with no contraindication to intravenous contrast, this modality may soon replace conventional arteriography as the initial imaging choice.

MR Angiography

MR angiography shows great promise in the evaluation of proximal RAS. Unlike conventional angiography, MR angiography can image blood flowing in the renal arteries without the need for intravenous contrast media (Fig. 2.24). Significant stenoses are depicted as

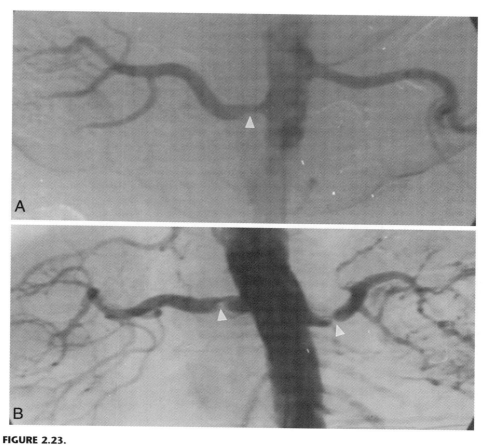

FIGURE 2.23.

Renal artery stenosis (RAS). **A.** Conventional arteriogram shows stenosis of the right renal artery *(arrowhead)*. Note the normal left renal artery. **B.** Bilateral renal artery stenosis is demonstrated *(arrowheads)*.

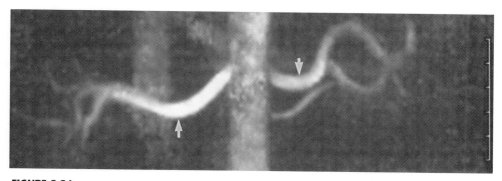

FIGURE 2.24.

Normal MR angiogram. Coronal projection demonstrates normal renal arteries *(arrows)*.

anatomic narrowings or as areas of signal loss. MR angiography is particularly well suited for patients with underlying renal insufficiency who then develop accelerated hypertension and worsening renal func-

tion. These patients are usually older and often have bilateral RAS, which can be difficult to diagnose with other noninvasive modalities such as captopril renography.

KEY POINTS

- CT angiography is a developing field that is proving useful in evaluation of RAS.

- Ultrasound is the safest method of examining the kidneys in a patient who cannot receive an intravenous contrast agent.

- Doppler imaging is useful for evaluating the renal veins for thrombosis, aiding in the diagnosis of inflammatory and neoplastic renal lesions, and assessing the vascular integrity of renal transplants.

- MRI is the method of choice for evaluating renal lesions suspected to be malignant in patients who have poor renal function or who are allergic to iodinated intravenous contrast material.

- Patients who have had a previous contrast reaction are clearly more prone to a second reaction and should only be given contrast media with great caution.

- Patients with preexisting renal insufficiency may be at increased risk for further kidney damage if administered an intravenous contrast agent.

- Most renal masses are detected on radiologic studies done for nonurologic reasons.

- Once a mass is detected on excretory urography, CT or ultrasound is usually needed to confirm its cystic or solid nature.

- Patients with hematuria are best studied with excretory urography, which provides an overall evaluation of the kidneys, collecting systems, and ureters but is insensitive in detecting small renal and bladder masses.

- Because of the risk of urosepsis and potential death, pyonephrosis is one of the few urologic emergencies.

- CT is extremely accurate at diagnosing the entire spectrum of renal injuries, including renal vascular trauma, replacing angiography for this purpose.

- RAS is the major cause of secondary hypertension.

- Excretory urography is the test most frequently used for the initial evaluation of stone disease.

- Approximately 85% of urinary calculi are calcified and can therefore be detected on the preliminary film.

- After administration of a contrast agent, the acutely obstructed kidney will appear fainter than the contralateral normal kidney. As time progresses, the affected kidney will appear denser and the dilated calyceal system will appear to be opaque.

- Ninety percent of stones less than 4 millimeters in diameter are likely to pass spontaneously, compared with 50% of stones 5 to 7 millimeters in diameter. Stones measuring greater than 8 millimeters are unlikely to be passed into the bladder.

- Contraindications to urography include a previous history of allergy to contrast material, renal insufficiency, and pregnancy. In these situations, ultrasound is the safest method to evaluate patients with renal stone disease or mass lesions.

SUGGESTED READINGS

Barbaric ZL. Principles of Genitourinary Radiology. 2nd ed. New York: Thieme, 1994.

Beregi JP, Elkohen ME, Deklunder G, et al. Helical CT angiography compared with arteriography in detection of renal artery stenosis. AJR 1996;167:495–501.

Cochlin DL, Dubbins PA, Goldberg BB, et al. Urogenital Ultrasound: A Text Atlas. Philadelphia: Lippincott, 1994.

Curry NS. Small renal masses (lesions smaller than 3 cm): imaging evaluation and management. AJR 1995;164:355–362.

Davidson AJ, Hartman DS. Radiology of the Kidney and Urinary Tract. 2nd ed. Philadelphia: Saunders, 1994.

Dunnick NR, McCallum RW, Sandler CM. Textbook of Uroradiology. Baltimore: Williams & Wilkins, 1991.

King BF. Diagnostic imaging evaluation of renovascular hypertension. Abdom Imag 1995;20:395–405.

Lowe LH, Zagoria RJ, Baumgartner BR, et al. Role of imaging and intervention in complex infections of the urinary tract. AJR 1994;163:363–367.

3

CHAPTER

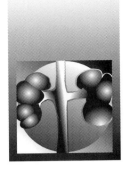

Nuclear Imaging of the Genitourinary System

Neil Katz

BASICS

Radioactive Tracers

Nuclear medicine uses a radioactive tracer that, when introduced into the body, targets a specific organ and emits a type of radiation that can be imaged for use diagnostically and therapeutically. Radioactive tracers usually consist of a radionuclide and a nonradioactive pharmaceutical.

The radionuclide is an isotope with an unstable nucleus, which seeks a more stable form through decay. Energy is produced in this decay process. The unit of measure of energy commonly used in nuclear medicine is kiloelectron volts (keV). Gamma radiation and x-rays emitted by the decay process can be imaged. Beta radiation cannot be imaged but is used in various nuclear medicine therapies, such as thyroid ablation and treatment of bone pain caused by metastatic carcinomas.

The radiopharmaceutical targets a specific organ. A radiopharmaceutical is composed of a radionuclide and a pharmaceutical. The most common radionuclide used in nuclear medicine is technetium-99m (^{99m}Tc). It has an energy level of 140 keV, which is near optimal for nuclear medicine cameras. As the energy levels of radionuclides increase or decrease from this level, image quality degrades.

Half-life of Radionuclides

Radionuclides have a physical half-life, the time needed for the agent to decay to half its initial value. Most radionuclides used in nuclear medicine have a relatively short half-life, ranging from hours to days. ^{99m}Tc has a physical half-life of approximately 6 hours.

The radiopharmaceuticals introduced into the body are metabolized and excreted; the time necessary to excrete half the introduced radioactivity from the body is termed the biologic half-life.

The effective half-life is a combination of the physical and biologic half-lives.

Half-lives become important when multiple nuclear medicine studies are done within a short time on the same patient because the studies may interfere with each other, and the tests need to be timed properly.

Nuclear Medicine Imaging

Nuclear medicine imaging does not provide the anatomic detail seen with computed tomography (CT) or magnetic resonance imaging (MRI). Although some anatomic information is obtained, nuclear medicine diagnostic procedures provide physiologic data about the function of the organ of interest. Nuclear medicine studies have an advantage over other radiologic procedures in that function of an organ, such as the kidney, can be quantified.

The cameras used in nuclear medicine are known as gamma cameras. They are designed to convert photons emitted from the radionuclide in the patient into a light pulse, which is eventually converted into a picture of the organ of interest.

The primary care physician should be familiar with single photon emission computed tomography (SPECT). A single- or multihead gamma camera is used in this imaging technique. The camera rotates around the organ of interest and an image is taken continuously, or every few degrees. The images are then computer processed, and views of the organ can be visualized in multiple planes, similar to the visualization allowed by MRI and CT. Smaller lesions can be detected with this technique, and, although sensitivity is increased, it is often at the expense of specificity.

RADIOPHARMACEUTICALS

The more commonly used radiopharmaceuticals in imaging of the genitourinary system are described here. Other agents that may be employed but are less specific for use in the genitourinary system are described as they are discussed in the text.

^{99m}Tc Diethylenetriamine Pentaacetic Acid (DTPA)

DTPA is approximately 90% filtered by the glomerulus and is useful in measuring the relative or absolute glomerular filtration rate (GFR). DTPA is used for measuring renal perfusion and is rapidly cleared by the kidneys, allowing an evaluation of renal excretion, or clearance. As renal function deteriorates, the uptake and clearance of DTPA decreases, and substitution by another agent should be considered.

Orthoiodohippurate (OIH)

OIH is an excellent agent for measuring effective renal plasma flow (ERPF). It is labeled with either iodine-131 (^{131}I) or iodine-123 (^{123}I); however, the latter is not available in the United States. In many institutions, the use of ^{131}I OIH has been supplanted by the use of ^{99m}Tc mercaptoacetyltriglycine (MAG$_3$).

^{99m}Tc Mercaptoacetyltriglycine (MAG3)

MAG$_3$ has properties similar to those of OIH but is labeled with ^{99m}Tc, which improves image quality.

Approximately 40 to 50% of the agent is cleared (primarily through the proximal tubules) with each pass through the kidney, a percentage better than that of DTPA but approximately half that of OIH. MAG$_3$ can also be used to measure relative and absolute ERPF, as well as provide information on renal blood flow, concentration ability, and excretion. It is often used as the imaging agent for captopril renal scintigraphy in assessing renal vascular hypertension.

Because more MAG$_3$ is cleared with each pass through the kidney than is DTPA, it is the preferred agent for patients with decreased renal function. However, it is significantly more expensive than DTPA (from a centralized unit-dose pharmac, approximately $110 for MAG$_3$ and $14.00 for DTPA).

^{99m}Tc Dimercaptosuccinic Acid (DMSA)

Approximately 40% of the injected DMSA dose is retained in the renal cortex several hours after injection, which makes this agent excellent for cortical imaging. Imaging is delayed 2 to 3 hours. Shelf life, which previously had been 30 minutes, has been extended to 4 hours, which means that this agent is available to most nuclear medicine departments.

DMSA is commonly used in pediatrics for evaluating pyelonephritis and renal scarring, but it can also be used in assessing space-occupying lesions to differentiate normal variants from pathologic lesions.

^{99m}Tc Glucoheptonate

This radiopharmaceutical is also used for delayed cortical imaging. Approximately 10 to 15% is retained in the renal cortex 1-2 hours postinjection, but up to 45% is excreted during the first hour.

Although the agent can be used to provide information on renal blood flow and supplies some excretory data, because of its cortical retention properties it is not the preferred agent for these purposes.

INDICATIONS FOR GENITOURINARY IMAGING

Table 3.1 lists the various indications for radionuclide imaging of the genitourinary system. Primary care physicians should consider these procedures as primary when physiologic information is needed and as alternatives to radiologic procedures in many situations. These procedures are available in most nuclear medicine departments; of course, the choice of test will depend partially on availability in a particular community and on the capabilities of the nuclear medicine service.

Summary of Diagnosis

- Radioactive tracers usually consist of a radionuclide and a nonradioactive pharmaceutical.
- The most common radionuclide used in nuclear medicine is ^{99m}Tc. ^{99m}Tc has a physical half-life of approximately 6 hours.
- The radiopharmaceuticals introduced into the body are also metabolized and excreted; the time necessary to excrete half the introduced radioactivity from the body is termed the biologic half-life.
- The effective half-life is a combination of the physical and biologic half-lives.
- The cameras used in nuclear medicine are known as gamma cameras.
- Radiopharmaceuticals, such as DTPA and OIH, are useful markers for GFR and ERPF, respectively.
- DMSA is commonly used in pediatrics for evaluating pyelonephritis and renal scarring, as well as for assessing space-occupying lesions.
- Renal scintigraphy is useful for determining asymmetrical disease or relative functional differences between the two kidneys. Diuretic-augmented renal scintigraphy is useful in differentiating a dilated, nonobstructed renal collecting system from a dilated urinary tract because of lower urinary tract obstruction.
- Gallium imaging is useful in assessing acute interstitial nephritis (AIN), renal abscess, and perirenal abscess.
- Renal imaging may be helpful to assess congenital anomalies such as horseshoe kidneys and ectopic kidneys.
- Radionuclide cystography plays an important role in the evaluation of vesicoureteral reflux.
- Testicular scintigraphy can be used to differentiate testicular torsion from acute epididymitis.
- ^{131}I metaiodobenzylguanidine (MIBG) imaging for the diagnosis of pheochromocytoma should be considered when CT or MRI has been unrevealing.

Evaluation of Renal Artery Flow

Renal artery flow, concentration, and excretion are evaluated by renal scan, using DTPA or MAG$_3$ (Fig. 3.1).

Indications for Radionuclide Imaging of the Genitourinary System	TABLE 3.1

Indications for renal imaging
   Obstructive uropathy
   Renovascular hypertension
   Renal transplant assessment
   Evaluation of mass lesions, cortical defects
   Infection (pyelonephritis)
   Evaluation of renal perfusion and function
      Absolute and relative measurements of GFR and ERPF
      Evaluation and localization of asymmetrical renal disease
   Renal trauma
   Assessment of functional recovery and prognosis
   Assessment of diffuse renal disease
   As alternative to contrast studies (CT, IVP)
      in patients with contrast allergy
Indications for radionuclide cystography
   Ureteral reflux
Indications for scrotal imaging
   Testicular torsion vs. epididymitis
Indications for adrenal imaging
   Localization of pheochromocytoma

CT, computed tomography; ERPF, effective renal plasma flow; GFR, glomerular filtration rate; IVP, intravenous pyelography.

The radiopharmaceutical is injected into the patient in a bolus fashion. Posterior images are obtained by gamma camera and the data are stored on a computer, which allows quantification and dynamic playback after the study is completed.

Renal artery flow (blood flow down the aorta and into the renal arteries) is visualized. The radiopharmaceutical then concentrates within the renal cortex; this process takes approximately 1 to 2 minutes, and relative GFR or ERPF is calculated from these data. Clearance is evaluated during the final phase of the study, which can take from 30 to 60 minutes depending on the protocol used. Using the data stored on the computer, regions of interest are drawn around each kidney, and time–activity curves are generated, which show the activity in each kidney during the course of the study (Fig. 3.2).

Evaluation of Renal Function

Measurement of GFR and ERPF

Relative and absolute measurements of GFR and ERPF can be made using nuclear medicine techniques. ^{99m}Tc DTPA is used to assess GFR, and OIH or ^{99m}Tc MAG$_3$ is used for ERPF. One advantage of nuclear medicine techniques over others is that the contribution by each kidney to total GFR or ERPF can be quantified.

The relative contribution from each kidney to GFR or ERPF can be determined from the isotope counts in each kidney at 1–2 minutes postdosing (Fig. 3.3). This information is useful in assessing asymmetrical renal disease and for monitoring changes in function over time.

Several methods are available for absolute measurement of GFR or ERPF; the specifics are beyond the scope of this chapter. GFR measurements using the nuclear medicine techniques correlate well with inulin clearance and 24-hour creatinine clearance measurements.

Renal Scintigraphy

Renal scintigraphy plays a limited role in the evaluation of diffuse renal disease, the injured kidney, and trauma to other parts of the genitourinary system because it is sensitive but not very specific. The study demonstrates poor uptake and excretion. It is useful for determining asymmetrical disease or the relative functional differences between the two kidneys. Renal scintigraphy should be considered as an alternative to contrast studies, especially for diabetics with renal insufficiency. It serves as an alternative to CT and other anatomic imaging modalities when those modalities are not available or when functional and prognostic information is desired. For example, prognostic information can be obtained for

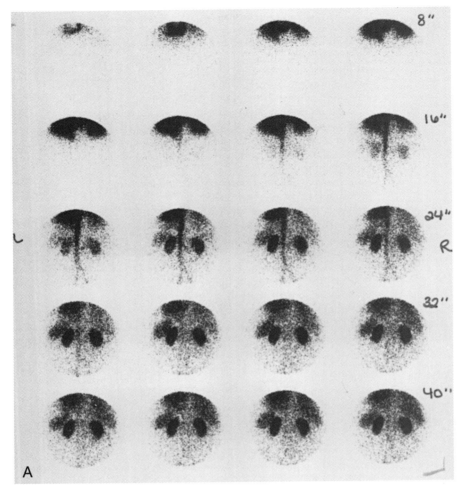

FIGURE 3.1.
Normal renal scan, posterior imaging. Flow study, 2 seconds per image. **A.** Symmetrical flow is seen to the kidneys.

patients with acute renal failure (ARF); renal function is likely to return if there is adequate hippuran uptake.

Gallium Imaging

Gallium imaging is useful in assessing AIN. Gallium-67 citrate is a radiopharmaceutical that accumulates in areas of inflammation, and it is used in situations of renal infection, such as renal abscess and perirenal abscess, and for tumor imaging. It is normally excreted by the kidneys 24 to 48 hours after injection. Gallium retention at 72 hours postinjection in the setting of ARF is suggestive of AIN. However, 72-hour retention may also be seen in other disease processes, such as nephrotic syndrome, acute tubular necrosis (ATN), ARF from causes other than AIN, and in patients receiving chemotherapy or nephrotoxic antibiotics.

Evaluation of Obstructive Uropathy

Diuretic-augmented Renal Scintigraphy

Diuretic-augmented renal scintigraphy is useful in differentiating a dilated, nonobstructed renal collecting system from a system dilated because of a lower urinary tract obstruction. The diuretic stimulates urine flow, clearing activity from a dilated, nonobstructed system. Anatomic imaging studies such as CT, ultrasound, and intravenous pyelogram (IVP) will show a dilated renal pelvis or collecting system, but the dilatation may have been caused by previous insults, such as reflux or previous obstruction, and not by a current obstruction.

Procedure for diuretic-augmented renal scintigraphy
1. Before the study, the patient is hydrated orally or intravenously.

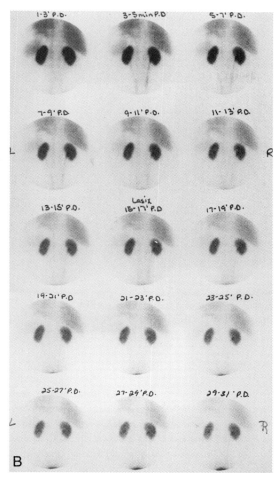

(FIGURE 3.1—continued)
B. Clearance phase, 2 minutes per image. Maximal radiotracer concentration usually occurs within the first 5 minutes postdosing, followed by excretion of the radiotracer from both kidneys.

2. A Foley catheter is inserted into the bladder of patients who cannot void on request.
3. A renal scan is done, consisting of a flow study and delayed static images.
4. The renal pelvis and collecting system should begin to clear approximately 15 to 20 minutes after injection of the radiotracer.
5. If there is retained activity, the patient is given furosemide intravenously (0.5 mg/kg up to 40 mg total; higher if there is renal failure). Imaging is continued for at least an additional 20 minutes.

Time–activity curves   Time–activity curves are then generated for each kidney. These curves demonstrate one of four patterns, as shown in Figure 3.4.

Calculating quantitative indices   The data can be analyzed visually, but quantitative indices may also be calculated. A clearance half-time ($t \frac{1}{2}$) is generated, which is the time taken for half the activity to clear after the diuretic has been given. If the $t \frac{1}{2}$ is greater than 20 minutes, the system is obstructed; if it is less than 10 minutes, the system is dilated but not obstructed; and if the $t \frac{1}{2}$ is between 10 and 20 minutes, the condition is equivocal. However, the generation of quantitative indices has not been standardized, and this type of measurement may actually give a false diagnosis, depending on when the diuretic was given and on the $t \frac{1}{2}$ to the rest of the curve. The author prefers qualitative analysis using time-activity curves.

Evaluation of Renal Anatomy and Mass Lesions

As mentioned earlier, the primary care physician should use nuclear medicine procedures for physiologic and

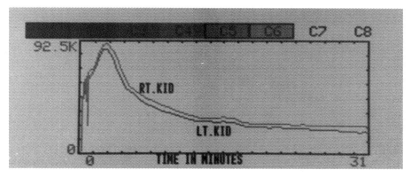

FIGURE 3.2.
Time–activity curves for the study shown in Figure 3.1. Peak concentration occurs at approximately 3 minutes for both kidneys. There is symmetrical and prompt clearance of the radiotracer from both kidneys.

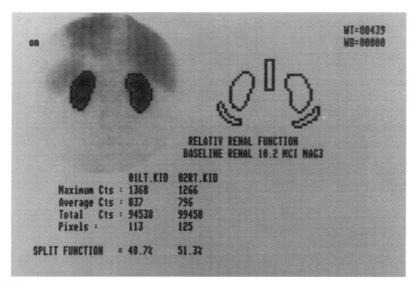

FIGURE 3.3.
The relative glomerular filtration rate (GFR) or effective renal plasma flow (ERPF) can be calculated for each kidney, depending on the radiopharmaceutical used. This figure shows the relative ERPF for each kidney for the study shown in Figures 3.1 and 3.2. *Left kidney,* 48.7%; *right kidney,* 51.3%.

functional evaluation of the kidneys. Ultrasound and CT provide better anatomic details, especially in the assessment of renal size and shape, as well as better visualization of intrarenal mass lesions. Renal defects, however, are often seen during renal nuclear imaging, and these defects must be correlated with findings via ultrasound and CT.

Renal imaging may be requested to assess congenital anomalies such as horseshoe kidneys and ectopic kidneys. Renal cortical imaging, using either DMSA or glucoheptonate, helps differentiate a true intrarenal mass from a renal column (columns of Bertin, hypertrophied renal columns, fetal lobulation). Cortical imaging should also be considered as an alternative to CT and ultrasound in the evaluation of renal anatomy, cortical infarcts, and scarring in patients with contraindications to contrast media or when ultrasound images are of poor quality.

Evaluation of Renal Vascular Hypertension

Secondary hypertension accounts for less than 10% of hypertensive cases; renal vascular hypertension accounts for up to 5% of the hypertensive population.

Renal artery stenosis (RAS), caused by atherosclerosis or fibromuscular dysplasia, causes a fall in renal perfusion, resulting in a fall in GFR. The body compensates for this by activating the renin angiotensin system. Increased levels of renin are released by the juxtaglomerular apparatus of the kidneys, which is a catalyst for the conversion of angiotensin I to angiotensin II. Angiotensin II is a powerful vasoconstrictor, causing constriction of the intrarenal efferent arterioles, increasing the pressure gradient across the glomerulus, and thus maintaining the GFR. However, angiotensin II causes hypertension by systemic arterial vasoconstriction and by stimulating the release of aldosterone, with resulting sodium retention.

Determining Hypertension Caused by RAS

Many patients have both RAS and hypertension, but the stenosis may not be the cause of the hypertension. Captopril renal scintigraphy is a physiologic test that evaluates the response of the kidneys to angiotensin-converting enzyme (ACE) inhibition, and it helps to predict in which patients hypertension is caused by RAS and thus will respond to a revascularization procedure.

ACE inhibitors such as captopril block the conversion of angiotensin I to angiotensin II, causing a fall in GFR in patients with renovascular hypertension. This can be imaged and measured using captopril renal

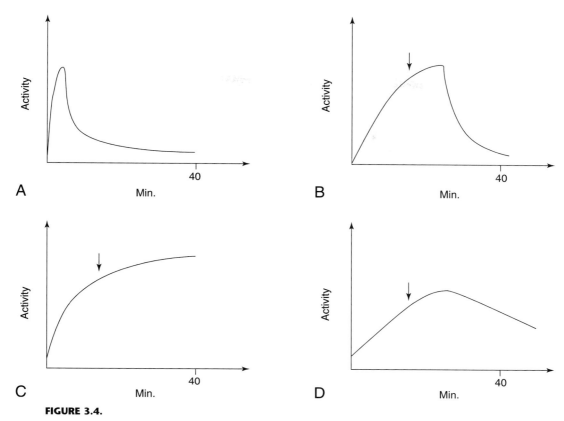

FIGURE 3.4.
Diuretic renogram time–activity curves. *Arrow* indicates when diuretic is injected. **A.** Normal time–activity curve in a nonobstructed, nondilated kidney. **B.** Nonobstructed kidney, with retention of radiotracer in a dilated renal pelvis that clears promptly with the diuretic. **C.** Obstructed kidney with a dilated renal pelvis and no response to the diuretic. **D.** Equivocal response. This may represent either a partially obstructed kidney or a kidney with a nonobstructed, dilated collecting system with slow washout of the radiotracer secondary to baseline renal insufficiency, a distended bladder, or lack of response to the diuretic. (Reprinted with permission from O'Reilly PH. Diuresis renography 8 years later: an update. J Urol 1986;136:994.)

scintigraphy. The test usually consists of two parts, a baseline renal scan followed by a captopril renal scan.

Procedure for captopril renal scintigraphy
1. The patient's blood pressure is taken before captopril dosing and is monitored for 1 hour thereafter.
2. The patient is administered 25 to 50 mg of captopril orally. (Some institutions use intravenous enalapril and then the protocol will be slightly different.)
3. Immediately afterward, a renal scan is done.
4. Renogram time-activity curves are generated for the baseline study and the captopril study, and the two are compared. The exact change in the curve

depends on the radiopharmaceutical used. In Figure 3.5, ^{99m}Tc DTPA demonstrates a reduction in uptake on the affected side, whereas the tubular agents, OIH and ^{99m}Tc MAG$_3$, demonstrate reduced time to peak activity and continued accumulation of the radiotracer within the kidney. The author recommends ^{99m}Tc MAG$_3$ in any patient with a creatinine level greater than 1.5 mg/dL.

Standardizing protocols for captopril renal scintigraphy
Protocols for doing captopril renal scintigraphy have not been standardized, although there is movement in the nuclear medicine community to do so. Readers are advised to familiarize themselves with the protocol

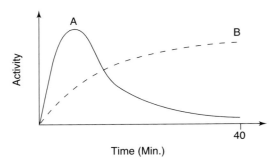

FIGURE 3.5.
Positive response to captopril in a patient with renal vascular hypertension (only affected kidney shown). Baseline study demonstrates normal uptake and excretion of the radiopharmaceutical *(curve A). Curve B* shows the same kidney as in *curve A,* but the study was done 1 hour after an oral dose of captopril. There is a delay in time-to-peak activity, and increasing activity over time.

used by their consulting nuclear medicine physicians. The author advises the following:

1. Before each study, the patient should be well hydrated with 500 to 1000 mL of fluid.
2. If the patient is already on an ACE inhibitor, it should be discontinued for several days before doing the study (captopril for 2-3 days; longer-acting ACE inhibitors, up to 7 days). There is some evidence that studies done on patients on chronic ACE inhibition demonstrate false–negative results because of some intrarenal accumulation mechanism.
3. Diuretics should be withheld.
4. Both studies can be done on the same day or 1-2 days apart. Doing the captopril portion of the study first is also acceptable. If the results are normal, a baseline study need not be done; and if they are abnormal, the baseline study is then done.

Indications for captopril renal scintigraphy   Appropriate patient selection is important for cost-effective use of this procedure. Secondary causes should be considered in any patient with early (less than age 30) or late (more than age 50) onset of hypertension. However, renovascular causes should be especially considered in patients with the following signs and symptoms:

- Worsening of preexisting hypertension
- Hypertension that is refractory to drug therapy
- Hypertension with abdominal bruits
- Abrupt onset
- Associated worsening of renal function

Figures 3.6 and 3.7 show pre- and postcaptopril studies, respectively, in a 46-year-old man. Several years earlier, the patient had suffered a hypertensive cerebral vascular event with resulting right hemiparesis. His blood pressure was poorly controlled, despite multiple medications. Physical examination revealed a right abdominal bruit. The study results are consistent with renin-dependent renal vascular hypertension from stenosis of the right renal artery. Contrast angiography revealed a 99% stenosis of the right renal artery; an angioplasty was done and a stent was placed. The patient's blood pressure was under good control with 25 mg atenolol for the first year after the stent placement, and since then it has been normal without any antihypertensive medications.

Captopril renal scintigraphy has reported sensitivity and specificity up to 95 and 94%, respectively. It is effective in lateralizing to the affected kidney, and, more importantly, it is a strong predictor of who will respond to a revascularization procedure (97% positive predicted value). There are limitations to the study, however. The study appears to be less accurate in patients with bilateral RAS and in those with renal failure.

Monitoring Renal Transplants

The assessment of patients with renal transplants is often left to the nephrologist and transplant surgeon. However, primary care physicians should be aware of the role renal imaging plays in monitoring the transplanted kidney for rejection, drug toxicity, renovascular disease, and other complications. Renal imaging is used to evaluate the following conditions:

- ATN
- Acute rejection
- Chronic rejection
- Cyclosporine nephrotoxicity

Unfortunately, the tests are nonspecific, require serial imaging, and need to be correlated with the clinical situation. A baseline renal scan is often done within 1 to 2 days after transplantation.

Acute Tubular Necrosis

ATN occurs in almost all patients with cadaveric transplants and is present almost immediately after transplantation. Renal imaging using ^{99m}Tc MAG$_3$ reveals a decrease in blood flow, reduction in ERPF, and retention of the radiopharmaceutical. This situation improves over time, as demonstrated by serial studies.

Acute Rejection

Findings in situations of acute rejection are similar to those of ATN, but renal function, as documented on serial renal studies, gets worse over time.

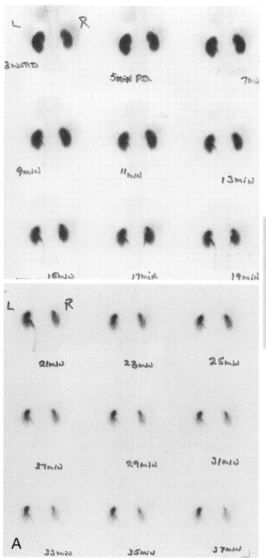

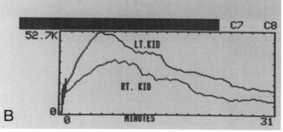

FIGURE 3.6.
Baseline renal scan in a 46-year-old man with suspected renal vascular hypertension. Flow study not shown. **A.** Clearance images show the right kidney to be smaller than the left kidney, but relatively normal excretion from both. **B.** Time–activity curves reveal overall less activity in the right kidney but symmetrical excretion.

Chronic Rejection

Chronic rejection occurs months to years after transplantation. The findings on the renal scan vary, depending on the degree of rejection. However, cortical thinning and decreased flow and transit, which worsen as renal function deteriorates, may be demonstrated.

Cyclosporine Nephrotoxicity

Findings associated with cyclosporine nephrotoxicity are similar to those of ATN, making it difficult to distinguish between the two. Diagnosis is often one of

exclusion, correlated with cyclosporine levels and serial renal scans.

Other Complications

Other complications associated with renal transplantation may be imaged using radionuclide techniques. These complications include:

- Vascular occlusion
- Renal vascular hypertension
- Ureteral obstruction
- Hematoma

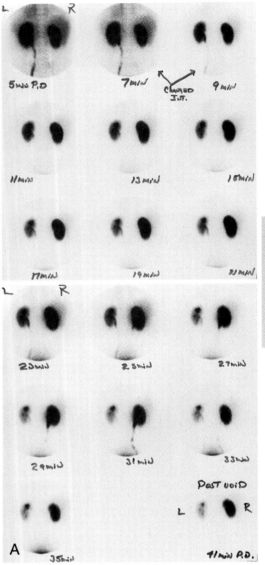

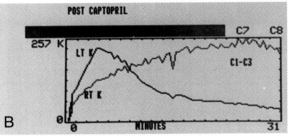

FIGURE 3.7.
Postcaptopril study, same patient as in Figure 3.6. The patient received 25 mg captopril orally, and the study was done 1 hour later. Clearance images show persistent activity in the right kidney. **A.** Excretion from the *left kidney* is unchanged from the baseline study. **B.** Time–activity curves demonstrate marked delay in time-to-peak activity for the right kidney, when compared with the baseline study, and increasing activity during the course of the study. This patient had a 99% stenosis of the right renal artery and an excellent response to a revascularization procedure.

- Lymphocele
- Urine leak

Renal vascular hypertension can be assessed by captopril renal scintigraphy, and obstruction can be evaluated by diuretic-augmented renal scintigraphy. Urine leaks appear as extravasation of radiotracer into the abdomen or pelvis. Hematomas and lymphoceles appear as photopenic ("cold") areas; however, lymphoceles appear several weeks after transplantation, in comparison to hematomas, which appear within days.

Evaluation of Vesicoureteral Reflux and Pyelonephritis

Nuclear medicine has an evolving role in the evaluation of children with urinary tract infections (UTIs) and is considered by many to comprise the procedures of choice for evaluation of these children. The procedures—direct radionuclide cystography for evaluating vesicoureteral reflux, and renal cortical scintigraphy for assessing renal scarring and pyelonephritis—may also be used in the evaluation of adults. It is currently recommended that all children have diagnostic imaging studies done after their first UTI to detect treatable conditions. The physician's goal is to prevent development of renal parenchymal injury caused by UTI.

Vesicoureteral Reflux

Vesicoureteral reflux involves the pathologic retrograde flow of urine from the bladder into a ureter and possibly into the pelvicaliceal system. It is caused by a failure at the ureterovesicular junction. Reflux provides a pathway for bacteria to reach the kidneys and is suspected of playing a role in pathogenesis of pyelonephritis and renal scarring. In fact, experimental models have shown that reflux of infected urine into the kidney can cause pyelonephritis. Patients with severe reflux are more likely to develop renal damage leading to reflux nephropathy, with associated hypertension and renal failure. Most cases of reflux resolve spontaneously, and the goal of therapy is to prevent renal damage until the reflux does not resolve. Imaging helps identify patients at risk (more females than males) and determine therapeutic intervention.

Imaging studies for evaluation of vesicoureteral reflux Two imaging studies are available for evaluation of vesicoureteral reflux: contrast cystography and direct radionuclide cystography.

CONTRAST CYSTOGRAPHY Contrast cystography provides better anatomic definition, especially in visualizing posterior urethral valves, in males than in females. Direct radionuclide cystography is as sensitive as, and possibly more sensitive than, contrast cystography for detecting reflux. Bladder filling and voiding can be continuously monitored using the radionuclide technique, and there is significant reduction in radiation exposure to the gonads when compared with the contrast cystography. This is an important concern when numerous studies are to be done. One approach is to initially do contrast cystography and follow serially with the radio-nuclide technique.

RADIONUCLIDE CYSTOGRAPHY To do the radionuclide cystogram, a Foley catheter is inserted and any residual urine is drained. A saline bag is attached to the Foley catheter. Bladder volume is estimated using the formula:

$$(\text{age} + 2) \times 30 = \text{bladder volume in mL}$$

The radiopharmaceutical commonly used is ^{99m}Tc sulfur colloid, a nonabsorbable colloid, which is the same agent used for liver-spleen scans. Continuous imaging of bladder filling and emptying is recorded, and several static images are taken as well. Figure 3.8 depicts bilateral reflux in a young girl with recurrent UTIs.

A radiologic grading system for reflux demonstrated on radionuclide cystography is as follows:

Grade I   Reflux into the ureter
Grade II Filling of the ureter, pelvis, and calyces
Grade III Mild to moderate dilatation or tortuosity of the ureter and renal pelvis
Grade IV More moderate dilatation of the ureter and renal pelvis
Grade V   Gross dilatation and tortuosity of the ureter with gross dilatation of the renal pelvis

Because the resolution provided by radionuclide cystography is not as good as that provided by a contrast study, some physicians will use a slightly different grading scheme that combines the grades given above: mild (grades I and II); moderate (grade III); and severe (grades IV and V).

Assessing Damage from Pyelonephritis, Scarring, and Infections

Renal damage from pyelonephritis and scarring may be assessed using cortical imaging agents. ^{99m}Tc DMSA is the agent of choice, but ^{99m}Tc glucoheptonate may also be used. These agents show decreased uptake in areas of renal parenchyma inflammation, as shown in Figure 3.9. DMSA is more sensitive in detecting cortical defects than either ultrasound or IVP, and sensitivity may be increased by using SPECT imaging. One set of recommendations for use of renal cortical imaging is presented in Table 3.2.

Renal infections may also be evaluated using gallium-67 citrate. Gallium-67 citrate is normally excreted by the kidneys 24 to 48 hours after injection, and delayed imaging is often required. Increased focal uptake in a kidney may represent an abscess or acute pyelonephritis. Also included in the differential diagnosis are tumor and focal bacterial nephritis. Pyelonephritis may also appear as unilateral or bilateral diffuse uptake.

Indium-111-labeled white cell imaging is an alternative to gallium, but it is not used in children because of the potential risk of oncogenesis. The technique requires obtaining approximately 50 mL of blood from the patient and labeling it with indium-111. Platelets and red cells are removed, leaving just white cells; the radiation dose is high enough to kill the lymphocytes, leaving neutrophils. The neutrophils are reinjected into the patient, and the white cells accumulate in acute pyogenic processes.

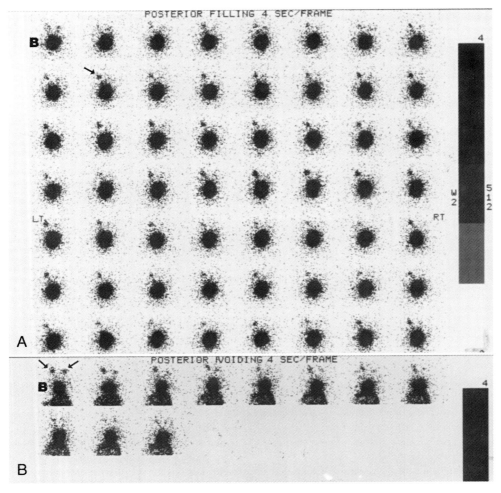

FIGURE 3.8.
Bilateral reflux in a young girl with pyelonephritis. **A.** Filling phase. **B.** Voiding phase. *Arrows* demonstrate reflux to the renal pelvis. Note that the reflux to the right kidney is worse during the voiding phase. *B,* bladder. (Courtesy of Childrens Medical Center, Dayton, Ohio.)

FIGURE 3.9.
DMSA scan, left posterior oblique view, demonstrating two abnormal cold areas *(arrows)* in a young girl with recurrent urinary tract infections. This finding indicates parenchymal damage. *L,* left; *R,* right. (Courtesy of Childrens Medical Center, Dayton, Ohio.)

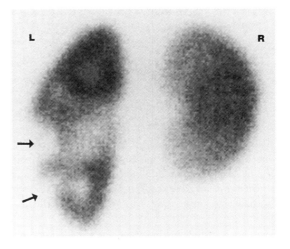

Modified with permission from Rosenfeld DL, Fleischer M, et al. Current recommendations for children with urinary tract infections. Clin Pediatr May 1995;34(5):261–264.

Indications for Renal Cortical Scintigraphy in Children	TABLE 3.2

Documented vesicoureteral reflux for which surgery is considered
Numerous urinary tract infections or suspected previous pyelonephritis
Breakthrough infections while on prophylaxis
Children older than age 6 with persistent moderate vesicoureteral reflux while on prolonged antibiotic prophylaxis
Hospitalized children with suspected acute pyelonephritis

Evaluation of the Acute Scrotum

Testicular Torsion

Testicular torsion is considered a surgical emergency requiring quick intervention (within the first 24 hours) to salvage the testicle. After 4 hours, the success rate decreases. Peak incidence occurs around puberty—although it may occur earlier in childhood—as well as in young adulthood.

The diagnostic dilemma is to differentiate torsion from nonsurgical or nonemergent causes of the acute scrotum, such as epididymitis. Clinically it is difficult to distinguish between epididymitis and torsion because there is significant overlap in the associated signs and symptoms. Torsion can be intermittent, making the diagnosis even more difficult.

Typically, testicular torsion presents with abrupt onset of pain and with nausea, vomiting, and an inability to walk. The onset of epididymitis is more gradual, not as intense, with dysuria, fever, and a positive urinalysis; symptoms may be relieved by elevation of the scrotum (Prehn's sign).

Diagnostic Tests

Two diagnostic tests may be used to help diagnose the cause of an acute scrotum: testicular scintigraphy and color Doppler ultrasound. Both have equal sensitivities (84-100% and 82-100%, respectively). Accuracy of Doppler ultrasound appears to be more operator dependent, improving with experience. The reader is advised to use the diagnostic test with which the consulting radiologist or nuclear medicine physician is most comfortable. Both techniques are less accurate in neonates and small children because of the small size of the testicles. If neither test is available, the patient should be taken to surgery.

Testicular scintigraphy Testicular scintigraphy takes only approximately 15 minutes; it consists of a continuous flow study followed by a series of static images. The nuclear medicine physician doing the study must first examine the patient to confirm the affected testicle. Testicular torsion shows decreased perfusion

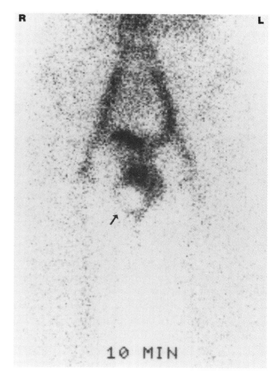

FIGURE 3.10.
Testicular torsion involving the right testicle. The patient is a 13-year-old boy with right scrotal pain for 24 hours. Findings were confirmed at surgery, and the torsion was successfully reduced. The testicle was thought to be viable. The *arrow* points to the right hemiscrotum with a photopenic (cold) defect, which corresponds to the torsed right testicle. There is normal activity in the left hemiscrotum. *R,* right; *L,* left. (Courtesy of Childrens Medical Center, Dayton, Ohio.)

and a cold area of decreased or absent activity on delayed images (Fig. 3.10). Increased perfusion on the flow images and increased activity on static images are seen in epididymitis.

Cold lesions may also be seen in abscess, trauma, hydrocele, inguinal hernia, tumor, and other conditions.

Clinical presentation and examination, as well as gray-scale ultrasound, should help in the diagnosis. However, a cold lesion in many of these conditions represents testicular ischemia, although not caused by torsion.

Evaluation of the Adrenal Gland

Adrenal imaging is possible using ^{131}I MIBG, a norepinephrine analog, or indium-111 pentetreotide. Both agents are taken up in tumors of neuroendocrine origin.

Pheochromocytomas are tumors of neuroectodermal origin, which secrete catecholamines—norepinephrine, epinephrine, and dopamine. They are a rare cause of hypertension. The hypertension is often paroxysmal and associated with pounding headache, sweating, palpitations, and flushing of the face. The diagnosis is suspected in patients with the appropriate symptoms and elevated urinary metanephrines or blood catecholamines. Approximately 10% of tumors are bilateral, 10% are extra-adrenal, and 10% are malignant. Approximately 20% of pheochromocytomas are associated with multiple endocrine neoplasia (MEN) II and III. Initial diagnostic workup should include CT or MRI of the abdomen, or both. When the lesion cannot be identified or extra-adrenal locations are suspected, an ^{131}I MIBG or indium-111 pentetreotide study should be done. Imaging for both of these studies take several days, and multiple imaging sessions may be needed.

MIBG Imaging

MIBG imaging compares favorably with both CT and MRI (sensitivity is 71-87% and specificity is 94-100% for ^{131}I MIBG). Some institutions use MIBGs as the initial imaging technique because it provides whole body images. Additionally, it may be more specific in patients who have had previous abdominal surgery. Before ^{131}I MIBG injection, the patient should be started on an iodine solution (e.g., oral potassium iodide solution 120 mg/day) to block any uptake of the radioiodine by the thyroid gland. Some medications interfere with uptake of ^{131}I MIBG and must be discontinued, some as much as 4 to 6 weeks in advance. These medications include:

- Antidepressants, tricyclics and others
- Labetalol
- Sympathomimetic agents (e.g., decongestants)
- Calcium channel blockers

If medications cannot be discontinued, the indium-111 pentetreotide study should be considered. Both studies are expensive, costing the patient approximately $2000.

MISCELLANEOUS PROCEDURES

Skeletal Imaging

Skeletal imaging can also provide information about the genitourinary system. The diphosphonate radiopharmaceuticals used in bone imaging are excreted through the kidney, and cortical defects, obstruction, bladder deformities, congenital abnormalities, ectopically located kidneys, failure to visualize a kidney, and asymmetrical renal disease may be incidentally seen on a bone scan and reported to the ordering physician. These abnormalities may require follow-up, with additional radiographic or nuclear medicine studies.

Perfusion Studies

The author has used upper extremity and subclavian perfusion studies to evaluate arteriovenous (A-V) grafts in patients on dialysis. Perfusion studies can also aid in the evaluation of gross obstruction to flow or delayed flow in patients being considered for A–V graft revision or replacement. Graft infection can be assessed using the indium-111-labeled white blood cell technique described previously. The indium-111 technique can also aid in the evaluation of graft infections or abscess in patients on chronic hemodialysis or ambulatory peritoneal dialysis.

KEY POINTS

- Nuclear imaging is a safe alternative to radiologic procedures for measuring renal blood flow and clearance.

- Nuclear imaging is useful in determining relative functional differences between the two kidneys.

- Nuclear imaging is an alternative to contrast studies for patients with contraindications to contrast media.

- Nuclear imaging is useful in differentiating between a dilated but nonobstructed renal collecting system and an obstructed system. This may not always be clear on anatomic studies such as ultrasound of the kidneys or IVP.

- Nuclear scintigraphy is useful in locating ectopic kidneys and for differentiating pathologic lesions from normal anatomic variants that cannot be distinguished by other anatomic studies.

- Captopril renal scintigraphy is a test that screens for physiologically significant renal vascular disease and helps to predict patient response to a revascularization procedure.

- Nuclear techniques often are the procedures of choice in the pediatric population. Radionuclide cystography is used serially to assess for changes in vesicoureteral reflux and to help determine those patients who may need surgery. Renal cortical imaging is more sensitive than either ultrasound or IVP in detecting renal cortical defects caused by scar tissue or focal pyelonephritis.

- Testicular scintigraphy and color Doppler ultrasound are two diagnostic tests used in diagnosing testicular torsion, which is difficult to distinguish clinically from epididymitis.

- Nuclear scintigraphy is used to assess neuroendocrine tumors, such as pheochromocytomas.

- Nuclear techniques are expensive, but they have equal or better sensitivities than CT or MRI.

SUGGESTED READINGS

Blaufox MD. Procedures of choice in renal nuclear medicine. J Nucl Med 1991;32:1301–1309.

Conway JJ, Cohn RA. Evolving role of nuclear medicine for the diagnosis and management of urinary tract infection. J Pediatr 1994;124:87–90.

Dubovsky EV, Russell CD, Erbas B. Radionuclide evaluation of renal transplants. Semin Nucl Med 1995; 25:49–59.

Eggli DF, Tulchinsky M. Scintigraphic evaluation of pediatric urinary tract infection. Semin Nucl Med 1993; 23:199–218.

Fine EJ. Nuclear medicine evaluation of hypertension. Urol Radiol 1992;14:85–95.

Fommei E, Volterrani D. Renal nuclear medicine. Semin Nucl Med 1995;25:183–194.

Francis IR, Gross MD, Shapiro B, et al. Integrated imaging of adrenal disease. Radiology 1992;184:1–13.

Goldraich NP, Goldraich IH. Update on dimercaptosuccinic acid renal scanning in children with urinary tract infection. Pediatr Nephrol 1995;9:221–226.

Lebowitz RL. The detection and characterization of vesicoureteral reflux in the child. J Urol 1992;148: 1640–1642.

Lutzker LG, Zuckier LS. Testicular scanning and other applications of radionuclide imaging of the genital tract. Semin Nucl Med 1990;20:159–188.

Majd M, Rushton HG. Renal cortical scintigraphy in the diagnosis of acute pyelonephritis. Semin Nucl Med 1992; 22:98–111.

McBiles M, Lambert AT, Cote MG, et al. Diuretic scintigraphy: past, present, and future. In: Freeman LM, ed. Nuclear Medicine Annual. New York: Raven Press, 1995:185–216.

Mettler FA, Guiberteau MJ, eds. Essentials of Nuclear Medicine Imaging. 3rd ed. Philadelphia: WB Saunders, 1991.

Middleton WD, Siegel BA, Melson GL, et al. Acute scrotal disorders: prospective comparison of color Doppler us and testicular scintigraphy. Radiology 1990;177:177–181.

Middleton ML, Bongiovanni JA, Blaufox D, et al. Evaluation of renovascular hypertension. Curr Opin Nephrol Hypertens 1993;2:940–948.

Nally JV, Black HR. State-of-the-art review: captopril renography—pathophysiological considerations and clinical considerations. Semin Nucl Med 1992;22:85–97.

Olsen JO, Pozderac RV, Hinkle G, et al. Somatostatin receptor imaging of neuroendocrine tumors with indium-111 pentetreotide (octreoscan). Semin Nucl Med 1995;25: 251–261.

O'Reilly PH. Diuresis renography 8 years later: an update. J Urol 1986;136:993–999.

Pedersen EB. Angiotensin-converting enzyme inhibitor renography: pathophysiological, diagnostic, and therapeutic aspects in renal artery stenosis. Nephrol Dial Transplant 1994;9:482–492.

Pickering TG. Renovascular hypertension: etiology and pathophysiology. Semin Nucl Med 1989;19:79–88.

Rosenberg AR, Rossleigh MA, Brydon MP, et al. Evaluation of acute urinary tract infection in children by dimercaptosuccinic acid scintigraphy: a prospective study. J Urol 1992;148:1746–1749.

Rosenfeld DL, Fleischer M, Yudd A, et al. Current recommendations for children with urinary tract infections. Clin Pediatr 1995;34:261–264.

Shapiro B, Copp JE, Sisson JC, et al. Iodine-131 meta-iodobenzylguanidine for the locating of suspected pheochromocytomas: experience in 400 cases. J Nucl Med 1985;26:576–585.

Taylor A, Datz FL, eds. Clinical Practice of Nuclear Medicine. 1st ed. New York: Churchill Livingstone, 1991.

Taylor A, Nally JV. Clinical applications of renal scintigraphy. AJR 1995;164:31–41.

4

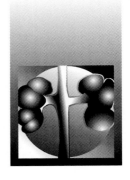

Evaluating Renal Function:
Acute and Chronic Renal Failure

Michael E. Falkenhain
William A. Wilmer

DETERMINATION OF KIDNEY FUNCTION

Many symptoms of renal failure are nonspecific and occur only after renal function is significantly impaired. Most cases of renal failure are first diagnosed when a chemistry profile identifies elevated serum levels of blood urea nitrogen (BUN) and creatinine. In the absence of symptoms, subtle changes in BUN and serum creatinine (SCr) must be considered significant, since:

1. A small increase above the patient's baseline value may reflect a marked decrease in glomerular filtration rate (GFR).
2. Elevated BUN and creatinine levels are rarely the result of laboratory error.
3. Arrest or delay of additional kidney injury can decrease significant morbidity or even mortality.

Glomerular Filtration Rate (GFR)

The most widely used determinant of renal function is the GFR. GFR is best measured using an exogenous substance (e.g., inulin or iothalamate) that enters the systemic circulation at a relatively continuous rate, is freely filtered at the glomerulus, and is not secreted or reabsorbed by the tubule. Serum creatinine levels and BUN provide only gross estimates of GFR, but because they are easily measured and reproduced, they are useful in measuring GFR. Serum creatinine more accurately reflects GFR, whereas measurements of BUN have better correlations with toxic symptoms of renal failure. Clearance of exogenous compounds such as inulin and iothalamate is a good marker of GFR, but measuring the compounds is cumbersome and requires a high level of technical skill that precludes their routine use in patient care. Urine output alone is an inadequate index of renal dysfunction.

Serum Creatinine

Creatinine is a product of muscle metabolism. It enters the circulation at a relatively constant rate and is excreted at a nearly constant rate by the kidney. This process provides stability in serum creatinine levels unless production, volume of distribution, or renal excretion acutely change. Because creatinine is both filtered and secreted by the renal tubules, serum creatinine and urinary creatinine clearance can overestimate actual GFR. When renal function is near normal, creatinine secreted by the renal tubule has a minimal effect on the GFR.

Despite the limitations of using creatinine secretion to measure GFR, serum creatinine measurement remains the most frequently used method to screen for renal disease. Although serum creatinine levels reflect GFR, more accurate estimates of renal function are obtained from urinary creatinine measurements.

To determine GFR, creatinine clearance (C_{cr}) can be calculated using any of three approaches:

1. Urine creatinine excretion divided by plasma creatinine concentration (UV/P).
2. Reciprocal of serum creatinine levels (1/serum creatinine).
3. Serum creatinine levels and a patient's anthropometric measurements (Cockcroft-Gault formula).

Urine Creatinine Excretion Divided by Plasma Creatinine Concentration. The clearance of creatinine from the circulation is equal to the amount of creatinine excreted in the urine divided by plasma concentration. C_{cr} (mL/min) is calculated by using a standard formula, UV/P. **U** is urine concentration of creatinine in milligrams per 100 milliliter (deciliter, or dL); **V** is the volume of urine per minute (24 hours = 1440 minutes); and **P** is the serum concentration of creatinine in milligrams per 100 milliliter (dL).

Although simple to calculate, a 24-hour urine collection requires the patient's understanding and cooperation. Incomplete collections commonly occur and, at times, overcollection results when the urinary bladder is not emptied at the start of collection. A guide for patients and for physicians regarding 24-hour urine collections is outlined in Table 4.1.

Urine C_{cr} is a useful marker of GFR only if the following limitations are kept in mind:

- The patient's creatinine excretion must be in steady state. For this to occur, the GFR cannot fluctuate during the 24-hour urine collection. Therefore, it is not useful to measure C_{cr} during an episode of acute renal failure (ARF).
- The clinician must check that the urine collection is adequate for measurement. This is done by comparing the total measured creatinine with the expected creatinine excretion. Expected creatinine excretion can be estimated using the equation:

Creatinine production/day (mg/day) = (140 minus age) × body weight (kg) divided by 5

- Urine creatinine collections that differ by more than 20% of the expected value should be considered as incomplete, unless muscle mass appears significantly reduced.
- As renal failure progresses, the proportion of the total creatinine that is excreted (creatinine that is excreted independent of filtration) progressively increases. Therefore, with severe renal impairment, C_{cr} is an overestimation of true GFR.

Reciprocal of Serum Creatinine Levels and Creatinine Clearance Per Minute. The equation for C_{cr} (UV/P) can be rewritten to show that the serum creatinine level is inversely proportional to the GFR:

1 / serum creatinine
or
1 / UV/GFR

In the steady state, when GFR is not acutely fluctuating, the renal excretion of creatinine ($U \times V$) is a constant that is equal to the amount of creatinine generated daily divided by the volume of distribution of total body water. With stable creatinine generation, a stable volume of distribution, and stable creatinine secretion, the serum creatinine level will increase

TABLE 4.1	Urine Collection for Creatinine Clearance

Technique	Example
24-hr urine collection starts at the time the patient empties his or her bladder. This first void is not saved.	Patient awakens at 8:00 AM, urinates, and discards the urine.
All urine voided throughout the next 24 hours is collected in a clean container.	Patient urinates at noon, at 4:00 PM, and at 11:00 PM. All urine is saved.
The urine is either refrigerated or kept on ice.	
The patient must empty the bladder at the end of the 24-hr urine collection period. This urine is saved and all urine is taken to the laboratory.	At 8:00 AM the following day, the patient urinates. With the saving of this urine, the collection ends.

Calculation

A 40-year-old male patient who weighs 70 kg collects a 24-hr urine sample with the following results:

Volume: 1.5 L
Creatinine: 1.5 g 24 hr, 100 mg/dL
Serum creatinine: 1 mg/dL

Expected creatinine production: $(140 - 40) \times 70/5 = 1500$ mg

Expected creatinine production agrees within 20% of calculated creatinine production, thus this is likely to be an adequate collection.

$$\text{Creatinine clearance} = \frac{100 \text{ mg/dL} \times 1500 \text{ mL}}{1 \text{ mg/dL} \times 1440 \text{ min}} = 104 \text{ mL/min}$$

proportionately as GFR falls. Therefore, the reciprocal of the serum creatinine level $(1/Cr)$ is an estimate of GFR (in milliliters/minute).

Because of this inverse relationship between serum creatinine and GFR, small increases of serum creatinine above baseline represent substantial changes in kidney function (Fig. 4.1). For example, a doubling of the serum creatinine concentration from a baseline of 0.6 mg/dL to a new steady state value of 1.2 mg/dL reflects a 50% reduction in GFR. A further increase from 1.2 to 2.4 mg/dL reflects only an additional 25% reduction, compared with the original renal function.

As this example demonstrates, serum creatinine measurements may be within the "normal range" provided by a reference laboratory when a patient actually has a markedly diminished GFR. Patients with lower than average creatinine generation include the elderly and those with muscle wasting as a result of chronic disease. Serum creatinine levels may also exceed a reference range if a patient's muscle mass is greater than normal. Additionally, excessive intake of overcooked meats, which contain large quantities of creatinine precursors, can increase levels of serum creatinine. Drugs that block tubular secretion of creatinine (trimetho-

prim, cimetidine) can increase serum creatinine levels without affecting true GFR.

The normal values for serum creatinine are not age-adjusted because, with advancing age, GFR falls in parallel to muscle loss. GFR falls on average 1.0 mL/min annually after age 30. By age 80, GFR will have fallen approximately 50 mL/min. A "normal" serum creatinine level of 1 mg/dL in a person 80 years old may reflect a GFR of only 50 mL/min. If the same 80 year old were cachectic (creatinine generation less than normal for age), the serum creatinine level would be even lower. This point is especially useful when considering drug dosing in the elderly. For these reasons, anthropometric calculations using serum creatinine values are recommended.

Serum creatinine and anthropometric measurements. The most widely used estimate of GFR from serum creatinine and anthropometric measurements is the Cockcroft-Gault formula. According to this formula, the C_{cr} for adults is calculated as follows:

$$\text{Creatinine clearance (mL/min)} = \frac{(140 \text{ minus age}) \times \text{weight (kg)}}{72 \times \text{serum creatinine (mg/dL)}}$$

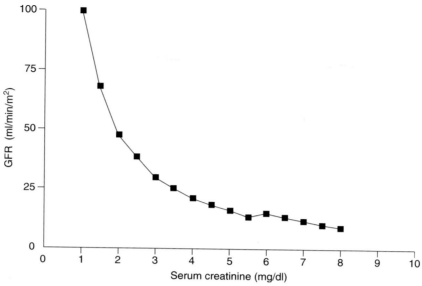

FIGURE 4.1.

An example of the relationship between serum creatinine (*x axis*) and the glomerular filtration rate *(GFR),* which is shown on the *y* axis. The shape of the *curve* should remain consistent among individuals; however, it may be shifted to the left or right, depending on the patient's muscle mass.

FEMALES, multiply by 0.85:

Creatinine clearance (mL/min) =

$$\frac{(140 \text{ minus age}) \times \text{weight (kg)}}{72 \times \text{serum creatinine (mg/dL)} \times 0.85}$$

This equation should be applied only to adults because estimates of GFR in children by this method are commonly in error. Cockcroft-Gault estimates of GFR should be routinely taken when prescribing medications that require adjustments for GFR and when muscle mass appears inappropriately low.

Blood Urea Nitrogen (BUN)

Urea is another metabolite that serves as a marker of kidney function. Measurements of urea are commonly expressed as the nitrogenated form of urea in blood. Because BUN is reabsorbed across the tubular wall after glomerular filtration, only 45 to 50% of filtered BUN is excreted in urine. As a result, both the clearance of BUN and serum BUN values poorly reflect GFR. BUN absorption increases when urinary flow declines or when protein catabolism increases (Table 4.2). Low urine flow allows the tubule more contact time with filtered BUN. This additional contact time permits increased absorption; as a result, less BUN enters the urine. If the serum creatinine is near normal and the ratio of BUN to serum creatinine exceeds 20, excessive protein catabolism or tubule resorption may occur.

Causes of Elevated BUN   **TABLE 4.2**

Normal BUN values = 10–20 mg/dL

Increased BUN to creatinine ratio:
Increased tubular reabsorption
Low urine flow
Dehydration
Low cardiac output
Low intravascular volume caused by third-
spaced fluids
Sodium depletion

Increased protein catabolism
Sepsis
Corticosteroids
Parenteral nutrition
GI bleeding (requires an intact colon)

BUN increases with creatinine increases =
acute or chronic renal failure

When excessive protein catabolism is absent, an increasing BUN to creatinine ratio is useful to identify renal insufficiency associated with low tubule flow. The BUN to creatinine ratio is less useful for identifying diminished tubular flow when a marked reduction in GFR is present.

Oliguria

Failure to excrete solutes is a definition of renal insufficiency. States of low urine output may suggest the presence of renal disease and be an initial marker of renal failure. Oliguria represents a urine output less than 500 mL/day, which for most patients is a volume too small to permit a normal amount of solute excretion. Because incomplete solute excretion may exist despite urine volumes in excess of 500 mL/day, oliguria is an insensitive marker of renal disease.

The healthy kidney can excrete its daily osmotic load as a concentrated or dilute urine. The typical osmotic load is approximately 10 Osm/L body weight/day. For a 70-kg patient, the 700 mOsm/day of obligatory solute can be excreted in as little as 0.5 L urine (1400 mOsm/L) or as much as 14 L (50 mOsm/L). The kidney cannot typically exceed these thresholds of concentration and dilution.

The diseased kidney often cannot produce maximally concentrated or dilute urine. An impaired kidney unable to produce concentrated urine requires greater volumes of urine output. For example, the 70-kg patient who can only maximally concentrate the urine to 350 mOsm/L must urinate at least 2 L daily to excrete his daily osmotic load. Patients with a urinary concentrating defect may quickly develop intravascular volume depletion when they are in a condition requiring volume conservation (e.g., diarrhea).

DIAGNOSIS: ACUTE VERSUS CHRONIC RENAL FAILURE

When approaching the patient with an abnormal GFR, the most effective means of assessing chronicity and etiology is a directed history and physical examination (see Tables 4.3 and 4.4, respectively). All patients should have a complete renal function and electrolyte evaluation:

- BUN
- Creatinine
- Calcium
- Phosphorous
- Urine electrolyte
- Urine creatinine
- Urinalysis
- Serum electrolyte

TABLE 4.3	**Historical Clues in the Diagnosis of Renal Disease**

Previous renal disease?
  Old creatinine measurements
  Previous radiologic evaluations (IVP, etc.)

History of related systemic disease?
  Diabetes mellitus
  Hypertension—duration and degree of control
  Pelvic radiation or surgery
  Sickle cell anemia
  SLE

Uremic symptoms and signs present? (see Table 4.11)
  Loss of appetite
  Nausea/vomiting
  Fatigue
  Somnolence
  Pleuritic chest pain

Urine output changed?
  Nocturia suggests an inability to concentrate the urine
  Anuria implies an acute process; consider obstruction
  Dysuria implies infection/inflammation of the urinary bladder, urethra

Hematuria—"tea-colored" urine is often gross hematuria, but may suggest rhabdomyolysis

Intravascular volume changed? (see Table 4.5)
  Recent dehydration
  Blood loss
  Overdiuresis
  New-onset edema—implies sodium retention

Medications
  NSAIDs
  Recent antibiotic administration?
  Antihypertensives

Family history
  Heritable kidney diseases
  Polycystic kidney disease
  Renal failure associated with hearing loss in males (hereditary nephritis)
  Atherosclerotic disease

Social history
  Illicit drug use
    Cocaine-associated vasomotor ARF
    Hepatitis-associated ARF
    Alcohol-cirrhosis and hepatorenal syndrome

IVP, intravenous pyelography; SLE, systemic lupus erythematosus; ARF, acute renal failure.

Physical Examination Findings in the Diagnosis of Renal Failure	TABLE 4.4

General	Weight loss; could suggest decreased appetite from uremia, presence of malignancy
	Weight gain; is weight gain secondary to volume expansion?
Skin	A recent rash may provide clues to allergic renal disease, connective tissue disease, vasculitis, or atheroembolic disease
HEENT	Hearing loss associated with hereditary nephritis
	Chronic sinusitis or nasal ulcers—Wegener's granulomatosis
	Oral ulcers—may suggest connective tissue disease
	Retinopathy—malignant hypertension, connective tissue disease
CV	Evidence of systolic dysfunction
	Acute pulmonary edema—suggests the presence of sodium retention by the kidney in association with cardiac dysfunction
Pulmonary	Hemoptysis—suggests pulmonary renal syndromes
	Pulmonary hypertension predisposing to right heart failure
Abdomen	Bladder distension
	Liver disease
	Abdominal bruits
Extremities	Claudication—suggests atherosclerotic disease
Musculoskeletal	Bone pain—associated with multiple myeloma or osteomalacia

HEENT, head, ears, eyes, nose, and throat; CV, cardiovascular.

Additional laboratory data, including autoimmune serologies, serum albumin, CPK, etc., should be obtained if the history, physical examination, and screening laboratory work suggest a particular cause. Anatomic assessment to determine the number, size, and symmetry of a patient's kidneys should be obtained by renal ultrasound or abdominal plain films.

ARF implies an abrupt (days to weeks) reduction in GFR; chronic renal failure (CRF) implies a more slowly progressing (months to years) reduction without the potential for improvement. These two processes are not mutually exclusive, and often acute failure will be superimposed on CRF. Differentiating ARF from CRF is critical because the focus in ARF is to establish a cause with hopes of promoting recovery. In CRF the emphasis shifts to slowing the progression of disease and preparing the patient for long-term renal replacement therapy.

When assessing chronicity of disease, it is helpful to compare current serum creatinine values with previous GFR measurements. Old records and previous screening urinalyses completed for employment or school enrollment may identify when a process started. A renal ultrasound assessing renal size and echogenicity is also useful. Small echogenic kidneys suggest chronic disease; however, the absence of echogenicity does not exclude a chronic process. In diabetic renal disease and in infiltrative processes such as amyloid-osis, kidney size is generally larger than normal. In these conditions, kidneys may appear "normal" despite serious injury.

Few laboratory markers other than a baseline serum creatinine are helpful in determining chronicity. Metabolic acidosis and abnormalities in potassium and water excretion develop acutely but may also exist chronically. Anemia secondary to erythropoietin deficiency is more common in CRF than in ARF. Despite the association of anemia with chronic renal disease, it is often difficult to conclusively distinguish acute from chronic disease on the basis of hemoglobin or hematocrit levels. Many ARF diseases are associated with nonrenal blood loss and systemic inflammation that likewise cause anemia. In addition, patients with certain chronic renal diseases, such as polycystic kidney disease, are slow to develop anemia or may not develop anemia at all.

The presence of secondary hyperparathyroidism is unreliable in establishing an estimate of chronicity because biochemical abnormalities can evolve abruptly. A marked elevation in serum parathyroid hormone (PTH), decreased serum calcium, and increased serum phosphorous suggest secondary hyperparathyroidism. Radiographic changes of secondary hyperparathyroidism are specific but insensitive. Generally, bone changes as visualized by routine radiograph require months or years to develop.

Summary of Diagnosis

- Serum creatinine is generally a useful marker of renal clearance in clinical practice.
- In the elderly population and in malnourished individuals, serum creatinine may grossly underestimate renal clearance.
- Twenty-four hour urine collection can be difficult in office practice. For adjustment of medication dosage, creatinine clearance (mL/min) can be estimated using the formula (for females, multiply by 0.85):

$$\frac{(140 \text{ minus age}) \times \text{weight (kg)}}{72 \times \text{serum creatinine (mg/dL)}}$$

- Blood pressure measurement, chest radiograph, blood count, and ultrasound of kidneys could help to distinguish acute from chronic renal failure. Elevated blood pressures, cardiomegaly, anemia, and appearance of small kidneys are supportive evidence of CRF.
- Spot urinary electrolytes and creatinine are helpful indices to differentiate pre-renal ARF from acute tubular necrosis (ATN). In pre-renal ARF, urinary sodium and chloride values are less than 20 mEq/L, and sometimes as low as < 10 mEq/L. Urinary creatinine is higher than 100 mg/dL. In ATN, although urinary sodium and chloride values are higher, urinary creatinine is lower.
- Lower urinary tract obstruction caused by benign hypertrophy of the prostate or cancer of the prostate is a common cause of acutely or chronically impaired renal function in the elderly.
- Nonsteroidal anti-inflammatory drugs (NSAIDs) and angiotensin-converting enzyme (ACE) inhibitors are two families of drugs that commonly give rise to ARF and hyperkalemia, particularly in the elderly population.
- On detection of a reduced GFR, the following questions should be asked:
  What is the chronicity of the problem?
  What is the etiology of the renal dysfunction?
  Can treatment be offered to restore GFR or prevent further loss?

ACUTE RENAL FAILURE (ARF)

Clinicians must determine if ARF is caused by an abnormality proximal to the kidney (pre-renal), distal to the kidney (post-renal), or the result of lesions within the kidney (intrinsic renal ARF).

Pre-renal ARF

Causes

Common causes of pre-renal failure are listed in Table 4.5. Pre-renal or "hemodynamic" ARF results when GFR is impaired as a result of diminished glomerular capillary pressure. The normal compensatory mechanism by which the glomerular capillary pressure can be maintained in the face of renal underperfusion is outlined in Figure 4.2. This compensation is evoked in states of renal underperfusion and when there is underlying intrinsic renal pathology. When the normal compensatory mechanisms to preserve GFR are already being used, patients are sensitive to hemodynamic insults. For example, patients with renovascular disease are more susceptible to ARF from hypotension and diminished intravascular volume. Medications such as ACE inhibitors, the angiotensin receptor blockers, and NSAIDs can inhibit compensation. These agents may therefore precipitate ARF when given to patients with preexisting renal disease or when given during states of renal underperfusion.

The hepatorenal syndrome evolves through progressive renal vascular resistance. In hepatorenal ARF, renal vascular resistance exceeds systemic vascular resistance, leading to marked renal underperfusion. Sepsis may cause a similar type of hemodynamic insult but, as discussed later, renal injury during sepsis usually is caused by renal tubule toxicity.

Signs and Symptoms

The effective arterial blood volume status of patients with pre-renal ARF can range from intravascular volume depletion to pulmonary edema. A detailed physical examination with attention to volume status is essential. The following symptoms are all suggestive of volume depletion:

- Decreased skin turgor
- Rapid weight loss (> 0.25 kg/day)
- Blood pressure that is less than usual
- Drop in the systolic blood pressure by more than 20 mm Hg, with an increase in pulse rate by more than 10 beats/min on upright posture

Diagnosis

The urine sodium and chloride concentrations reflect the concentrations in circulating blood. The renal re-

Diminished cardiac output
   MI/cardiomyopathy/CHF
   Pericardial disease: tamponade, pericarditis
   PE

Decreased circulating volume
   Hemorrhage
   Diminished intake
   Excessive diuresis
   GI loss
   Skin loss
   Third-space sequestration

Systemic vasodilation
   Anaphylaxis/sepsis
   Antihypertensives

Systemic/renal vasoconstriction
   General anesthesia

Alpha agonists/pressers
Hepatorenal

Renovascular obstruction
   Renal artery stenosis (atherosclerotic or
      fibromuscular dysplasia)
   Renal artery dissection
   Renal artery embolism (large vessel)
   Renal vein thrombosis

Impaired renal vascular regulation
   ACE inhibitors
   NSAIDs
   Cyclosporine

Hyperviscosity syndromes
   Multiple myeloma
   Macroglobulinemia

ARF, acute renal failure; MI, myocardial ischemia; CHF, congestive heart failure; PE, pulmonary embolism; ACE, angiotensin-converting enzyme; NSAIDs, nonsteroidal anti-inflammatory drugs.

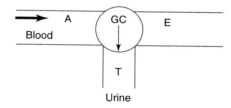

GFR is dependent on the pressure in the glomerular capillary (GC).

$$GFR = K\,[(GC_P - T_P) + (T_O - GC_O)]$$

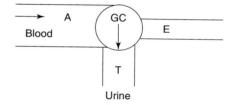

Glomerular capillary pressure can be maintained in response to a reduction in renal flow by vasodilation of the afferent arteriole (A) and vasoconstriction of the efferent (E) arteriole.

FIGURE 4.2.
Schematic of blood arriving through the afferent arteriole and entering the glomerular capillary (GC), where an ultrafiltrate is produced that eventually becomes urine. K, filtration coefficient; $_P$, pressure; $_t$, tubule; $_o$, oncotic pressure.

sponse to underperfusion is to decrease sodium and chloride excretion. Thus, urine sodium less than 20 mEq/L or urine chloride less than 15 mEq/L suggests below-normal renal blood flow. Clinicians commonly use only the urine sodium concentration to diagnose pre-renal ARF. When metabolic alkalosis is present and an alkaline urine produced, urine sodium concentrations may be inappropriately high in relation to the volume. Such high concentrations of sodium occur because bicarbonate excretion, as a correction of meta-

bolic alkalosis, causes obligatory sodium loss (as the cation for bicarbonate). In the presence of metabolic alkalosis, with an alkaline urine and a normal urine sodium concentration, a low urine chloride concentration suggests volume depletion. A fractional excretion of sodium (FE_{Na}) (FE_{Na} = spot urine $[Na] \times$ Scr/spot urine $[cr]$) provides the added benefit of correcting for the urine concentration (see Tables 4.3 and 4.4). A sodium excretion less than 1% strongly suggests the presence of renal underperfusion. As mentioned previously, if the GFR is not markedly impaired, a BUN to creatinine ratio exceeding 20 may provide an additional clue to diagnosing a pre-renal state. The urinalysis in pre-renal ARF should be normal, without an active sediment, significant proteinuria, or hematuria. The renal ultrasound is normal in pre-renal ARF.

Treatment

Patients with pre-renal ARF need improvement in their glomerular capillary pressure, which usually requires an increase in the effective circulating volume and renal blood flow. The patient with hemodynamic compromise secondary to intravascular volume depletion will require different therapy from the patient with hemodynamic compromise and pulmonary edema secondary to impaired cardiac function.

If the pre-renal ARF requires intravascular fluid replacement, isotonic fluids or colloidal agents should be used. The rate of fluid replacement should be dictated by the degree of hemodynamic compromise and by cardiac and renal impairment. If orthostatic hypotension is present, replacement of losses should be provided within a few hours. Half of estimated losses should be replaced within 24 hours, with the remaining half replaced within 48 hours. Evidence of cardiac compromise should be monitored. When in doubt about a patient's intravascular volume, Swan-Ganz catheter measurements may be beneficial. Even with Swan-Ganz catheter measurements, frequent clinical assessment of volume status during aggressive replacement is advised. Repeated monitoring of orthostatic blood pressure and pulse measurements, along with frequent chest auscultation to rule out a diagnosis of pulmonary edema, is advisable. Patients who have progressed to oliguric ATN benefit greatly from this monitoring.

Medications that lower vascular resistance and promote renal hypoperfusion should be discontinued whenever possible. Continued use of antihypertensives, NSAIDs, and negative inotropic medications may exacerbate pre-renal ARF. Improving systemic vascular resistance with the use of pressor agents or improving cardiac output with positive inotropes and afterload reduction may be useful in the proper clinical setting. Although ACE inhibitors may improve renal perfusion by improving cardiac output, they may worsen glomerular hemodynamics. If this occurs, the authors prefer switching to a non–ACE inhibitor afterload-reducing agent such as hydralazine.

Toxicity to kidney cells from contrast agents and aminoglycosides is increased in pre-renal states. Limiting these and other direct toxins is prudent.

Treatment of the hepatorenal syndrome primarily involves prevention, because once this syndrome develops there is little hope of reversing the process. GFR is maintained in patients with severe liver disease caused by compensatory increases in renal vasodilating prostaglandins. Therefore, use of NSAIDs, intravascular dehydration caused by diuretics, or sepsis may precipitate a rapid and irreversible deterioration of kidney function. In hepatorenal syndrome and in other forms of renal hypoperfusion, low-dose dopamine infusions have been suggested to stimulate renal blood flow. Although beneficial in some forms of pre-renal disease, renal-dose dopamine cannot override the effect of a diminished circulating volume on the renal blood flow and GFR, especially in hepatorenal syndrome. A patient's failure to respond to renal-dose dopamine should indicate its discontinuation.

Post-renal ARF

Causes

Obstruction to urine flow anywhere within the urinary system can cause acute impairment of GFR and result in ARF. Obstruction results in elevated back pressures within the kidney, and if left uncorrected can result in CRF. The most common causes of obstruction are stones, malignancy, and, in males, prostatic hypertrophy (Table 4.6). Prostatic disease, either benign or malignant, can result in obstruction of the urethra or of the bladder outlet, independent of urethral involvement in the disease.

Signs and Symptoms

The most sensitive test for obstruction of the urethra or bladder is renal ultrasound to determine the presence of pelvicalyceal dilatation. False–positive results can occur in patients with chronic obstruction. Chronic pelvicalyceal disease can result in fibrosis and chronic dilatation of the proximal urinary system, despite unobstructed urine flow. Nevertheless, pelvicalyceal dilatation on ultrasound should be considered obstruction until proven otherwise. Confirmation of obstruction, when necessary, can be made by cystoscopy with retrograde pyelography, nuclear renal scans, or computed tomography (CT) scans.

Because of hyperfiltration of nondiseased nephrons, a rise in serum creatinine does not occur unless obstruction is bilateral, or unilateral obstruction occurs with preexisting contralateral renal disease. Post-renal ARF may be present despite normal urine volumes, as partial obstruction may increase intrarenal pressure but permit urine flow. Pain does not frequently occur with obstruction unless marked bladder or renal capsule disten-

	Causes of Urinary Obstruction	TABLE 4.6
Type of Obstruction	**Causes**	
Pelvicalyceal obstruction	Nephrolithiasis	
	Papillary necrosis	
	Pelvic cysts	
Urinary bladder obstruction	Bladder tumors	
	Lymphadenopathy	
	Bladder stones	
	Blood clots	
Urethral obstruction	Prostatic hypertrophy	
	Prostate cancer	
	Blood clots	
	"Flaccid" bladder or diabetes	
Ureteral obstruction	Intra-ureteral	
	Nephrolithiasis	
	Tumors	
	Extra-ureteral	
	Retroperitoneal fibrosis: idiopathic, cancer (prostate, gyn), drugs (methysergide)	
	Pregnancy	
	Aortic aneurysmal disease	

sion develops. Fever and hemodynamic collapse should prompt concerns for urosepsis associated with urinary obstruction.

Diagnosis

A history of dysuria or changes in urinary frequency and strength of stream provide important clues to the diagnosis. An enlarged urinary bladder should be sought on physical examination. A palpable suprapubic mass may be overlooked on general inspection. Bladder distension may increase sympathetic activity, causing hypertension or cardiac ectopy. The presence of tenderness near the spine and pain in the low back or pelvis should alert the physician to the possibility of bone disease associated with pelvic malignancy.

Residual urine in the bladder after voiding (postvoid residual) is a marker of incomplete bladder emptying. High postvoid residuals are seen in patients with urethral obstruction, in diabetics with autonomic insufficiency, and in patients with spinal cord injury. Patients with very high postvoid residuals are at increased risk for developing renal failure, but large postvoid bladder volumes (up to 1 liter) can occur without causing obstructive uropathy. Patients with high postvoid residuals are additionally at risk for urinary infection. Postvoid residual can be assessed easily through ultrasonography or bladder catheterization after voiding.

Post-renal ARF may coexist with oliguric pre-renal ARF. Patients with coexisting disorders may present with fluid loss as a result of diuretic use or vomiting and may not exhibit pelvicalyceal dilatation on renal ultrasound. After the pre-renal condition is reversed, it is prudent to reevaluate patients with unresolved ARF for urinary tract obstruction.

The urinalysis in obstructive nephropathy is generally normal, with low-grade proteinuria or hematuria occasionally present. Sometimes the spot urine sodium will be low, mimicking that of pre-renal ARF.

Treatment

Removal of urethral obstruction can lessen pressure in a dilated urinary bladder, decrease intrarenal pressure, and increase GFR. As a markedly dilated urinary bladder is decompressed, gross hematuria may develop as a result of rupture of bladder vessels. Gradual decompression by removing only one liter of urine every few hours via bladder catheterization is advised to prevent this phenomenon. Unilateral obstruction or bilateral obstruction that remains after bladder catheterization suggests disease proximal to the bladder. Cystoscopy with retrograde stent placement in an obstructed ureter is frequently indicated. If the ureter orifice cannot be accessed for retrograde stent placement, percutaneous nephrostomy tubes with antegrade studies are needed.

Intrinsic Renal ARF

When tests for pre-renal and post-renal ARF prove negative, parenchymal kidney disease is likely present. Intrinsic renal ARF is more accurately evaluated when the workup addresses four anatomically distinct kidney regions:

1. Glomerulus
2. Tubule
3. Interstitium
4. Vasculature

Glomerular ARF

Most glomerular diseases cause a slow loss of renal function, although several forms of glomerular injury can be associated with an acute loss of renal function. An acute or subacute rise in the serum creatinine and the presence of a nephritic urine sediment defines a rapidly progressive glomerulonephritis (RPGN). Diseases that frequently present as an RPGN are listed in Table 4.7. The finding of red blood cell (RBC) casts and urinary acanthocytes in the presence of ARF strongly suggest an RPGN. RBC casts are not consistently present, and often white blood cell or white cell casts are the only urinary clue to the diagnosis. Proteinuria in modest amounts (100 mg/dL by urine dipstick, 1–3 g/24 hr) is usually present.

When an RPGN is suspected, a renal biopsy is indicated to provide a definitive diagnosis and important prognostic information. Laboratory data that should be ordered when one suspects an RPGN include:

- Antineutrophilic cytoplasmic antibody (ANCA)
- Antinuclear antibody (ANA)
- Serum complements (C3 and C4)
- Hepatitis serology
- Rheumatoid factor
- Serum cryoglobulins
- C-reactive protein

Prompt referral to a nephrologist should be made, even before all serologies have returned. Often therapy with immunosuppressive and cytotoxic agents is immediately indicated.

Tubulointerstitial ARF

Of the intrinsic renal causes of ARF, tubulointerstitial damage is most common. Tubulointerstitial damage may be divided into two categories: ATN and AIN (acute interstitial nephritis).

The major cause of ARF in patients in a hospital setting is ATN, which occurs as a result of damage to renal tubular cells. ATN may appear as a nonoliguric or oliguric ARF that may or may not be reversible. Table 4.8 lists the most common causes of ATN. It should be stressed that any hemodynamic stress, at its extreme, may result in ATN. Hemodynamic stress will also lower the threshold of developing ATN following toxin exposure. The classic example of this is contrast-induced ATN (Table 4.9).

TABLE 4.7	Glomerular Causes of ARF

Immune complex-mediated
  Systemic lupus erythematosus
  Poststreptococcal glomerular nephritis
  Cryoglobulinemia glomerular nephritis
Anti–GBM-mediated glomerulonephritis
  Goodpasture's syndrome
Pauci-immune glomerulonephritis
  ANCA-associated
    Wegener's granulomatosis
  ANCA-negative
    Idiopathic pauci-immune GN
    FGS/collapsing glomerulopathy of AIDS

ARF, acute renal failure; GBM, glomerular basement membrane; ANCA, antineutrophilic cytoplasmic antibody; GN, glomerulonephritis; FGS, focal glomerular sclerosis.

TABLE 4.8	Causes of Acute Tubular Necrosis (ATN)

Type	Causes
Ischemic	Hypoperfusion
	Hypoxia
Exogenous toxic	Contrast dye
	Antibiotics
	Chemotherapeutics
	Solvents (e.g., ethylene glycol)
	Cyclosporine
	Heavy metals
	Systemic infection (sepsis)
Endogenous toxic	Myoglobin
	Hemoglobin
	Calcium phosphate ppt.
	Uric acid
	Paraprotein
	Hypokalemia
	Hypercalcemia

Contrast-induced ATN	**TABLE 4.9**

Patients at risk for contrast-induced ATN
  Age more than 65 years
  Diabetic with impaired renal function
  Dehydration
  Impaired GFR
  Multiple myeloma
  Tubular toxins (e.g., gentamicin, myoglobin)
  Near end-stage liver or heart disease

Avoidance of contrast-induced ATN
  Establish or maintain normal intravascular volume with increased urinary flow rates
  Hydration with 0.9% NS at rate dependent on patient's cardiac and renal function
  Risk of injury correlates with amount of dye used; venous studies typically require
    more dye than arterial studies

ATN, acute tubular necrosis; GFR, glomerular filtration rate; NS, normal saline.

The hallmark of acute tubular injury is an inability to concentrate the urine; urine sodium wasting may cause the kidneys to excrete a greater urine volume. In ATN, a random urine sodium measurement will be high (> 40 mEq/L), as will be FE_{Na} ($> 2\%$). The urinalysis usually reveals only low-grade proteinuria without significant hematuria or pyuria. The urinary sediment often will show shed tubular cells, hyaline casts, and broad muddy brown casts. The renal ultrasound is usually normal in ATN.

AIN has many similarities to ATN in that it is a reversible form of tubulointerstitial injury that is often drug-mediated (Table 4.10). The urinary findings include proteinuria, which may exceed 1 g/day. Hematuria may occur. The urine sediment may show pyuria, including urinary eosinophils. White cell casts are common. As with ATN, there is an inability to concentrate the urine, and the random urine sodium and FE_{Na} may both be elevated. AIN associated with medication use may be accompanied by fevers and rashes. NSAID-associated AIN does not classically manifest with fevers and rashes, and often the proteinuria is in a nephrotic range.

In both conditions the care is supportive. The cause of the insult should be sought and eliminated. Most patients will show some improvement within 2 weeks and recover completely in 1 month. In patients with severe tubular injury, recovery can require months. In these patients a nuclear renal scan can be used to assess renal perfusion. If renal perfusion is absent, prognosis for early recovery is poor. If dialysis support is needed, the use of a biocompatible membrane dialyzer may speed renal recovery. Avoiding hemodynamic insults or

Causes of Allergic Interstitial Nephritis	**TABLE 4.10**

Drug-induced
  Methicillin
  Sulfa-containing antibiotics
  NSAIDs—all
  Allopurinol
  Cimetidine
  Phenytoin
Immune-mediated
  Sarcoidosis
  Sjögren's syndrome
  SLE
Infection-mediated
  Pyelonephritis
  Legionella

NSAIDS, nonsteroidal anti-inflammatory drugs; SLE, systemic lupus erythematosus.

other nephrotoxin exposure is prudent. Attention to volume status and avoidance of NSAIDs and ACE inhibitors during the recovery phase of tubular interstitial injury are advisable.

As oliguric ATN or AIN resolves, a polyuric phase may occur because of the kidney's inability to adequately concentrate the urine. Patients manifesting a polyuric phase should drink sufficient fluid to offset intravascular depletion; in cases of massive loss, intravenous fluids consisting of isotonic fluid should be administered.

Vasculature

Vascular cause of intrinsic renal failure cannot be conveniently discussed as though it is one topic. Vasculitis, such as Wegener's vasculitis, is best considered under the topic of glomerular disease because it commonly presents with a nephritic urine.

Atheroembolic disease is a unique, under-recognized cause of vascular-mediated ARF. Atheromatous plaques may break loose spontaneously, following an intra-arterial procedure or during thrombolytic or anticoagulant therapy, causing occlusion of distal capillary beds. The symptoms that follow an embolic "shower" depend on which capillary beds are affected. A typical course is a rise in the serum creatinine 2 days to 2 weeks following angiographic intervention that is slow to reverse or that culminates in end-stage renal disease (ESRD). The urinary findings may include pyuria, white cell casts, and urine eosinophils. Atheroemboli are inflammatory, and elevations of the sedimentation rate and consumption of serum complements may occur. Other symptoms may also be present, including:

- Bluish discoloration of the toes (cyanotic)
- Bluish discoloration surrounding pale central areas on extremities and trunk (livedo reticularis)
- Abdominal pain
- Bloody stools

The renal ultrasound may be normal or, if previous disease has occurred, show a nodular distortion of the renal capsule. None of the signs and symptoms of atheroembolic disease are sensitive, and often the diagnosis is one of exclusion.

Malignant hypertension can cause a vascular-mediated acute renal injury. Histologically, this takes the form of "onion-skinning," in which endothelial damage followed by endothelial repair results in a thickened endothelium that can obliterate the arteriole lumen. This vascular trauma can lead to renal ischemia and ARF. The urinalysis may indicate benign hypertension or hematuria. Malignant hypertension can result in a microangiopathic hemolytic anemia and thrombocytopenia mimicking the hemolytic uremic syndrome/thrombotic thrombocytopenia (HUS/TTP).

HUS/TTP often presents with ARF, accompanied by evidence of microangiopathic hemolytic anemia and thrombocytopenia. The renal injury results from thrombin formation in renal arterioles. Secondary causes of renal injury include but are not limited to cyclosporine, FK506, estrogen-containing birth control pills, and diarrhea caused by certain strains of *Escherichia coli*. Prompt referral to a nephrologist for consideration of plasma exchange is warranted when HUS/TTP is suspected.

Oliguric Versus Nonoliguric ARF

The morbidity and mortality of patients with oliguric ARF ($<$ 500 mL daily urine output) significantly exceeds that of patients with nonoliguric ARF. The excessive morbidity and mortality is ascribed to an increased rate of infection and cardiovascular events. Failure to excrete metabolites and water may increase the tendency toward cardiovascular stress. Despite improvements in dialytic treatment of oliguric ARF, the prognosis remains poor.

Attempts to force an oliguric state into nonoliguria by the aggressive use of intravenous loop diuretics may not necessarily reduce mortality. Use diuretics to control fluid balance, which may delay or prevent the need for dialysis. If a patient fails to respond to a high dose of an intravenous loop diuretic, discontinue the effort.

Conditions Associated with ARF

Diabetes

Diabetic nephropathy is a chronic renal disease that manifests as interstitial and glomerular scarring, as well as arteriolar damage, in the form of arteriolar hyalinosis. ARF frequently exacerbates the chronic fibrosing process. Arteriolar disease places a diabetic patient at increased risk for hemodynamic ARF. Accordingly, diabetic patients are more likely to have a rise in the serum creatinine in response to ACE inhibitors, NSAIDs, or dehydration. The presence of diabetes with macrovascular disease (e.g., coronary disease, peripheral vascular disease) increases the possibility of ARF mediated by renal artery stenosis (RAS). RAS should be sought if a diabetic develops acute or subacute worsening in the serum creatinine or if refractory hypertension is present. The diabetic with autonomic insufficiency is also at risk for urinary retention with overflow incontinence from a neurogenic bladder. The patient with diabetic glomerulosclerosis and an elevated serum creatinine is at increased risk for contrast–induced ATN.

Heart Disease

Impaired cardiac output causes not only acute but also chronic forms of pre-renal disease. The compensatory mechanisms protecting GFR in cardiomyopathies place patients at risk of hemodynamic or drug-induced ATN. Overdiureses, excessive use of ACE inhibitors, or NSAIDs may precipitate ARF in cardiac disease. Patients with cardiac disease may have peripheral vascular disease, and therefore are at risk of RAS. The combination of RAS and diminished cardiac output makes the cause of ARF in cardiac patients particularly difficult to define.

HIV/AIDS

Patients infected with the HIV virus are at high risk for developing renal disease. The most common finding is a chronic glomerular disease with nephrotic-range proteinuria, normal-size or enlarged echogenic kidneys, and a noninflammatory urine sediment. Patients with HIV nephropathy are at risk for acute renal insults from nephrotoxic medicines, contrast media, and hemodynamic insults (e.g., diarrhea). A classic pathologic correlate to HIV nephropathy is a collapsing focal segmental glomerular sclerosis that is most commonly experienced by HIV-positive African-Americans. Many other glomerular lesions have been described in association with HIV nephropathy, including TTP, which may herald the diagnosis of AIDS. Some medications that combat HIV have unique tendencies to cause tubulointerstitial toxicity; urinalysis suggesting ATN or interstitial nephritis should prompt a thorough reevaluation of a patient's medications. Coinfection with hepatitis B and hepatitis C may also cause renal disease.

NSAID Complications

Nonsteroidal agents are well tolerated in patients with normal kidney function. Patients with even mild renal impairment or diminished effective circulating volume may develop a hemodynamic form of pre-renal ARF caused by antagonism of the protective and compensatory effects of renal prostaglandin (Fig. 4.2). An allergic interstitial nephritis can occur in patients with normal kidney function. AIN caused by nonsteroidal agents is not typically associated with fevers, rash, or eosinophilia, unlike other forms of AIN (e.g., AIN caused by antibiotics). White blood cells or white cell casts are usually present on the urinalysis. Proteinuria may be mild but commonly is in the nephrotic range because of the coexistence of NSAIDs-induced minimal-change lesions in primary glomerular disease. Hyperkalemia in NSAID users is caused by temporary hyporeninemia hypoaldosteronism brought on by antagonism of renin release. Likewise, accentuation of vasopressin in the collecting ducts of the kidneys may promote excessive water reabsorption that leads to hyponatremia.

Multiple Myeloma

Myeloma and other paraprotein diseases may cause ARF through an associated hypercalcemia, from direct

tubular or interstitial damage, and from glomerular insults. Low GFR caused by hypercalcemia often can be reversed with hydration and loop diuretic use. GFR improves slowly after the serum calcium level is normalized. Tubulointerstitial disease caused by precipitated paraprotein may present as ATN. Unexplained ATN in the elderly (the age group more likely to be affected by paraprotein diseases) should include a workup for myeloma and related diseases.

CHRONIC RENAL FAILURE (CRF)

CRF represents a permanent decrease in GFR. If CRF is detected early enough and the primary insult is eliminated, ESRD can often be mitigated. An example would be the patient with a GFR of 50 mL/min as a result of hypertensive nephrosclerosis. Keeping the patient's blood pressure under control may minimize the injury and prevent further decline in GFR. In cases such as diabetic glomerulosclerosis, the underlying disease cannot be totally eliminated and often the best hope is to delay, rather than thwart, ESRD progression.

In patients with CRF, three main interventions slow the progression of disease. Although these interventions have not been critically and prospectively evaluated for all patient populations, it is the authors' practice to recommend them for most patients with CRF, particularly for those with proteinuric diseases.

1. **Control systemic blood pressure.** The higher the blood pressure, the faster a given renal disease will progress.
2. **Use ACE inhibitors if proteinuria is present.** ACE inhibitors (and perhaps ACE-II receptor blockers) decrease glomerular capillary pressure and reduce proteinuria. In patients with CRF in whom ACE inhibitors decrease proteinuria, progression to ESRD is delayed.
3. **Limit dietary protein.** Amino acid loads increase filtration, which is often injurious to nephrons. Additionally, diets high in protein will usually contain high levels of phosphorous, which increases the risk of CRF progression. Although controversial, it is the authors' practice to recommend that patients with CRF follow a 0.6 to 0.8 g/kg protein diet under the supervision of a nutritionist.

Treatment

Erythropoietin Therapy

Treatment with recombinant erythropoietin should be offered to patients when the hematocrit falls below 25%. Improvements in cardiac disease and overall well-being are the benefits of such therapy. Correction of anemia in diabetics may improve macular edema. Improving the hematocrit may halt the bleeding tendency associated with CRF. Evidence also suggests that immune responses to inoculations may be boosted by the effects of erythropoietin.

Erythropoietin therapy is administered two to three times weekly by subcutaneous injection. Local pain with the injections is common and may be caused by the suspension solution used in the preparation. The dose of erythropoietin needed to successfully increase a patient's hematocrit varies between 50 to 75 U/kg, three times weekly. A recommended starting dose is 50 U/kg three times per week. A maximal response may take 8 to 12 weeks, and the dose should be adjusted depending on the hematocrit response. Target hematocrit values should generally be 30 to 36%. In patients with ischemic coronary disease, hematocrit values may need to be higher. Hemoglobin and hematocrit values should be ordered at least monthly to assist with dose titration. (Many third-party payers have a threshold hematocrit above which the medication costs will not be covered.) Patients receiving erythropoietin therapy often need iron replacement; thus, all patients should have iron profiles measured monthly. Baseline vitamin B_{12} and folate levels must be measured at least twice yearly. Diminished responsiveness to subcutaneous erythropoietin occurs most commonly in patients with iron deficiency.

Other causes of diminished responsiveness include chronic inflammation (either infections or inflammatory diseases), aluminum overload, and secondary hyperparathyroidism. Secondary hyperparathyroidism may cause an irreversible bone marrow fibrosis that chronically impairs erythropoiesis.

Debate exists regarding the best measurement of iron stores in patients with azotemia. Uremia may impair the bone marrow response to erythropoietin and it is possible that, with worsening renal function, larger doses of erythropoietin are needed. Rarely, erythropoietin replacement therapy has been associated with severe hypertension and seizures. Serum ferritin level and transferrin saturation index are dependable measures of iron stores and utilization respectively.

Transfusions

Transfusions should be reserved for patients with symptoms attributable to anemia, such as gastrointestinal bleeding, and those failing to respond to properly administered erythropoietin therapy. Transfusions should be restricted in potential renal transplant candidates. Consultation with a nephrologist before elective transfusion is advisable because older patients and those with extensive comorbid medical conditions are increasingly becoming transplantation candidates.

Calcium, Phosphorous, and Bone Health

All CRF patients should have serum calcium, phosphorous, and intact parathyroid hormone values measured. The most common form of renal bone disease is osteitis fibrosa cystica, a manifestation of chronically elevated PTH. The parathyroid gland releases PTH into the circulation if serum calcium levels are low, if serum 1,25–dihydroxyvitamin D_3 levels are low, or if serum phosphorous levels are elevated. Low serum calcium levels may result from impaired synthesis of vitamin D by the diseased kidney, resulting in diminished calcium absorption. Low circulating calcium levels trigger PTH release, which removes calcium from bone. Excessive PTH release indicates secondary hyperparathyroidism, a condition that is often reversible early in renal disease but which may progress to an autonomous, unrestrained state. Serum phosphorous levels are elevated in CRF because of impaired GFR; however, another cause of elevation is the onset of secondary hyperparathyroidism, indicating phosphorous release from bone.

Serum PTH levels should be followed at least biannually and therapy offered as follows:

- **Correct low serum calcium levels with oral calcium supplementation.** This is accomplished by instructing patients to increase calcium in their diet, by adding calcium supplements, or by offering oral 1,25–dihydroxyvitamin D_3. Of the calcium preparations available, calcium carbonate 650 mg three times daily, given between meals, is well-absorbed and generally well tolerated.

- **Reverse hyperphosphatemia.** A nutritionist should advise the patient to adhere to a well-balanced, low protein, low phosphorous diet. Binding dietary phosphorous should be taken if the serum phosphorous levels remain elevated despite dietary manipulation. Two forms of phosphorous binders are available, aluminum compounds and calcium products. Aluminum binds phosphorous well, but absorption of aluminum places a patient at risk for the deposit of aluminum into bones and its subsequent inability to be mineralized (osteomalacia). The calcium preparations used most frequently are calcium acetate and calcium carbonate. Calcium acetate binds phosphorous well and is less likely than calcium carbonate to cause hypercalcemia. Oral binders should be ingested just before or during a meal (e.g., calcium acetate 667 mg with meals), in contrast to calcium supplementation for hypocalcemia, which is taken between meals on an empty stomach. Calcium citrate preparations, although successful in binding dietary phosphorous, stimulate aluminum absorption from the gastrointestinal tract and should be avoided because aluminum may be present in sufficient quantities in food and water to cause osteomalacia.

- **1,25–(OH₂) D₃ Supplementation.** When serum PTH values are elevated or when hypocalcemia is resistant to oral supplementation, 1,25–dihydroxyvitamin D_3 therapy should be prescribed. Biologically active vitamin D stimulates calcium absorption from the gastrointestinal tract, and through binding to specific parathyroid gland receptors limits PTH release. It is the authors' practice to initiate 1,25–(OH₂) D₃ replacement therapy when the intact PTH is greater than three times normal (e.g., calcitriol, 0.5 μg daily). Oversuppression of the parathyroid gland resulting in normalized or even low PTH values may promote a form of "low bone turnover" disease. In azotemia, PTH actions on bone are somewhat attenuated, and greater levels of PTH in the bones are needed for normal bone remodeling. Impairment of normal bone remodeling leads to stress fractures that manifest clinically as bone pain and pathologic fractures. Low bone turnover has been associated with aluminum precipitation and with blockage of bone mineralization. Judicious use of aluminum-containing medications has diminished the prevalence of osteomalacia, and the new type of low bone turnover has been more frequently diagnosed. A clue to a low bone turnover state is hypercalcemia that develops rapidly after calcium supplementation. Diabetics appear particularly vulnerable to low bone turnover states. If serum phosphorous levels are elevated, aggressive normalization of serum calcium levels should not be attempted unless symptomatic hypocalcemia is present. Calcium replacement in the milieu of hyperphosphatemia may result in calcium–phosphate precipitation in the lungs, skin, and other organs.

End-stage Renal Disease (ESRD)

If renal damage is severe and a patient cannot maintain normal metabolic balance or excrete enough toxins to prevent uremic symptoms (Table 4.11), renal replacement therapy in the form of dialysis or transplantation must be initiated. When renal replacement therapy is needed, ESRD has been reached. ESRD may precede CRF months or years after the primary insult has passed, suggesting that the permanent loss of renal function promotes secondary changes in remaining nephrons that allow ESRD to evolve. ESRD may occur after a single renal insult or after continual or recurrent injury by systemic disease. Common causes of ESRD include:

- Diabetes mellitus
- Hypertension
- Polycystic kidney disease
- Urinary tract obstruction
- Renal vascular disease
- Unknown causes

Dialysis

Patients with CRF should have serial measurements of GFR. If the patient's muscle mass is stable, plotting 1/Scr is a useful way to follow disease progression (Fig. 4.1). Patients who experience changes in muscle mass and weight must have urinary creatinine clearances measured. Following serial urinary creatinine clearances or a 1/Scr plot is useful because most renal disease progresses at a constant rate. This allows the physician to anticipate when the GFR will be less than 10 mL/min, the point at which time renal replacement therapy is needed. If the slope of the 1/Scr plot changes abruptly, the clinician should suspect an acute insult superimposed on the chronic disease process. Serial GFR measurements also allow one to anticipate when renal replacement will be needed. This allows a nephrologist time to schedule surgery for dialysis access or preemptive renal transplantation.

Uremic Signs	TABLE 4.11
System	**Signs and Symptoms**
Gastrointestinal	Decreased taste sensation
	Nausea
	Vomiting
	Gastric inflammation
Cardiac	Pericarditis
	Worsening hypertension
	Accelerated atherosclerosis
Neurologic	Asterixis
	Peripheral neuropathy: sensor and motor
	Decreased concentration/ mental alertness
Endocrine	Hypogonadism
	Impotence
	Hypoglycemia

Dialysis is generally done when the patient's GFR is 10 mL/min or less and uremic symptoms have appeared (Table 4.11). When GFR approaches 15 to 20 mL/min, the patient begins to experience fatigue followed by an abnormal taste sensation. This abnormal taste has been described as metallic and ammonia-like and often precedes nausea and vomiting. Weight loss may coincide with the gastrointestinal complaints.

Signs and symptoms of congestive heart failure caused by increased intravascular volume may be the initiating factors to recommend dialysis in some patients. Most patients in whom circulating volume overload becomes the primary factor in initiating dialysis have systolic cardiac dysfunction. It is rare that hyperkalemia or acidosis is a sole reason to initiate dialysis. Uremic pericarditis and the development of uremic peripheral neuropathy are absolute indications for renal replacement therapy. Both may evolve independent of other uremic signs; therefore, detailed and serial physical examinations are prudent as the GFR falls. Although most uremic changes will resolve with dialysis, neuropathy may be irreversible.

If hemodialysis is the modality chosen for renal replacement therapy, establishment of intravascular access should be planned as the GFR falls to 20 mL/min, or as GFR rapidly decreases. Referral to a nephrologist should be arranged early in the course of CRF because of the complexity of diagnosing and managing uremic signs and symptoms.

Conditions Associated with CRF

Multiple metabolic and endocrine changes occur with CRF. Observation, diagnosis, and treatment of these associated comorbid conditions can increase patient survival.

Anemia

The most common cause of anemia in renal disease is diminished erythropoietin production by diseased kidneys. Other causes of anemia, particularly gastrointestinal bleeding, must be excluded before initiating erythropoietin treatment for renal anemia.

Acidosis

As GFR declines, the ability to excrete acid is impaired. The acids that accumulate are "mineral acids" (e.g., phosphoric, sulfuric acids) rather than organic acids. This accumulation predisposes the patient with CRF to a high anion gap metabolic acidosis. Typically this

form of chronic acidosis is well tolerated. When serum bicarbonate levels fall below 16 mEq/L, some patients will be uncomfortable with the rapid, shallow breathing that is a result of the degree of respiratory alkalosis necessary to compensate for the acidosis. Patients with a limited ability to compensate, such as those with pulmonary or musculoskeletal diseases, may not tolerate even mild acidosis. Chronic metabolic acidosis may additionally promote bone demineralization and adversely affect hepatic albumin synthesis. Therefore, correction of acidosis when the serum bicarbonate has fallen below 16 mEq/L is advisable.

Besides the level of renal function, the main determinant of acidosis severity is protein intake. High protein diets may cause excessive acid generation and overwhelm renal compensation. The protein intake of a patient with metabolic acidosis should be evaluated and reduced if excessive.

If protein intake is not excessive, bicarbonate therapy is prescribed. Oral sodium bicarbonate therapy is the best tolerated treatment for acidosis. Initial treatment should target the correction of acidosis while preventing alkalosis. Correction of acidosis is calculated from the bicarbonate distribution space, which is approximately 50% body weight. Correcting a serum bicarbonate from 12 to 20 mEq/L in a 70-kg patient would require approximately 280 mEq bicarbonate (8 mEq/L increase in bicarbonate $\times$ [70 kg (50%]), which can be taken over several days. To offset ongoing acidosis, approximately 0.5 to 1.0 mEq bicarbonate/kg body weight should be prescribed to compensate for the daily acid load of approximately 1 mEq/kg/day. Sodium bicarbonate tablets (650 mg) offer 8 mEq bicarbonate. Bicarbonate therapy is best tolerated when taken in two to three separate doses (e.g., 1300 mg of sodium bicarbonate [$Na\ HCO_3$] three times daily). Despite a high sodium content, sodium bicarbonate therapy does not increase intravascular volume or cause edema because absorption of sodium into veins requires a reabsorbable anion such as chloride, as opposed to bicarbonate. Evidence of sodium and water retention in patients taking sodium bicarbonate should alert the physician to reexamine the patient's dietary history.

Modified Shohl's solution (sodium citrate 500 mg with citric acid 334 mg/5 mL) corrects acidosis by providing the hepatic bicarbonate substrate. Shohl's solution is most often used in patients who cannot swallow large pills, such as patients requiring enteral feeding. Each milliliter of the solution provides 1 mEq bicarbonate. Shohl's solution is palatable and hence is tolerated better than taking several bicarbonate tablets.

Hypertension

Renal failure is frequently associated with the development or exacerbation of hypertension. Volume retention is a major component in CRF hypertension. Even when a patient appears to have normal volumes, diuretic therapy will often improve the effects of other antihypertensive agents. Hypertension and anemia often accompany CRF, causing a high incidence of left ventricular hypertrophy (LVH). LVH creates a risk for high mortality, and reversal of LVH should be one of the goals of blood pressure management.

Gastrointestinal Conditions

Dyspepsia is a common problem in renal failure. Gastrin levels are elevated and rates of peptic ulcer disease are increased in renal failure patients. Gastrointestinal bleeding occurs because of defective platelet functions, a complication of azotemia. Arteriovenous malformations in the small bowel and colon also occur more commonly in renal disease and often require procoagulant therapy or surgery.

Reproductive Conditions

As renal disease progresses, endocrine disturbances may cause impotence in males and anovulation in women. Serum prolactin levels are generally elevated in renal failure, suggesting that end-organ compromise occurs as uremic toxin accumulation occurs. The effects of low testosterone levels in males with CRF or ESRD have been alleviated with topical testosterone in some patients. The long-term benefits of testosterone therapy are not known, however. Intermittent ovulation as renal disease progresses may cause sporadic menstrual bleeding and "hot flashes." Gynecologic referral, particularly for routine pelvic examinations, is advisable. Despite anovulatory changes in some women, others are able to conceive when CRF is less severe. Premenopausal patients should be informed that pregnancy increases the risk of renal failure progression, preeclampsia or eclampsia, and the possibility of fetal death. Appropriate contraceptive intervention may be required. Often, with aggressive dialysis or renal transplantation, the likelihood of conception is improved.

Hypoglycemia

Hypoglycemia results from impaired carbohydrate metabolism in CRF patients. Insulin clearance decreases as kidney disease progresses, requiring periodic adjustments in the amount, frequency, and type of insulin or oral hypoglycemic prescribed. Very long-acting preparations of insulin may not be appropriate, and often smaller doses of regular insulin may be needed. Likewise, oral hypoglycemic preparations may need to be limited.

Hypoglycemia can occur in diabetics and in nondiabetics, caused by altered hepatic glucose metabolism. In some patients, agents that impair hepatic glucose metabolism (rifampin, isoniazid, propranolol) are implicated in hypoglycemia, but in other patients history of ingestion of those drugs is absent. Most cases of hypoglycemia in CRF occur in patients undergoing dialysis, although hypoglycemia in predialysis has been described.

Pruritus

Pruritus in CRF can be intense and difficult to control. The most common cause of pruritus is hyperphosphatemia. The serum level of phosphorous that elicits itching varies among patients, with some patients tolerating significant elevations of serum phosphorous levels and others manifesting debilitating symptoms at lower levels. Lowering the serum phosphorous with diet and phosphate binders, as described previously, is effective. The temporary use of aluminum compounds may be required to lower serum phosphorous levels quickly, as these compounds are more effective than calcium compounds. Limited aluminum use (2 weeks) with subsequent resumption of calcium-containing products is advocated to reduce the risk of aluminum bone disease. Control of serum PTH values with phosphorous restriction, calcium supplementation when indicated, and 1,25–dihydroxyvitamin D_3 therapy may help resolve the pruritus.

Systemic histamine levels may be elevated in CRF, resulting in pruritus. Use of antihistamine compounds may therefore be useful. In patients with pruritus and anemia, histamine levels may increase and pruritus may resolve with the initiation of erythropoietin therapy.

Occasionally pruritus occurs in the absence of hyperphosphatemia and is not readily responsive to antihistamine therapy. Dermatitis attributed to CRF has been responsive to ultraviolet phototherapy administered by a dermatologist in some patients. In all patients with pruritus and renal disease, the use of skin moisturizing compounds is advised. In patients with intractable pruritus, parathyroidectomy has resulted in complete remission of itching.

KEY POINTS

- Serum creatinine level is generally considered as an acceptable substitute of creatinine clearance (GFR) in adults.

- Serum creatinine measurements may underestimate creatinine clearance in the elderly and in malnourished individuals.

- BUN is a poor predictor of renal function abnormality.

- Acute impairment of renal function results from drug-induced renal disease, volume loss, or lower urinary tract obstruction.

- Elevated serum potassium level out of proportion to the degree of azotemia is a strong clue for acute or chronic lower urinary tract obstruction.

- 2+ to 4+ protein and presence of many different types of cast in urine analysis suggest glomerular disease.

- Straight bladder catheterization and ultrasound of kidneys can rule out lower urinary tract obstruction in the majority of patients.

- Urinary sodium and chloride concentrations in a spot urine sample are sensitive markers for initiation and maintenance of fluid therapy.

REFERRAL

When to refer a patient to a nephrologist is subjective, depending on the generalist's comfort in dealing with renal disease. The authors recommend prompt referral in the following situations:

- **Rapidly progressive glomerular nephritis (RPGN).** If the patient has ARF and a nephritic urine sediment, he or she needs an immediate renal biopsy and often initiation of aggressive immunomodulating treatment.
- **ARF secondary to HUS/TTP.** If the patient has ARF and a microangiopathic hemolytic anemia with thrombocytopenia, the patient may require plasma exchange.

- **Impaired renal function** and evidence of increased intravascular volume unresponsive to diuretic therapy.
- **Persistent hyperkalemia** in a patient with marginal urine output or evidence of an increased intravascular volume.
- **Uremic pericarditis**
- **Uremic neuropathy**
- **Dialysis support.** Any cause of ARF in which the clinician anticipates the need for dialysis support.
- **Unexplained chronic renal insufficiency.** Less urgent but still important, unexplained chronic renal insufficiency calls for nephrology referral. In the authors' opinion, referral to a nephrologist early in the course of unexplained CRF is necessary to confirm or establish a diagnosis, offer the most current therapy to prevent or delay the need for dialysis, and counsel the patient on renal replacement therapy options. Referral to a nephrologist before dialysis is imminent allows renal replacement therapy to be started on an outpatient basis before cardiovascular or pulmonary injury. Often, timely referral can allow a preemptive renal transplant to be done before or soon after dialysis is initiated.

COMMONLY ASKED QUESTIONS

Patients may be overwhelmed after learning of their kidney disease. Many may show disinterest in their diagnosis. As with most chronic diseases, patient education and family participation may be the most successful long-term approach. All patients deserve an explanation of their underlying kidney disease, and most will have questions in the realm of "Why me?" Topics routinely include:

Will my kidney failure improve?
Patients must know when improvement in kidney failure is expected and, conversely, when little hope of improvement exists. Education about the cause and treatment of renal disease enables patients to accept their disease. Acceptance will then promote better personal involvement in their care.

What foods should I eat?
Diets limited in protein and sodium or restricted in calories may be difficult for the patient to tolerate. Professional counseling, preferably by a nutritionist who routinely deals with CRF, is advisable.

Can my family get kidney failure?
Many patients realize that kidney diseases are genetic and will inquire about disease in other members of their family. If not initiated by the patient, the physician should discuss the likelihood that his or her form of kidney impairment is inheritable to allay the unspoken concerns of family.

What is dialysis and can transplantation help me?

The widespread use of dialysis and renal transplantation has, to some extent, lessened the concern of many patients with kidney disease. However, morbidity and in many instances mortality is greater in patients requiring either modality, compared with age- and sex-matched controls. Patients with even modest CRF must be informed that they often can affect the rate of disease progression through lifestyle modifications presented by their physicians. Once ESRD occurs, the patient must also know that he or she must adhere to these modifications. Noncompliance with dialysis schedules and immunosuppressive agents will result in dialysis failure and premature loss of a renal transplant, respectively. Patients with CRF who are progressing toward ESRD can often quickly recruit family and friends willing to donate a kidney for transplantation.

Conversely, the workup for transplantation can be prolonged and patient anxiety may mount because a "quick remedy" does not occur. Referral to a nephrologist to address most of these concerns is advisable.

SUGGESTED READINGS

Brenner B, Brady H, Brenner B, et al. Acute renal failure. In: Brenner B, ed. The Kidney. 5th ed. Philadelphia: Saunders, 1996.

Massry SG, Glassock RJ, eds. Uremia and the effects of dialysis. In: Textbook of Nephrology. 3rd ed. Baltimore: Williams & Wilkins, 1995.

Thadhani R, Pascual M, Bonventre J. Acute renal failure. New Engl J Med 1996;334(22):1448–1460.

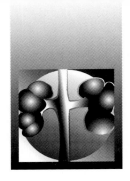

5

Hyponatremia and Hypernatremia

Anil K. Mandal

HYPONATREMIA

Basics

Hyponatremia by definition is a serum sodium concentration of less than 136 mEq/L (the normal level is 136 to 145 mEq/L). The serum sodium concentration is largely a reflection of total body water; therefore, changes in the concentration of serum sodium essentially reflect changes in body water.

Hyponatremia is a common abnormality detected by laboratory tests and found in 15 to 25% of patients in general hospital settings. However, in most instances patients are asymptomatic or only minimally symptomatic. Conversely, it is not uncommon to see a patient brought to the hospital emergency room because of neurologic manifestations, such as gross alterations in state of mind, convulsions, or coma, that are directly attributable to hyponatremia. In psychiatric wards of general hospitals, and more often in psychiatric institutions, symptomatic hyponatremia is a common occurrence.

Associated Conditions

Hyponatremia can be associated broadly with three major types of conditions:

1. Conditions associated with excessive accumulation of extracellular fluid. In these settings, hyponatremia usually is chronic and causes no symptoms. Typical examples include:
   - Congestive heart failure
   - Cirrhosis of the liver
   - Nephrotic syndrome
2. Excessive loss of sodium in the urine. Typical causes include:
   - Large doses of loop diuretics
   - Medullary cystic disease of kidney
   - Chronic kidney disease
   - Hypertension
3. Inability to excrete free water, which is probably the most common cause of acute and symptomatic hyponatremia. Typical causes include:
   - Syndrome of inappropriate antidiuretic hormone (SIADH)
   - Compulsive water drinking (water intoxication)
   - Overzealous use of potent diuretics
   - Acute alcoholism
   - Postsurgery conditions
   - Drugs (a list of drugs that may produce hyponatremia mimicking SIADH are listed in Table 5.1.)

Less typical examples include:

- Severe dehydration from vomiting
- Nasogastric suction
- Diarrhea
- Moderate to severe exercise
- AIDS and AIDS-related complex

Glucocorticoid Deficiency

Glucocorticoid deficiency results in a clinical picture almost indistinguishable from that of SIADH. Persistent arginine vasopressin (AVP) secretion in this condition is caused by loss of hypotonic suppression of AVP release, which may be occasioned primarily by glucocorticoid deficiency per se and aggravated secondarily by multiple nonosmotic stimuli, including nausea, hypotension, and hypoglycemia.

Acute Brain Disease

Three theories explain the origin of hyponatremia in acute brain disease:

1. Cerebral salt wasting syndrome, in which excessive natriuresis caused by some unknown cerebral natriuretic factor lowers the total body sodium concentration, and, hence, the sodium plasma concentration.
2. SIADH, in which an increase in total body water is caused by unphysiologic secretion of AVP, lowering the concentration of sodium in the plasma.
3. Sodium shift (i.e., a displacement of sodium from the extracellular to the intracellular space with a simultaneous movement of potassium in the opposite direction).

In acute brain disease, such as occurs in association with intracranial bleeding, urinary sodium excretion is increased despite hyponatremia, with urinary osmolality exceeding plasma osmolality. These findings are supportive of SIADH. However, in some of these patients, a water loading test showed no impairment in diuresis, and replenishment of sodium without water restriction improved the hyponatremia as well as the clinical conditions. Plasma AVP levels relative to plasma osmolality in these patients are consistently elevated. Another study on patients with tuberculous meningitis associated with hyponatremia demonstrated elevated levels of atrial natriuretic peptide (ANP) in some of them. In these hyponatremic patients, a moderate negative correlation was obtained between plasma levels of ANP and sodium. The elevated ANP concentration could account for cerebral salt wasting syndrome, which is distinct from SIADH in acute or chronic central nervous system injury or disease.

Drugs Associated with Hyponatremia	**TABLE 5.1**
Anticancer agents	Cyclophosphamide
	Vincristine
Antidepressants	Tricyclics
	Fluoxetine
Antipsychotics	Chlorpromazine
Antidiabetics	Chlorpropamide
	Glyburide
Natriuretic agents	Diuretics
Central nervous system depressants	
Anticonvulsants	Morphine
	Carbamazepine (5%)

In summary, all hyponatremic states have vasopressin elevation in common. Without this increase, the loss of salt would be followed by appropriate diuresis and normonatremia. If the initial event is inappropriate antidiuretic hormone (ADH) secretion (whether caused by cerebral disease, neoplasm, a pulmonary lesion, or drugs), there is no related signal for salt retention and urinary sodium levels and tonicity are high, the latter usually higher than the plasma tonicity. If salt loss is caused by intrinsic renal disease, diuretics, or adrenal failure, the urinary sodium concentration varies depending on the magnitude of the response to the volume of salt-retaining factors. Because hyponatremia often occurs with major illness and because more than one factor may be involved in its pathogenesis, establishing its origin and appropriate treatment remain a diagnostic and therapeutic challenge.

Patients at Risk

Psychiatric and Alcoholic Patients

The mechanisms associated with acute hyponatremia in psychiatric inpatients and in alcoholics have not been well defined. The risk factors that have been investigated include medications, basic demographic variables, and medical comorbidities. Certain psychiatric diagnoses are also associated with an increased risk. The following medications are associated with the development of hyponatremia in psychiatric and alcoholic patients but are not limited to those patient groups.

- Diuretics
- Fluoxetine
- Tricyclic antidepressants
- Calcium antagonists

  Important comorbidities include:

- Elevated creatinine levels
- Chronic obstructive pulmonary disease (COPD)
- Hypertension
- Diabetes

Although elderly psychiatric inpatients appear to develop hyponatremia more often than do younger patients, once drug use and comorbidities are taken into account, age does not appear to be a significant risk factor for this population.

Postsurgery Patients

Hyponatremia is common in postsurgery patients, particularly when operated on transsphenoidally for pituitary tumors. Hyponatremia occurs most commonly (61%) in patients operated on for Cushing's disease. Neither the size and operability of the tumor nor transient postoperative polyuria can predict the development of hyponatremia. High urinary osmolality and elevated plasma AVP concentration during the hyponatremic state indicate that SIADH is involved in the pathogenesis of hyponatremia after transsphenoidal surgery.

Other types of surgery associated with hyponatremia include:

- Adult spinal fusion surgery
- Transurethral resection of the prostate
- Hysterectomy
- Labyrinthectomy
- Abdominal surgery (such as cholecystectomy)

Signs and Symptoms

Patients with acute hyponatremia are usually symptomatic, whereas those with chronic hyponatremia are either asymptomatic or minimally symptomatic. *The rate of development of hyponatremia and its severity are the sole determining factors for the appearance of symptoms, for the severity of central nervous system symptoms and signs, for morbidity and mortality, and for the urgency of treatment.* The signs and symptoms of hyponatremia, especially those associated with the central nervous system, develop mainly as a result of plasma hypo-osmolality and migration of free water from extracellular space to intracellular space. In this respect the most vulnerable organ is the brain, which tends to become edematous. Osmotic swelling of the brain is maximal in the first few hours of hyponatremia and is commensurate with the appearance of neurologic symptoms and signs. Gradually the brain adapts to this process by generating solutes, which apparently help in dissipation of the swelling. Pathologic examination of the brains of patients who died shortly after the onset of hyponatremia has shown cerebral edema and brainstem herniation. However, the incidence of dramatic and frequently catastrophic clinical consequences of acute hyponatremia culminating in seizures and respiratory arrest is unknown.

Some factors predispose patients to neurologic damage. For instance, postoperative hyponatremia complicated by respiratory arrest and leading to hypoxia is reported mostly in women. In men, the incidence of neurologic complications with a comparable degree of postoperative hyponatremia is much lower. A similar female predisposition is apparent in thiazide-associated hyponatremia and may even lead to neurologic complications in elderly women.

Severity of Symptoms and Rate of Decrease of Serum Sodium

The symptoms and signs of hyponatremia are unusual unless the serum sodium concentration has decreased to or below 125 mEq/L and has reached this level rapidly (in less than 24 hours). Severity of symptoms and signs varies in direct proportion to the rate of decrease of the serum sodium concentration. A slow decrease even to a very low (110 mEq/L) level may give rise to mild symptoms such as apathy, lethargy,

Summary of Diagnosis: Hyponatremia

- Inability to excrete free water is probably the most common cause of acute and symptomatic hyponatremia. Associated conditions include SIADH, compulsive water drinking, a postsurgical state, and the use of some drugs.
- Diuretics, fluoxetine, tricyclic antidepressants, and calcium antagonists are all associated with development of hyponatremia.
- Hyponatremia is common in postsurgical patients, particularly those who have been operated on transsphenoidally for pituitary tumors.
- All hyponatremic states have in common elevation of plasma vasopressin levels.
- Signs and symptoms of hyponatremia are unusual unless the serum sodium concentration has decreased to or below 125 mEq/L and has reached this level rapidly (in less than 24 hours).
- A slow decrease of the serum sodium concentration to even a very low level (110 mEq/L) may give rise to mild symptoms (i.e., apathy, anorexia), whereas a rapid decrease of even 5 to 6 mEq/L is likely to result in central nervous system symptoms.
- Hyponatremia is an important cause of seizure in infants younger than 6 months.
- The presence of signs and symptoms is the sole determining factor for the type of treatment and rapidity of initiating treatment.
- Hypertonic saline is the treatment of choice in acute symptomatic hyponatremia.
- Central pontine myelinolysis (CPM) occurs in asymptomatic chronically hyponatremic patients treated with saline infusion.

anorexia, nausea, and muscle cramps. Conversely, a rapid decrease from 140 to 125 mEq/L or lower in less than 24 hours will likely result in headache, confusion, disorientation, obtundation, and, in some patients, stage IV coma, convulsions, Cheyne-Stokes respiration, pathologic reflexes, and pseudo-bulbar palsy.

Diagnostic and Laboratory Tests

The diagnosis of hyponatremia involves the following diagnostic and laboratory tests:

- Neuropsychological and behavioral testing: mental flexibility, verbal fluency, short-term memory, and attention
- Serum and urine osmolality
- Spot testing for urinary electrolytes
- Serum uric acid level
- Arterial blood gas analysis
- Water loading test
- Magnetic resonance imaging (MRI)

Neuropsychological testing Paired neuropsychological and behavioral testing was done on a patient once during a state of hyponatremia (serum sodium level was less than 130 mEq/L) and once during a state of normonatremia (serum sodium level was 136 mEq/L). The testing revealed significant deficits associated with the hyponatremia involving complex information-processing skills. The neuropsychological effects of hyponatremia are remarkably consistent across patients. Furthermore, the Virginia Polydipsia Scale (VPS) can distinguish the patient drinking patterns associated with psychosis, intermittent hyponatremia, and polydipsia from those of controls.

Serum uric acid level The serum uric acid concentration is typically low in patients with SIADH and in patients with hyponatremia associated with hypopituitarism. A low serum uric acid concentration has also been observed in patients with poly-dipsia–hyponatremia and adrenal insufficiency syndrome.

Anion gap A similar study demonstrated that 50% of individuals with SIADH presented with an anion gap less than 11 mEq/L. In patients with adrenal insufficiency, hyponatremia is typically associated with a low bicarbonate concentration but a normal anion gap. In patients with hyponatremia associated with cardiac failure or cirrhosis, the anion gap is usually normal despite mild hypoproteinemia.

Water loading test   The water loading test is administered to determine the kidney's ability to excrete water load. The test is conducted in the morning, according to the following procedure:

1. A control-collection of urine is taken, and blood samples are drawn.
2. Urinary sodium and osmolality are measured, and blood samples are analyzed for sodium and osmolality.
3. A water load consisting of 20 mL/kg per body weight is given to the patient to drink within 15 to 20 minutes.
4. Urine collection begins every hour for 4 hours (although the test can be extended to 5 hours). Vigilant attention must be paid to the patient to make certain that there is no drinking of additional fluid.
5. After 4 (or 5) hours, the total urine volume is measured, and the urine sample of the first hour and the last hour are measured for sodium and osmolality.
6. At the final hour, blood samples are again drawn and analyzed for serum sodium and osmolality.

The normal response is a decrease in serum osmolality. The osmole sends a blunted signal to the hypothalamus, resulting in slight or no release of AVP. Therefore, a large volume of free water (dilute urine) is excreted. After giving water load to a subject who is in normal fluid-electrolyte balance, serum osmolality in a control study decreases from 293 to 285; urine osmolality decreases from 775 to 77 in two hours associated with excretion of free water. Compare this with the increase in urinary osmolality in a patient with SIADH as shown in Table 5.2.

In the case of SIADH, although the water load will decrease the plasma osmolality, resulting in a particularly blunted hypothalamic release of AVP, the urinary osmolality concentration remains unchanged. The excretion of concentrated urine despite dilution of plasma osmolality suggests action of AVP, which may be released from a source other than the hypothalamus (e.g., from a tumor).

Differential Diagnosis

Diagnosis of hyponatremia becomes more challenging when a patient has repeated seizures or is suffering from respiratory arrest and hyponatremia, and the determination must be made if the symptoms are in fact associated with hyponatremia or with another condition. A systematic approach should be used in a patient with suspected hyponatremia and the following information elicited:

- Age
- Sex
- History of diuretic use
- History of recent surgery, especially transsphenoidal surgery
- Presence of polyuria/polydipsia
- Alcohol intake
- Presence of infection

Pseudohyponatremia

In every case of suspected hyponatremia, factors other than excess body water should be considered as causes

---

TABLE 5.2   Water Loading Test: Case Example

Hour	Urine Volume (mL)	Urine Sodium (mEq/L)	Urine Osmolality (Osm/kg)	Serum Sodium (mEq/L)	Serum Osmolality (Osm/kg)
0 (control hour)	Water load (20 mL/kg) 1680 mL to drink	39	401	139	293
1	0				
2	260[a]	61	431		
3	0				
4	0				
5	150	58	428	134	284

[a]Volume replaced.

of the signs and symptoms. These factors are hyper-globulinemia, hyperglycemia, and hyperlipidemia, which can be associated with a low serum sodium concentration. This condition is called pseudohyponatremia and commonly is observed in patients with uncontrolled diabetes mellitus. Lowering the elevated blood glucose levels with insulin results in a prompt increase of the serum sodium level to normal.

In pseudohyponatremia, measured serum osmolality is normal to high, precluding the possibility of dilutional hyponatremia. Hyponatremia can be associated with contracted extracellular fluid, which characteristically gives rise to postural hypotension (>10-mm decrease in systolic blood pressure on standing) and low urinary sodium (<20 mEq/L in a spot test urine sample).

Management

"Hyponatremia which develops fast should be treated fast; whereas hyponatremia when developed slowly should be corrected at a proportionately slower pace" (Berl, 1990).

The presence of signs and symptoms is the sole determining factor for the type of treatment and the rapidity of initiation of treatment in a patient with hyponatremia. Thus, there is slight or no disagreement about aggressive treatment in patients with symptomatic hyponatremia; however, a more conservative approach is generally recommended for patients with asymptomatic hyponatremia.

Treatment of Acute Symptomatic Hyponatremia

A patient is brought to the emergency room with confusion, disorientation, and seizure activity; his serum sodium level is 105 mEq/L. Most clinicians agree that a patient with these signs must be treated with hypertonic saline.

The ideal rate of administration of hypertonic saline and the safe limit of increase of serum sodium levels are highly controversial. Hypertonic saline may be administered at a rate to increase serum sodium concentration by 1 mEq/L/hour safely up to 10-12 mEq/L total in the first 24 hours or until the neurologic symptoms and signs have abated. Furosemide at 1 mg/kg should be given intravenously to facilitate free water excretion and promote steady increase of serum sodium. Increase of serum sodium up to 25 mEq/L on day 1 in a severely symptomatic patient may be considered.

Guidelines for use of hypertonic saline   Guidelines for appropriate use of hypertonic (3%) saline for the treatment of acute hyponatremia are ill-defined. Hypertonic saline should be reserved for symptomatically hyponatremic patients, most of whom become acutely symptomatic. A target level for the serum sodium concentration should be determined and a time course for correction set. The infusion should be started promptly and monitored frequently for the effect on the serum sodium level and for patient symptoms.

PROCEDURE FOR HYPERTONIC SALINE INFUSION

1. To increase serum sodium by 5 mEq/L from baseline:

Total body weight × 5 mEq/L = 5 × 60 kg × .6 = 180 mEq/L total sodium to be infused (60% of body weight is water)

2. Hypertonic saline (3%) contains 513 mEq sodium/L (isotonic saline contains 154 mEq sodium/L)
3. 180 mEq sodium/L = 350 mL hypertonic saline
4. In severely symptomatic patients, hypertonic saline may be infused at a rate of 50 to 100 mL/hour and symptoms and serum sodium levels should be monitored hourly or every 2 hours

Central pontine myelinolysis (CPM)   Although overcorrection or rapid correction of hyponatremia has been incriminated for causing CPM, this hypothesis is not well founded. CPM is characterized by insidious progressive development of flaccid quadriplegia, cranial nerve abnormalities manifesting as pseudobulbar palsy, and alteration in mental status including behavior changes. There is some consensus that the absolute magnitude of correction rather than the rate of correction may increase the risk of this demyelination syndrome. Correction rates exceeding 2.5 mEq/L/hour or an absolute increase of more than 25 mEq/L on day 1, or both, have been associated with a high incidence of CPM. Evidence from studies in experimental animals is more supportive of absolute overcorrection than rate of correction as a cause of CPM. Also, there is some consensus that correcting hyponatremia of shorter duration (acute onset) carries no untoward consequences regardless of the treatment regimen. The hazards of seizures, coma, and respiratory arrest clearly outweigh the risks of rapid rate of correction and complete reversal of the neurologic manifestations.

PREDISPOSING CONDITIONS   CPM is more likely to occur in patients with chronic asymptomatic hyponatremia and in those with preexisting abnormalities, such as chronic alcoholism, malnutrition, or chronic hypokalemia, if they are treated with hypertonic saline infusion. Hypokalemia may predispose patients to develop CPM following correction of hyponatremia. In neurologically stable patients with severe hyponatremia, it may be beneficial to correct hypokalemia before correcting serum sodium levels.

PROGRESSION OF CPM Neurologic disorders developing after correction of severe symptomatic hyponatremia were studied in several patients. No patient had hypoxic events or other identifiable cause for the neurologic illness. Neurologic deterioration began approximately 3 days after correction and often followed a period of improvement in hyponatremic encephalopathy. Typically, spastic quadriparesis, pseudobulbar palsy, and impairment in the level of consciousness progressed for up to 7 days. Improvement generally began 2 weeks after correction and continued for up to 1 year in some patients. Routine spinal fluid analysis was normal. Electroencephalograms commonly showed nonfocal slowing. Brain imaging was normal in the initial weeks, but later showed pontine or symmetric extrapontine lesions. Although CPM typically occurred following an elevation in serum sodium greater than 18 mEq/L/24 hours, it sometimes developed following a rise in serum sodium level of 21 mEq/L/48 hours.

Treatment of Chronic or Recurrent Hyponatremia

Any one of the following regimens may be recommended for treatment of chronic or recurrent hyponatremia:

- Water restriction
- Salt tablet 1 g orally twice or three times daily, plus furosemide 40 mg orally once or twice daily
- Demeclocycline 600 to 1200 mg in two divided doses
- Urea 30 to 60 g in two divided doses, dissolved in water before drinking
- Phenytoin

Treatment of Asymptomatic Hyponatremia

The physician must make a therapeutic choice between saline infusion and water restriction in the treatment of asymptomatic hyponatremia.

Treatment of Hyponatremia in Postsurgery Patients

Fluid restriction alone is adequate treatment for post-transsphenoidal surgery patients. When treatment is limited to water restriction, patients do not develop progressive neurologic symptoms or other morbidity. The differences between transsphenoidal surgery–associated hyponatremia and other acute postoperative hyponatremia are presented in Table 5.3.

Demeclocycline is the recommended therapy for noncompliant patients with chronic or recurrent hyponatremia (e.g., in SIADH). The drug is a tetracycline derivative and inhibits adenylate cyclase, thus impeding the action of ADH on the collecting tubules and producing a picture of vasopressin-resistant diabetes insipidus. Demeclocycline has also been used successfully in the prophylaxis of carbamazepine-induced hyponatremia. Adverse effects include photophobia and malabsorption syndrome. Nephrotoxicity may occur in patients with abnormal liver function.

Referral

Hyponatremic patients should be referred for diagnosis and treatment to a nephrologist; referral to a neurologist may be advisable as well, depending on the central nervous system manifestations.

Prevention

- Hyponatremia is common in postsurgery patients, particularly when the surgery was done transsphenoidally for pituitary tumors. Hyponatremia is mild and takes 1 week to develop in patients who have undergone intracranial surgery. Fluid restriction

TABLE 5.3   Differences Between Transsphenoidal Surgery-associated Hyponatremia and Other Acute Postoperative-associated Hyponatremias

Transsphenoidal Hyponatremia	Other Postoperative Hyponatremias
Not iatrogenic	Frequently iatrogenic (induced by hypotonic fluid infusion)
One-week delayed onset	Rapid (36- to 48-hour) onset
Fluid restriction is adequate treatment	Hypertonic saline is treatment of choice
No associated morbidity or mortality	High rates of morbidity and mortality

alone could mitigate the development of hyponatremia in these patients.

- Infusion of hypotonic fluids, such as 5% dextrose in water, should be avoided in postsurgery trauma patients in whom the AVP level is high because of the danger of development of severe symptomatic hyponatremia.
- Close monitoring of compulsive water drinkers, many of whom have psychiatric illnesses, is necessary to prevent water intoxication.
- Correction of serum potassium levels, even before correction of serum sodium levels, could reduce the incidence of CPM in hyponatremic patients.

HYPERNATREMIA

Basics

Hypernatremia is a disorder of sodium and water metabolism defined by elevation of serum sodium levels higher than 145 mEq/L. Hypernatremia develops mainly because of deficient water intake; however, excessive water losses may contribute to the problem. Hypernatremia resulting from sodium excess occurs less frequently, and fatal hypernatremia caused solely by ingestion of table salt is rare.

Three important factors that frequently predispose a patient to hypernatremia are:

1. Hypodipsia caused by decreased thirst perception
2. Decreased renal ability to conserve water
3. Inappropriately low plasma vasopressin level for the degree of hyperosmolality, resulting in loss of free water and causing free water depletion syndrome

A patient who has a disability as a result of stroke or injury and thus lacks access to water is also a candidate for hypernatremia. A recent (Palevsky PM, et al.) report showed that 86% of patients with hospital-acquired hypernatremia lacked free access to water.

Cause

In the case of severe water depletion, initially the extracellular fluid space becomes contracted and hypertonic. The intracellular fluid space, with two-thirds of body water, then tries to minimize extracellular fluid hypertonicity by allowing the migration of water from its space to the extracellular fluid space; thereby, the intracellular fluid space rapidly shrinks. The target organ in this process is the brain, which bears the brunt of hypernatremic dehydration. The brain cells contract, which may cause rupture of the intercellular capillaries, resulting in intracerebral and subarachnoid hemorrhage.

The major factor determining the degree of volume depletion in hypernatremia of any cause is, of course, the severity of water deficit. When water deficit occurs rapidly without an opportunity for sodium to be retained, serum sodium concentration mathematically reflects the degree of water loss. However, when water loss occurs chronically and sodium intake continues, volume depletion causes renal sodium retention, and hypernatremia is then the result of sodium retention as well as water loss. Sodium retention continues until the natriuretic effect of hypernatremia overcomes the salt-retaining effect of volume depletion. At equilibrium, the patient will remain volume-depleted and hypernatremic. Because the natriuretic effect of hypernatremia is positively correlated to its magnitude, the degree of volume depletion is also a function of the degree of hypernatremia. The pathophysiology of hypernatremia is depicted in Figure 5.1.

Signs and Symptoms

The severity of signs and symptoms depends on:

- Rapidity of free water loss
- Duration of the disorder
- Magnitude of the osmotic stress

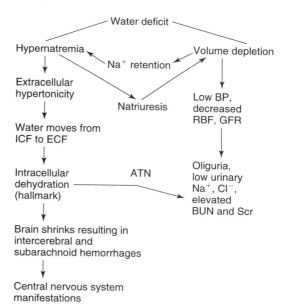

FIGURE 5.1.

Pathophysiology and clinical manifestations of hypernatremia. *ATN,* acute tubular necrosis; *BP,* blood pressure; *BUN,* blood urea nitrogen; *Cl⁻,* chloride; *ECF,* extracellular fluid; *GFR,* glomerular filtration rate; *ICF,* intracellular fluid; *Na⁺,* sodium; *RBF,* renal blood flow; *SCr,* serum creatinine.

The signs and symptoms of hypernatremia are mainly ascribed to the central nervous system. Therefore, in less acute or chronic hypernatremia, nausea, muscle weakness and fasciculations, and an altered sensorium are the only manifestations likely to be observed. In acute hypernatremia, the resulting intracerebral and subarachnoid hemorrhages frequently give rise to coma, convulsions, or cognitive dysfunction. The serum sodium level at hospital admission and the peak serum sodium level have not been found to be significant factors for the hypernatremic signs and symptoms, although central nervous system symptoms are more common when the serum sodium level is above 165 mEq/L. Serum osmolality is more significantly related to the symptoms of hypernatremia than is the serum sodium level; however, investigations by the author have shown that a persistently elevated serum sodium level is significantly related to the high mortality rate in hypernatremic patients.

The author has also noted that the incidence of cognitive dysfunction, consisting of confusion, obtundation, and speech abnormalities, was significantly higher in those patients who eventually died of hypernatremia than in those who survived. The admission and peak serum sodium levels were not different between the two groups.

Signs and symptoms of hypernatremia are not limited to the brain. Other organs that share the brunt of hypernatremic dehydration include the liver and kidneys, which may show signs and symptoms of acute hepatic necrosis and acute tubular necrosis (ATN), respectively. Thus, a hypernatremic patient may develop hyperbilirubinemia, overt jaundice, and elevated levels of hepatocellular enzymes. Renal function is initially diminished from a depleted extracellular fluid volume, resulting in a high blood urea nitrogen (BUN): serum creatinine (SCr) ratio, low urinary volume, and a low urinary sodium value (<20 mEq/L). There may be marked reduction (>20 mm Hg) in systolic blood pressure when an upright posture is assumed, often associated with dizziness. If hypernatremia remains untreated, renal failure may become sustained or progressive because of the development of ATN.

Hypodipsia–Hypernatremia Syndrome (Essential Hypernatremia)

Essential hypernatremia is persistent hypernatremia not explained by any apparent extracellular volume loss. It is characterized by the absence or attenuation of thirst and the intactness of the normal renal response to AVP. Some patients may have signs and symptoms of partial diabetes insipidus; these patients consistently respond normally to nonosmolar AVP release. All these observations suggest that the osmoreceptor neurons

Summary of Diagnosis: Hypernatremia

- Hypernatremia occurs with increased frequency in elderly patients and is associated with mortality rates ranging from 40 to 60%.
- Intracerebral hemorrhages resulting from acute hypernatremia give rise to coma, convulsions, and cognitive dysfunction.
- Signs and symptoms are not limited to the brain but may include the kidneys and liver, which may undergo necrosis and manifest features of acute renal failure or hepatic failure.

that regulate vasopressin secretion are not totally synonymous with those that regulate thirst.

Management

The treatment of choice for hypernatremia is free water replacement orally or in the form of 5% dextrose in water in severely symptomatic patients.

The goal of treatment is to restore serum tonicity to normal. This can be achieved by administration of fluid; therefore, fluid is the principal line of treatment. The type of fluid to be administered depends on the severity of extracellular fluid volume depletion. The rate of fluid administration depends on the rate at which hypernatremia has developed. The same principle applies here as in hyponatremia. Thus, acute hypernatremia, wherein fatal brain shrinkage is the likely event, warrants rapid fluid therapy. When hypernatremia develops gradually, however, the brain is "protected" from the generation of brain osmoles and the hypernatremia should be corrected at a much slower pace. Therefore, if extracellular fluid volume depletion is mild, with slight or no change in postural blood pressure, and renal function is normal or slightly impaired, the fluid of choice is 5% dextrose in water. Dextrose is metabolized, allowing repletion of pure water. Small doses of insulin may be given to control hyperglycemia.

In a situation of severe extracellular fluid volume depletion accompanied by oliguria, severe postural hypotension, and a markedly elevated BUN:SCr ratio, the initial fluid should be normal saline for volume expansion to occur. With normal saline infusion, blood pressure rises and urine output increases, but serum sodium and chloride concentrations may also increase. Therefore, after initial normal saline infusion, the author recommends maintenance fluid therapy with 5% dextrose in water.

The amount of fluid to be administered may be calculated by using the following formula:

Estimated total body water = 60% of body weight

A patient under consideration is estimated to weigh 70 kg, and his serum sodium concentration is 165 mEq/L (normal is 140 mEq/L). His actual body weight, and hence his estimated total body water, is unknown. Thus, his observed body water equals 70 × 60/100, or 42 L.

**Total body water = observed body water ×
actual plasma sodium/normal plasma sodium**

Or, in this case:

$$42 \times 165/140 = 49.5 \text{ L}$$

Therefore, the total body water in this patient is 49.5 L. The difference between observed body water (42 L) and total body water (49.5 L) in this patient is 7.5 L. Hence, 50% of 7.5 L (3.75 L) should be administered over a period of 12 hours, or 1 L every 3 to 4 hours. The remaining volume should be given at a rate of 1 L every 12 to 16 hours, for 48 to 72 hours.

For example, if a patient has a serum sodium concentration greater than 160 mEq/L and demonstrates confusion, disorientation, tremulousness, nystagmus, and Babinski's sign, fluid should be administered at a rapid rate to repair 50% of the deficit in 12 hours. The remaining deficit may be corrected slowly over a period of 48 to 72 hours.

Lateral pontine and extrapontine myelinolysis can be associated with rapid correction or overcorrection of hypernatremia and hyperosmolality. Rapid correction may lead to grand mal seizures caused by rapid decrease of extracellular fluid osmolality and shift of water from the extracellular fluid space to the intracellular fluid space, and result in cerebral edema. Potassium chloride should be added to the saline or dextrose solution bag from the beginning to prevent development of hypokalemia.

When treating a patient with hypernatremia associated with central diabetes insipidus, aqueous vasopressin (5 U subcutaneously) or desmopressin (1 to 2 μg intravenously or 10 to 20 μg intranasally twice daily) should be administered. Serum electrolytes should be monitored to prevent development of acute hyponatremia and cerebral edema.

Referral

A symptomatic patient with hypernatremia should be referred to a nephrologist for appropriate treatment of sodium and water imbalance.

Prevention

Access to free water is all that is required to prevent hypernatremia. Because deficient water intake is the major cause of water deficit and the target population is elderly, disabled, and ill, ensuring regular fluid intake will offset fluid loss and prevent hypernatremia. In hospitalized patients, the cause of hypernatremia may not necessarily be deficient fluid intake: too much normal saline and too long a period of infusion may be the cause more so than deficient fluid intake.

KEY POINTS

- Hyponatremia of variable severity is a common laboratory abnormality among hospitalized patients.

- Hyponatremia often produces mild symptoms, or no symptoms; however, it can give rise to serious signs and symptoms such as coma, convulsion, and respiratory failure.

- Brain swelling and herniation of the brainstem are the pathophysiologic hallmarks of acute hyponatremia.

- Acute symptomatic hyponatremia is commonly a result of SIADH, water intoxication, intravenous boluses of furosemide, and postsurgical states.

- Glucocorticoid deficiency results in a clinical picture almost indistinguishable from that of SIADH.

- Postoperative hyponatremia complicated by respiratory arrest and permanent brain damage is reported mostly in menstruant women.

- A female predilection is apparent in thiazide-associated hyponatremia, possibly leading to neurologic complications in elderly women.

- The serum uric acid level is typically low in SIADH and in hyponatremia related to hypopituitarism.

- In hyponatremia as a result of transsphenoidal surgery, fluid restriction alone is the treatment of choice.

- Demeclocycline should be tried in non-compliant patients in whom fluid restriction may not be successful.

- Although total fluid restriction and salt tablets are adequate treatment in mildly symptomatic patients, infusion of hypertonic (3%) saline with 1 mg/kg furosemide intravenously is the treatment of choice in severely symptomatic hyponatremic patients.

- Hypernatremia occurs with increased frequency in elderly patients, mainly as a result of hypodipsia and chronic disability, in that they often do not have access to free water.

- Hypernatremia can be severely symptomatic or asymptomatic. Central nervous system signs and symptoms are common.

- Impaired cognitive function observed in elderly patients could be caused by chronic or recurrent hypernatremia.

- Prevention is key for hypernatremia. Availability of and access to free water are the only requirements necessary to prevent hypernatremia.

SUGGESTED READINGS

Ayus JC, Krothapalli RK, Armstrong DL, et al. Symptomatic hyponatremia in rats: effect of treatment on mortality and brain lesions. Am J Physiol 1989;257:F18–F22.

Ayus JC, Arief AI. Pulmonary complications of hyponatremic encephalopathy. Noncardiogenic pulmonary edema and hypercapnic respiratory failure. Chest 1995;107:517–521.

Berl T. Treating hyponatremia: damned if we do and damned if we do not. Kidney Int 1990;37:1006–1018.

Berl T. Treating hyponatremia: what is all the controversy about? Ann Intern Med 1990;113:417–419. [Editorial]

Berl T, Schrier RW. Disorders of water metabolism. In: Schrier RW, ed. Renal and Electrolyte Disorders. 3rd ed. Boston: Little, Brown & Company, 1986.

Black RM. Diagnosis and management of hyponatremia. J Intensive Care Med 1989;4:205–220.

Culpepper RM, Clemente BD, Pence SR. Hypertonic saline: patterns of and guidelines for use. South Med J 1994;87:1203–1207.

Feig PU. Hypernatremia and hypertonic syndromes. Med Clin North Am 1981;65:271–290.

Harris CP, Townsend JJ, Baringer JR. Symptomatic hyponatremia: can myelinolysis be prevented by treatment? J Neurol Neurosurg Psychiatry 1993;56:626–632.

Helwig FC, Schutz CB, Curry DE. Water intoxication. Report of a fatal human case, with clinical, pathologic, and experimental studies. JAMA 1935;104:1569–1575.

Helwig FC, Schutz CB, Khun FP. Water intoxication. JAMA 1938;110:644–645.

Karp BI, Laureno R. Pontine and extrapontine myelinolysis: a neurologic disorder following rapid correction of hyponatremia. Medicine 1993;72:359–373.

Kroll M, Juhler M, Lindholm J. Hyponatremia in acute brain disease. J Intern Med 1992;232:291–297.

Lohr JW. Osmotic demyelination syndrome following correction of hyponatremia: association with hypokalemia. Am J Med 1994;96:408–413.

Mandal AK, Saklayen MG, Hillman NM, et al. Predictive factors for high mortality in hypernatremic patients. Am J Emerg Med 1997;15:130–132.

Palevsky PM, Bhograth R, Greenberg A. Hypernatremia in hospitalized patients. Ann Intern Med 1996;124:197–203.

Panayiotou H, Small SC, Hunter JH, et al. Sweet taste (dysgensia). The first symptom of hyponatremia in small cell carcinoma of the lung. Arch Intern Med 1995;155:1325–1328.

Raskind M, Barnes RF. Water metabolism in psychiatric disorders. Semin Nephrol 1984;4:316-324.

Shutty MS Jr, Briscoe L, Sautter S, et al. Neuropsychological manifestations of hyponatremia in chronic schizophrenic patients with the syndrome of psychosis, intermittent hyponatremia, and polydipsia (PIP). Schizophr Res 1993;10:125–130.

Siegler EL, Tamres D, Berlin JA, et al. Risk factors for development of hyponatremia in psychiatric inpatients. Arch Intern Med 1995;155:953–957.

Snyder NA, Feigel DW, Arief AL. Hypernatremia in elderly patients: a multifactorial, heterogeneous and iatrogenic entity. Ann Intern Med 1987;107:309–319.

Sterns RH, Thomas DJ, Herndon RM. Brain dehydration and neurologic deterioration after rapid correction of hyponatremia. Kidney Int 1989;35:69–75.

Williams AV. Hyponatremia: manifestations and treatment (review). J South Carolina Med Assoc 1992;88:285–290.

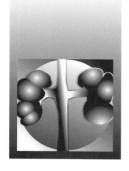

CHAPTER 6

Hypokalemia and Hyperkalemia

Michael E. Falkenhain
Amir Alamir

BACKGROUND

Potassium is the principal intracellular cation, with only 2% of total body potassium being found in the extracellular space. Despite serum potassium concentration not indicating total body stores, its measurement is useful because the amount of potassium in the extracellular space is critical for proper cellular depolarization. Normal serum potassium is 3.6 to 5.3 mEq per liter. Disturbances in serum potassium, both low (hypokalemia) or high (hyperkalemia), can therefore be life-threatening. Concentration of serum potassium is part of most chemistry profiles, and thus abnormal-

ities are often discovered in time to prevent adverse events. A disturbance in serum potassium is not a diagnosis in and of itself but a finding that requires further investigation.

The normal daily intake of potassium is 60 to 80 mEq per day (2340 to 3120 mg/day). In a steady state, urine voiding eliminates approximately 80 to 90% of potassium intake, 10 to 15% is excreted via the stool, and the remainder is lost through perspiration. The potassium content of various foods is listed in Table 6.1. Maintenance of potassium homeostasis involves two main steps:

TABLE 6.1	Potassium Content of Various Foods

High: Avoid completely when following a low potassium diet

Apricots	Nectarines
Artichokes	Nuts
Avocado	Plantain
Butter beans	Potatoes (baked, french fries, chips)
Cantaloupe	Sweet potato
Chocolate candy	Tangelos
Dried peas, beans, lentils	Tomato paste
Honeydew melon	Winter squash
Molasses	Yams

Moderately High: Limit to $1/2$–1 serving per day when following a low potassium diet

Asparagus	Orange, orange juice
Banana	Peach, fresh
Beets	Pear, fresh
Blackberries	Potato, leached
Boysenberries	Plum
Brussels sprouts	Prune juice
Carrots, raw	Pumpkin
Cherries	Raspberries
Collard greens	Spinach
Corn	Strawberries
Dried fruit (figs, prunes, raisins)	Tomato juice
Grapefruit	Turnips
Kiwi fruit	Watermelon
Mixed vegetables	Zucchini
Mushrooms	

1. Extrarenal handling of potassium
2. Renal handling of potassium

Extrarenal Handling of Potassium

Ingested potassium is driven into the cells by insulin. The alkaline tide that occurs with eating also shifts potassium into cells. Likewise, catecholamines play a role: stimulation of the α-receptor causes a nonsustained release of potassium from cells, while stimulation of the β-receptor causes cellular uptake. The net result of an epinephrine surge is an increase in potassium uptake by cells. An imbalance in any of the three main processors of potassium—insulin, catecholamine, acid-base—affects serum potassium concentration. A large potassium load, such as four glasses of orange juice (40 mEq of potassium), without normal extrarenal handling would nearly double the amount of potassium in the extracellular space. Life-threatening hyperkalemia may result before renal excretion. With normal extrarenal functioning, this is unlikely to occur because the potassium load is "shifted" into the intracellular space.

Rapid changes in serum osmolality may also influence potassium homeostasis. Infusion of an osmotically active substance will result in mild increases in serum potassium. This increase becomes clinically important in the patient with renal impairment who has a mildly elevated serum potassium and then receives ionic contrast. The contrast results in movement of water and ionic solvents out of cells, leading to the increase in serum potassium concentration.

Patients with end-stage renal disease (ESRD) often have an impairment in the extrarenal handling of potassium. Cellular uptake varies in response to both catecholamine and bicarbonate infusion in patients with ESRD. Sensitivity to insulin remains intact. Impaired extrarenal handling of potassium contributes to the hyperkalemia often seen with ESRD.

Renal Handling of Potassium

After a potassium load is shifted into cells, the kidney becomes the major organ effecting its excretion. The kidney has the ability to either conserve potassium or excrete it. Secretion occurs in the distal nephron in response to aldosterone. In the presence of aldosterone, flow rates to the distal tubule effect potassium excretion. Aldosterone and the flow rate in the distal tubule work together to effect potassium homeostasis. For example, a patient who is in steady state on a high salt diet will not become hypokalemic, even though flow rates to the distal tubule are high, because aldosterone activity is minimal. The patient who is dehydrated will not necessarily become hyperkalemic, even though distal flow rates are minimal, because aldosterone is stimulated to maintain electrolyte and water balance.

The amount of potassium in a 24-hour urine collection indicates the kidneys' response to disturbances in serum potassium. Urine potassium less than 30 mEq in 24 hours (Table 6.2) constitutes low urine potassium. On a normal potassium diet, a low urinary potassium of less than 30 mEq would reflect renal potassium conservation, whereas a high urine potassium of more than 40 mEq would reflect renal potassium excretion. A spot urine potassium or fractional excretion of potassium is not as useful as a 24-hour collection.

HYPOKALEMIA

Causes

When confronted with a low serum potassium, the clinician is faced with two principal questions:

1. What is the etiology of the low serum potassium?
2. How do you return the serum potassium to normal?

Because treatment is influenced by diagnosis, it is essential to investigate the etiology of hypokalemia.

Often this requires no additional testing. For example, if a patient has a normal serum potassium concentration and is then initiated on a diuretic that results in hypokalemia, potassium replacement therapy is sufficient to normalize levels. Obtain a 24-hour urine measurement for potassium excretion if the hypokalemia preceded diuretic therapy, if the cause is not readily obvious, or if serum potassium concentration remains low following corrective measures. The 24-hour urine potassium measurement distinguishes hypokalemic patients who are inappropriately losing potassium through the urine from those in whom the kidney is appropriately saving potassium (Fig. 6.1).

Diet

Because potassium is found in most diets and the kidney is very efficient in conserving potassium, dietary factors alone are unlikely to result in hypokalemia.

Transcellular Shifts

Transcellular shifts in potassium are a common cause of hyperkalemia but must also be considered in assessing hypokalemia, especially in an intensive care setting where the patient is likely to be receiving intravenous catecholamines or intravenous insulin. Respiratory alkalosis is less likely to cause hypokalemia than the same degree of metabolic alkalosis. A rare form of transcellular shift is autosomal dominant hypokalemic periodic paralysis, in which patients experience a sudden shift of potassium into cells, resulting in flaccid paralysis. These attacks are likely to occur after a carbohydrate meal or in response to an epinephrine surge.

Etiologies of Hypokalemia in Patients With an Appropriately Low 24-Hour Urine Potassium   **TABLE 6.2**

Decreased intake
   Low potassium diet
   Geophagia
Shifts
   Excess insulin (e.g., insulin-secreting tumor, kidney–pancreas transplant, exogenous insulin)
   Excess catecholamines (e.g., stress, pheochromocytoma, exogenous administration)
   Alkalosis
   Hypokalemic periodic paralysis
      Autosomal dominant
      Acquired (e.g., patients of Asian descent who develop thyrotoxicosis)
Nonrenal loss
   Diarrhea
   Massive sweating in well-conditioned athletes

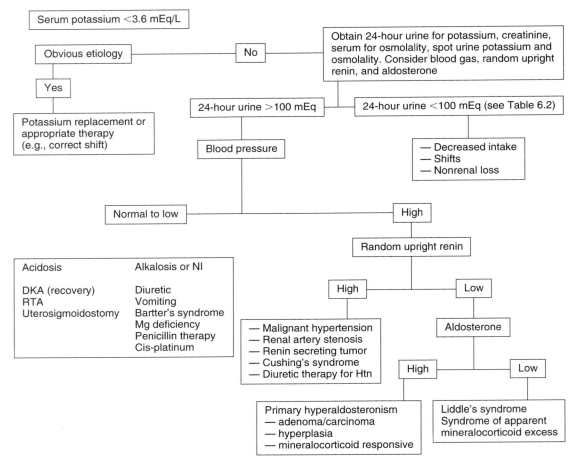

FIGURE 6.1.
General diagnostic scheme for approaching the patient with *hypokalemia*. *NI,* normal intake; *DKA,* diabetic ketoacidosis; *RTA,* renal tubular acidosis; *Htn,* hypertension.

Diarrhea

Diarrhea is the most common form of extrarenal potassium loss. Diarrheal stool contains approximately 10 to 40 mEq/L of potassium; thus, patients with large stool volumes from either osmotic or secretory diarrhea may develop hypokalemia. Dehydration that accompanies diarrhea will stimulate aldosterone but because flow rates in the distal tubule are low, concomitant renal loss of potassium usually does not contribute to the hypokalemia. In addition to hypokalemia, patients with diarrhea also have a non-anion gap metabolic acidosis secondary to bicarbonate losses. Distinguishing these patients from those with renal tubular acidosis (RTA) can usually be done with the history or with the urinary anion gap.

Renal Loss of Potassium

Urine potassium greater than 100 mEq in a 24-hour period constitutes high urine potassium. Renal loss of potassium is the most common cause of hypokalemia. Proper assessment of a hypokalemic patient with inappropriately high urine potassium should include measuring the patient's volume status as reflected by his or her blood pressure (Fig. 6.1). Renal loss of potassium may be caused by diuretic therapy, vomiting, the rare disorder known as Bartter's syndrome, or RTA.

Diuretic therapy   Both loop and thiazide diuretics promote urinary potassium loss by increasing flow rates to the distal nephron in the face of normal levels of aldosterone. A patient on a loop or thiazide diuretic who develops increased aldosterone levels (either primary or secondary) will become markedly hypokalemic. One-third (33%) of patients taking thiazides on a regular basis develop hypokalemia, compared with only 5% of patients on loop diuretics. This difference is accounted for by the shorter half-life of the loop diuretics. Hypokalemia associated with thiazides is dose-dependent, with a threshold between 25 and 37.5 mg/day. Mild baseline hypokalemia in patients on diuretics becomes a problem if the patient has a stress that lowers the potassium further. For example, in the patient on a diuretic who has an acute myocardial infarction, catecholamine release further decreases serum potassium, and in the presence of ischemia, the hypokalemia increases the risk of malignant arrhythmia.

Vomiting The potassium concentration of gastric fluid is low (5-10 mEq/L); however, vomiting is often accompanied by renal loss of potassium. The combination of renal loss with alkalosis initially accounts for the hypokalemia that is seen with upper gastrointestinal fluid loss.

Signs and Symptoms

The cardiovascular and neuromuscular systems are most likely to be affected by hypokalemia. ECG changes as a result of hypokalemia include:

- Flattening of the T wave
- Increase in amplitude of the P wave
- Prolongation of the P-R interval
- Prominent U waves

Hypokalemia may induce or enhance digitalis toxicity and increases the likelihood of both atrial and ventricular arrhythmia. In the face of acute myocardial infarction, hypokalemia increases morbidity and mortality.

Lower extremity cramps followed by diffuse muscle weakness and even paralysis may occur with hypokalemia. Rhabdomyolysis is a rare complication of severe hypokalemia; renal tubulointerstitial infiltration results in reduced ability to concentrate urine manifested by polyuria.

Because potassium is necessary for insulin secretion, hypokalemia may blunt insulin release, causing hyperglycemia.

Diagnosis

Bartter's Syndrome

Bartter's syndrome should be considered in the differential diagnosis when the clinician suspects a patient of taking diuretics. The syndrome includes urinary potassium wasting, hypokalemia, low to normal blood pressure, and elevated serum levels of renin and aldosterone indistinguishable from surreptitious diuretic use. Surreptitious diuretic use can be excluded by random urine testing. The presence of diuretics is detected using urine spectrometry followed by assays for specific diuretic agents.

Renal Tubular Acidosis

Both distal (type I) and proximal (type II) RTA can result in hypokalemia. RTA should be considered in any patient with a non-anion gap metabolic acidosis. The differential diagnosis often is between stool loss of bicarbonate versus an inability of the kidneys to appropriately save bicarbonate or to excrete acid. (Saving bicarbonate or excreting acid is the same function, but in discussing RTA, it is conceptually useful to make a distinction between them.)

Calculating urinary anion gap If it is unclear from the history whether acidosis is the result of renal or gastrointestinal causes, calculating a urinary anion gap is helpful. The spot test urinary chloride concentration is subtracted from the sum of the spot test urinary sodium plus spot test urinary potassium.

$$(UNa + UK) - UCl = \text{urinary anion gap}$$

In a state of hyperchloremic metabolic acidosis caused by diarrhea, the urinary anion gap should be negative, with the unaccounted for positive charge being ammonium (NH_4^+). In the presence of RTA, the urinary anion gap will be positive, reflecting the inability to secrete hydrogen ions as evidenced by a decrease in ammonium production.

Proximal RTA, type II An exception to a negative urine anion gap occurs with proximal RTA (type II) in steady state. In type II RTA, the proximal tubule cannot reclaim all the filtered bicarbonate, resulting in transiently alkaline urine and urinary potassium wasting until the serum bicarbonate falls low enough to enable all the filtered bicarbonate to be reclaimed by the distal tubule. When this occurs, the urine pH can fall to less than five and the patient enters a steady state in which the serum bicarbonate is below normal (12-18 mEq/L). The urine anion gap becomes negative at this point. Infusion of bicarbonate will result in marked bicarbonturia (elevated urine pH) before the serum bicarbonate becomes normal.

Distal RTA, type I In type I RTA, the distal tubule cannot properly excrete hydrogen ions. Patients with type I RTA have a urine pH that is greater than 5.5 and often have an extremely low serum bicarbonate concentration. Because of their propensity toward severe metabolic acidosis, these patients develop increased urinary calcium and phosphorous. This is a result of buffering the excess hydrogen via bone with resultant release of calcium and phosphorous into the circulation. Increased urinary calcium and phosphorous coupled with persistently alkaline urine commonly results in stone formation and nephrocalcinosis for patients with distal RTA. Because of hypokalemia and a tendency toward stone formation, patients with distal RTA may benefit from receiving their potassium supplementation in the form of potassium citrate rather than potassium chloride.

Evaluation of a patient with evidence of urinary potassium wasting and an elevated blood pressure should include a random upright renin and aldosterone level. Angiotensin-converting enzyme (ACE) inhibitor therapy will increase serum renin levels, making the interpretation of random renin levels more difficult.

Hyperaldosteronism

Regardless of etiology, most cases of malignant hypertension cause a hyperrenin or hyperaldosterone state. It is on the basis of secondary hyperaldosteronism that renal potassium wasting occurs, leading to mild hypokalemia. Likewise, bilateral renal artery stenosis (RAS) results in elevated aldosterone levels that may lead to mild hypokalemia. A normal serum potassium does not exclude the diagnosis of RAS, a condition discussed in Chapter 12.

The patient with hypokalemia, high urinary potassium, low renin, and increased aldosterone has hyperaldosteronism. The clinician should do an anatomic imaging study (e.g., CT scan) to look for an adenoma or carcinoma of the adrenal gland. If an adenoma greater than 5 cm is found, surgery is recommended to exclude carcinoma. Adrenalectomy is not usually indicated for patients with adrenal hyperplasia. Spironolactone in doses of 200 to 400 mg/day or amiloride 20 to 40 mg/day is the medical therapy of choice. Often, additional antihypertensive medications are necessary.

Uncommon Hypokalemic Disorders

Patients with low renin and low aldosterone have uncommon disorders in which potassium is lost through the urine. Liddle's syndrome, a disorder of the sodium channel in the distal tubule, has been linked to chromosome 16 and is inherited in an autosomal dominant fashion. The syndrome of apparent mineralocorticoid excess can be inherited or acquired through the ingestion of glycyrrhizic acid contained in products such as certain brands of chewing tobacco or licorice. In the state of mineralocorticoid excess, the enzyme that converts cortisol to cortisone (11-β-HSD) is inactivated, allowing normal levels of cortisol to function as a mineralocorticoid excess.

Summary of Diagnosis: Hypokalemia

- Diarrhea is the most common form of extrarenal potassium loss.
- Both loop and thiazide diuretics promote urinary potassium loss. However, one-third of patients taking thiazides chronically develop hypokalemia, compared with only 5% of patients on loop diuretics.
- In evaluating patients with high urinary potassium loss in the absence of diuretic therapy and elevated blood pressure, it is essential to obtain a random upright renin and aldosterone level.
- A combination of hypokalemia, high urinary potassium, low plasma renin activity, and high serum aldosterone levels strongly suggest primary hyperaldosteronism. The next important test is a CT scan of the abdomen to look for adrenal adenoma.

Treatment

When prescribing potassium, the clinician must decide the route—oral versus intravenous—via which to administer the replacement. As a rule, it is safer to administer potassium in oral form, reserving intravenous administration for patients with cardiac arrhythmia, neuromuscular changes, or an inability to take or absorb oral medication.

If given intravenously, a monitor should be employed if the potassium infusion rate exceeds 10 mEq/hour. The infusion rate should not exceed 40 mEq/hour because faster rates may precipitate life-threatening arrhythmia. Potassium infusion can cause phlebitis and therefore is preferably administered through a central vein in concentrations less than 60 mEq/L. Saline solutions are the preferred vehicle for potassium administration because dextrose infusion increases insulin levels, leading to intracellular shift of potassium.

KEY POINTS: HYPOKALEMIA

- Hypokalemia is more common in patients who use thiazide, rather than loop, diuretics. This difference is mainly related to the shorter half-life of the loop diuretics.

- As a rule, oral potassium is the safest form of replacement. Potassium chloride is the preparation of choice.

- On a normal potassium diet, a low urinary potassium (<30 mEq in 24 hours) would indicate renal potassium conservation. A 24-hour urinary potassium in excess of 150 to 200 mEq indicates renal potassium wasting.

- Respiratory alkalosis is less likely to cause hypokalemia than the same degree of metabolic alkalosis.

- Hypokalemia may induce or potentiate digitalis toxicity and increases the propensity to atrial and ventricular arrhythmias.

- In the presence of acute myocardial infarction, hypokalemia increases the risk of serious arrhythmias.

- Hypokalemia is frequently associated with hyperglycemia resulting from blunted insulin release.

- Potassium-sparing diuretics are an acceptable therapeutic option in patients with excessive urinary loss of potassium.

- Magnesium depletion often will cause renal potassium wasting, preventing potassium replacement from being effective. In patients with high risk for magnesium depletion or with refractory hypokalemia, measurement of serum magnesium and replacement of magnesium is advised.

Potassium Preparations **TABLE 6.3**

Preparation	Form	Dose (mEq)
Potassium chloride		
K-Dur Extended Release	Tab	10, 20
K-Tab Extended Release	Tab	10
Klotrix Sustained Release	Tab	10
K-Norm Extended Release	Capsule	10
Klor-con Extended Release	Tab	8, 10
Micro-K Extencaps	Capsule	8, 10
Slow-K Extended Release	Capsule	8
Ten-K Extended Release	Capsule	8
Klorvess 10%	Liquid	20 mEq/15 mL
K-Lor	Powder	15, 20
Kato	Powder	20
K-Lyte/CL	Effervescent tab	25, 50
Potassium citrate		
Polycitra K	Liquid	30 mEq/15 mL
K-Lyte DS	Effervescent tab	50
Urocit-K	Tab	5
Potassium gluconate		
Kolyum	Liquid	20 mEq/15 mL
Kaon	Elixir	20 mEq/15 mL
Potassium phosphate		
Neutra-Phos-K	Powder	14.25 mEq/pkg

When potassium is prescribed orally, the clinician has a choice of anion to accompany the potassium. Table 6.3 lists the various forms of potassium replacement available. When potassium is given with a readily reabsorbable anion such as chloride, it increases the total body potassium to a greater degree than potassium administered with a nonreabsorbable anion, such as citrate found in fruit. Ten mEq of potassium given as KCl is more likely to increase the serum potassium than eating a banana containing 10 mEq of potassium. Potassium citrate is reserved for those patients in whom it is desirable to provide a bicarbonate base and potassium phosphate when phosphate supplementation is needed.

The amount of potassium prescribed depends on the total body deficit. Because potassium deficit is difficult to estimate based on serum potassium concentration, a general guide is that a 1-mEq decrease in serum potassium reflects a greater than 300 mEq decrease in total body potassium. As a general rule, providing 40 to 80 mEq of potassium per day is more than adequate to safely replace potassium stores. In the event renal losses of potassium are extraordinarily high, replacing urinary potassium losses as measured by a 24-hour urine potassium is indicated. Potassium-sparing diuretics are an acceptable therapeutic option for patients with urinary loss of potassium. In the presence of renal insufficiency, potassium replacement should be more conservative (10-20 mEq/dose) and potassium-sparing diuretics should be avoided.

Magnesium depletion often will cause renal potassium wasting, rendering potassium replacement ineffective. In patients with high risk for concomitant magnesium depletion or with refractory hypokalemia, measurement and replacement of serum magnesium is advised.

HYPERKALEMIA

Determining ECG Changes

When confronted with a patient with hyperkalemia (Fig. 6.2), the first question should always be: *Are resultant ECG changes present?* The ECG changes of hyperkalemia are demonstrated in Figure 6.3. If ECG changes are present, the patient should receive intravenous calcium to provide immediate cardiac protection. Calcium therapy does not alter the serum potassium but does stabilize cardiac membranes, allowing time for more definitive therapy and a search for the etiology of the high

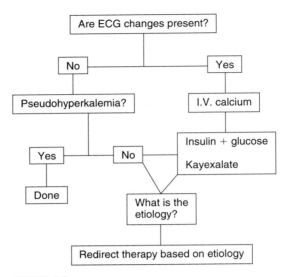

FIGURE 6.2.
General scheme for approaching the patient with *hyperkalemia*.

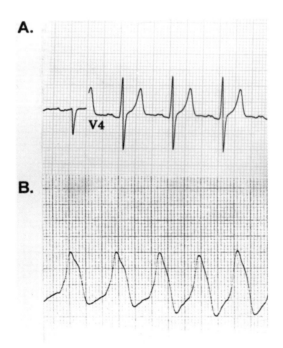

FIGURE 6.3.
A. Patient with *peaked T waves* secondary to hyperkalemia. **B.** Patient with *sine wave* (marked prolongation of QRS complex).

Immediate: does not change the serum potassium, but protects against life-threatening depolarization
    Calcium gluconate: 20 mL of 10% solution
    Calcium chloride: in code situation or if central line available
Intermediate: does not rid the body of excess potassium, but transiently lowers the serum potassium by
    shifting it into cells
    50% glucose (1 amp) + 10 units of IV insulin
    Sodium bicarbonate (1 amp = 44 mEq)
    β agonist (albuterol 10 mg − 20 mg nebulized or 0.5 mg SQ or IV)
Long-term: rids the body of excess potassium
    Diuretics
    Ion-exchange resin (Kayexalate)
        Oral
        Retention enema
    Dialysis (hemodialysis > peritoneal dialysis)

SQ, subcutaneous.

serum potassium. Even if it appears that the hyperkalemia is not real (pseudohyperkalemia) (e.g., hemolysis, severe leukocytosis, or thrombocytosis can resemble hyperkalemia), an ECG should be obtained and, if indicated, appropriate therapy initiated (Table 6.4). For example, if the serum potassium is reported as 7 mEq/L and grossly hemolyzed, the actual serum potassium may still be high, necessitating immediate intervention.

Pseudohyperkalemia

Pseudohyperkalemia is an artificially elevated potassium concentration resulting from potassium leakage from the cells during blood drawing or after blood collection. Hemolysis that occurs during a traumatic blood draw is the most common cause of pseudohyperkalemia. A prolonged, tight tourniquet and repeated fist clenching may also result in an artificially elevated potassium concentration. If the leukocyte count is greater than 100,000 or the platelet count is greater than 1,000,000, an abnormally high amount of potassium will leak out of these cells during coagulation, artificially raising the serum potassium. With good blood drawing technique and analysis of blood before clotting (plasma potassium as opposed to serum potassium), a true measure of extracellular potassium can be obtained. A normal plasma potassium concentration and an elevated serum potassium level along with an absence of ECG changes confirms the diagnosis of pseudohyperkalemia.

Hyperkalemia as a Result of Shifts   TABLE 6.5

Lack of insulin
    Diabetic ketoacidosis
    Fasting in a patient with ESRD
Interference with catecholamines
    Nonspecific β-blocker therapy
    ESRD
Acidosis
    Inorganic metabolic acidosis
    Respiratory acidosis
Rapid increase in serum osmolality
    Infusion of mannitol
    Infusion of ionic contrast
    Uncontrolled diabetic state with severe
        hyperglycemia
Loss of cell integrity
    Tumor lysis syndrome
    Compartment syndrome
    Tissue ischemia

ESRD, end-stage renal disease.

Causes

Hyperkalemia Secondary to Shifts

Shift of potassium out of cells commonly contributes to hyperkalemia (Table 6.5). Shift alone will not result in persistent hyperkalemia, unless the shift is concomitant with renal under excretion.

Lack of Insulin

Shifts may result from a lack of insulin. Insulin promotes cellular potassium uptake independent of its effect on glucose. Baseline levels of insulin are important in maintaining potassium homeostasis. An absolute decrease in insulin as occurs in type I diabetics or in a fasting patient with ESRD may provoke hyperkalemia. The latter condition is complex, involving not only a fasting-induced decrease in baseline insulin levels but also an insensitivity to catecholamine-driven potassium uptake by cells.

Inorganic metabolic acidosis   Inorganic metabolic acidosis also results in shift of potassium out of cells. Organic acidosis, such as that seen with lactic acidosis or diabetic ketoacidosis, is less likely to cause shifts of potassium on the basis of acidosis alone. A lack of insulin in diabetic ketoacidosis and the release of potassium from ischemic cells in lactic acidosis contribute to the hyperkalemia more than the acidosis per se.

The absence of aldosterone or interference with its activity invariably leads to hyperkalemic metabolic acidosis (Table 6.6). Along with electrolyte abnormalities, volume depletion with resultant hypotension may be present.

TABLE 6.6	Hyperkalemia Secondary to Limited Renal Excretion

Diminished aldosterone activity
    ACE inhibitor
    Heparin
    Primary hypoaldosteronism
    Type IV RTA
    Spironolactone
    NSAIDs
    Triamterene
    Amiloride
    Trimethoprim
Diminished glomerular filtration rate (GFR)
    GFR < 25 mL/min (for any reason)
Diminished flow rates[a]
    Dehydration
    Third-spacing of fluid
    Poor systolic function

[a]Anything that limits effective circulating volume may limit flow rates to the distal tubule. When this occurs in conjunction with diminished aldosterone activity or diminished GFR, hyperkalemia may occur.
RTA, renal tubular acidosis; NSAIDs, nonsteroidal anti-inflammatory drugs.

Tissue ischemia   Tissue ischemia that results in cell death will release intracellular potassium (140 mEq/L) and, combined with renal underexcretion, can result in marked hyperkalemia. The more common clinical examples include tumor lysis, compartment syndrome, and overwhelming shock with global decrease in tissue perfusion.

Muscle relaxants   Depolarizing muscle relaxants such as succinylcholine can result in hyperkalemia by promoting shift of potassium out of cells. Patients with neuromuscular diseases are especially sensitive to the hyperkalemic effects of succinylcholine. Severe digitalis toxicity, by interfering with the Na/K adenosine triphosphatase (ATPase) pump, may lead to severe hyperkalemia. At therapeutic levels, digoxin has little effect on the extrarenal handling of potassium. Rarely, nonselective β-blocker therapy can cause hyperkalemia by interfering with catecholamine-mediated cell uptake of potassium.

Hereditary hyperkalemia   Hereditary hyperkalemia periodic paralysis is a rare cause of hyperkalemia as a result of potassium shift out of cells. It is inherited in an autosomal-dominant pattern. High potassium diets do not result in hyperkalemia unless the extrarenal or renal handling of potassium is impaired.

RTA, Type IV

Type IV RTA results from primary nonproduction of renin, leading to both a hyporenin and hypoaldosterone state. It is most commonly seen in diabetics with renal impairment in whom metabolic acidosis and hyperkalemia are out of proportion to the loss of glomerular filtration rate (GFR). Type IV RTA may be seen with any chronic tubulointerstitial nephropathy or as a result of renal transplant, nonsteroidal anti-inflammatory agents (NSAIDs), or cyclosporine therapy.

ACE Inhibitors

ACE inhibitors can result in hyperkalemia in patients with impaired renal function. The mechanism of the hyperkalemia with ACE inhibitors involves a decrease in aldosterone production as a result of decreased angiotensin II levels.

Because this class of drugs benefits patients with impaired GFR, the risk of hyperkalemia should not be viewed as prohibitive but as requiring close monitoring of the serum potassium. The angiotensin II receptor-blocking agents may be less likely than ACE inhibitors to promote hyperkalemia; however, there is not enough data on this new class of drugs in the setting of renal impairment to make a firm recommendation for their use over ACE inhibitors.

Heparin Therapy

Prolonged heparin therapy has been reported to interfere with aldosterone release, resulting in hyperkalemia. Spironolactone limits potassium excretion by preventing aldosterone from binding to the mineralocorticoid receptor.

Decreased Number of Functioning Nephrons

In a steady state, a normal dietary intake of 60 mEq of potassium is shifted into cells (extrarenal potassium handling). Eighty percent of the potassium eventually is excreted in the urine, with 10 to 15% excreted in stool, and the remainder in perspiration. The normal kidney has the capacity to excrete in excess of 400 mEq of potassium per day; thus, it is unlikely an individual will become chronically hyperkalemic without some degree of renal impairment. The kidneys' ability to maintain homeostasis on a normal potassium diet is preserved until GFR is markedly diminished (Cr greater than 3 mg/dL). Once a critical number of nephrons have been lost, the remaining nephrons cannot excrete a normal potassium load. To prevent hyperkalemia at this point, dietary potassium must be restricted (<60 mEq/day).

Decreased Distal Flow

Renal underperfusion alone will not result in hyperkalemia unless the underperfusion leads to a marked reduction in GFR or is accompanied by insufficient aldosterone. If a patient with mild renal impairment on an ACE inhibitor becomes dehydrated, the decreased flow rates in the distal tubule may be enough to result in hyperkalemia. Likewise, if the renally impaired patient becomes volume depleted, hyperkalemia may ensue. Potassium-sparing diuretics such as amiloride and triamterene do not limit distal flow but instead prevent potassium excretion by their action on the ATPase. High-dose trimethoprim can also cause hyperkalemia because, like triamterene and amiloride, it is a cation that interferes with the sodium channel in the distal nephron.

Signs and Symptoms

Hyperkalemia is a life-threatening condition because of its potential to precipitate asystole or ventricular fibrillation. ECG changes (Fig. 6.3) are the principal sign by which the clinician guides therapy (Fig. 6.2). No direct correlation exists between the level of serum potassium and the ECG changes present, but, in general, sine wave will not result unless the serum potassium exceeds 7 mEq/L. Hyperkalemia may also result in marked muscle weakness.

Diagnosis

In assessing true hyperkalemia, it is useful to determine whether the potassium is elevated as a result of a potassium shift or renal underexcretion. This determination can often be made by completing a history and routine laboratory data. A 24-hour urine potassium may be helpful if some question remains.

Summary of Diagnosis: Hyperkalemia

- Extrarenal handling of potassium is important with a large potassium load. Without normal extrarenal handling, potassium load may result in life-threatening hyperkalemia before renal excretion.
- Patients with ESRD often have impairment in the extrarenal handling of potassium.
- In cases of hyperkalemia, pseudohyperkalemia must be ruled out. In general, if hyperkalemia is the only isolated finding, in all probability it is pseudohyperkalemia. In case of doubt, an electrocardiogram may be helpful.
- In assessing true hyperkalemia, determine whether the potassium is elevated as a result of a potassium shift or because of renal underexcretion.
- Diabetic nephropathy with chronic renal failure (CRF) and treatment with ACE inhibitors are probably the most common causes of hyperkalemia in primary care.
- In patients with CRF with persistent hyperkalemia, it is safe to prescribe Kayexalate (Winthrop, New York, New York) in sorbitol on a long-term basis.

Treatment

Short-term Therapy

Calcium therapy (Table 6.4) provides immediate cardiac protection for 30 minutes after administration. Calcium does not alter serum potassium concentration but permits time to initiate definitive therapy. Calcium gluconate is preferred if a peripheral vein is used for administration because extravasation of calcium chloride is toxic to the dermal tissue. For a patient in cardiac arrest, treatment with calcium chloride is preferred because of a slight delay in the action of calcium gluconate. Liver perfusion is essential for conversion of calcium gluconate to an active form of calcium to counteract potassium at the cellular level.

Intermediate Therapy

Insulin and glucose therapy   The cornerstone of intermediate therapy is insulin and glucose. Insulin (10 units intravenous) given with one amp of 50% dextrose solution to prevent hypoglycemia shifts potassium into cells, lowering the serum potassium within one hour (Fig. 6.4). The authors do not recommend giving glucose without insulin because the glucose may transiently increase serum osmolality, resulting in an elevation in serum potassium.

Sodium bicarbonate therapy   Sodium bicarbonate therapy shifts potassium into cells but not as effectively as insulin and glucose, especially in patients with renal failure. Likewise, adrenergic agonist (albuterol or albuterol sulfate 10-20 mg by nebulizer or 0.5 mg intravenous) may shift potassium into cells. Figure 6.4 shows that the use of albuterol is additive to that of insulin plus glucose because they effect potassium shifts by metabolically independent mechanisms.

Cation exchange resins   Cation exchange resins exchange potassium for sodium in the colon, ridding the body of potassium through the gastrointestinal tract. The resultant increase in sodium may expand the intravascular volume and precipitate pulmonary edema. Thus, these agents should be used with caution in the hyperkalemic patient with expanded vascular volume and renal insufficiency.

Kayexalate is the primary cation exchange resin in clinical use that can be given orally or as a retention

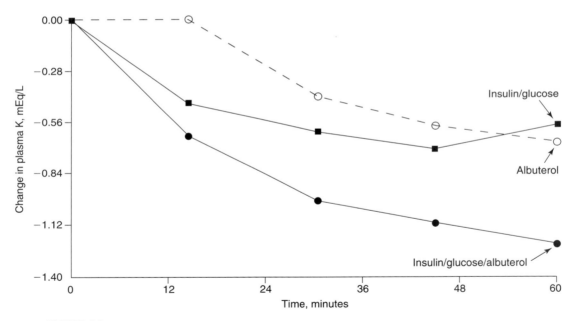

FIGURE 6.4.

A patient with ESRD response to potassium-lowering measures. (■), insulin + glucose; (○), albuterol; (●), insulin + glucose + albuterol. (Adapted with permission from Allon M, Copkney C. Albuterol and insulin for treatment of hyperkalemia in hemodialysis patients. Kidney Int 1990;38:869–872.)

KEY POINTS: HYPERKALEMIA

- The kidney has the ability to either conserve potassium or excrete it.

- Aldosterone and the flow rate in the distal tubule work together to effect potassium homeostasis.

- A normal plasma potassium (whole blood) in the presence of elevated serum potassium concentrations confirms the diagnosis of pseudohyperkalemia.

- Review of medications taken by patients with hyperkalemia is critical, particularly those patients with renal insufficiency.

- In all patients with hyperkalemia, the possibilities of adrenal insufficiency and selective hypoaldosteronism should be considered. Based on other clinical findings, a decision should be made whether to obtain plasma cortisol, renin, and aldosterone levels, respectively.

enema. Oral doses are administered in quantities of 30 to 60 g in a sorbitol-based solution. The sorbitol promotes rapid gastric transfer and prevents constipation. When orally administered, the onset of action is 1 to 2 hours. The response is quicker if the Kayaxelate is given as a retention enema in a dose of 60 to 120 g. A higher dose in enema form is recommended because it is not as efficacious as the oral form. It should be retained in the rectum for 30 to 60 minutes.

Diuretics and hemodialysis Diuretics will cause renal potassium wasting but are somewhat limited in use in the patient with advanced renal insufficiency. Hemodialysis corrects hyperkalemia rapidly if the aforementioned treatments fail.

COMMONLY ASKED QUESTIONS

Can I eat a banana instead of taking a potassium pill?
A high potassium diet (Table 6.1) may diminish the need for potassium replacement, but often pharmacologic therapy is needed because of the day-to-day variability in dietary potassium. Also, potassium in the form of potassium chloride is more likely to increase the total potassium pool, compared with the potassium found in organic anions, as in fruit. Salt substitute in the form of potassium chloride can be used on a daily basis as a replacement for KCl tablets or capsules.

As part of my low salt diet I have been told to use potassium chloride as a salt substitute. Is this okay?
Most salt substitutes are KCl, containing 33 to 55 mEq of potassium per tablespoon. Using a salt substitute is advisable if the patient has normal renal function or if potassium replacement therapy is needed. They cannot be used if the patient has oliguric renal failure.

What can I do to keep my potassium from being elevated?
See a nutritionist to initiate a low potassium diet. Avoid hidden sources of potassium such as salt substitute (KCl). Avoid NSAIDs that have the potential for diminishing GFR and interfering with potassium excretion. Avoid dehydration. If vascular volume status and blood pressure are not elevated, restricting water and sodium are not necessary even if renal insufficiency is present.

Do I need to start dialysis because of my elevated potassium?
It is rare that hyperkalemia is the sole indication for initiation of dialysis. If there is an increased volume status that is unresponsive to diuretics, hyperkalemia must be corrected with dialysis.

My potassium has gone up since I started an ACE inhibitor, but I have been told ACE inhibitors may delay my need for dialysis. Can I still take the ACE inhibitor?
The benefit of ACE inhibitors in slowing the progression of renal disease is well documented in type I diabetics. The potential for causing hyperkalemia increases as GFR is diminished. If one becomes hyperkalemic and there is no other obvious cause, the risk of the increased potassium would outweigh any potential benefit and the agent must be discontinued. There is hope that the angiotensin II receptor-blocking agents would be useful in this setting, although there is not enough data to make a firm recommendation.

SUGGESTED READINGS

Allon M. Treatment and prevention of hyperkalemia in end-stage renal disease. Kidney Int 1993;43:1197–1209.

Brown RS. Extrarenal potassium homeostasis. Kidney Int 1986;30:116–127.

Rose BD. Clinical Physiology of Acid-Base and Electrolyte Disorders. 4th ed. New York: McGraw-Hill, 1994.

7
CHAPTER

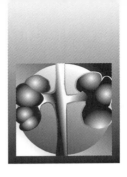

Hypomagnesemia and Hypermagnesemia

Anil K. Mandal
Abdulla Khan
Sucharita Nalagatla

BACKGROUND

Properties and Role of Magnesium

Magnesium (Mg) is the fourth most abundant cation in the human body and second only to potassium (K) as the major intracellular cation. Magnesium is bound mainly in bone and muscle tissue. It is found in various foods, but its richest stores are found in liver, nuts, leafy green vegetables, legumes, and whole grains. The normal serum concentration of magnesium is 1.7 to 2.2 mg/dL and is present in two forms: diffusible and protein-bound. The diffusible form constitutes 75% of the total amount; this fraction is filtered at the glomerulus and reabsorbed by the tubules. The reabsorption of magnesium differs from that of sodium and calcium. Approximately 20 to 30% of filtered magnesium is reabsorbed in the proximal tubule, compared with 50 to 70% of filtered sodium or calcium. The major portion of filtered magnesium (60–70%) is reabsorbed in the ascending thick limb of the loop of Henle. The absorptive rate of magnesium, as for other cations, is highly load dependent; that is, absolute magnesium absorption

94

increases with enhanced delivery to the ascending thick limb of Henle's loop. Delivery could be enhanced by either an increase in tubule fluid magnesium concentration or an increase in tubule fluid flow rate.

Besides tubule fluid magnesium concentration, a number of factors control renal magnesium absorption, urinary magnesium excretion, and serum magnesium levels. The factors are presented in Table 7.1. The main factors altering magnesium reabsorption in Henle's loop include parathyroid hormone, changes in serum magnesium, and calcium concentrations and the loop-acting diuretics. Clinically, osmotic diuresis, as in diabetes mellitus, diuretics, alcoholism, and chronic mineralocorticoid excess, is significant for hypomagnesemia. Serum magnesium in and of itself is also an important factor determining tubular reabsorption and urinary excretion of magnesium. Thus, hypermagnesemia is associated with diminished magnesium reabsorption and increased urinary excretion of magnesium. Certain drugs, including gentamicin, cisplatin, and cyclosporine, inhibit magnesium reabsorption in the loop and cause magnesium wasting.

HYPOMAGNESEMIA

Causes

Hypomagnesemia, defined as serum magnesium level less than 1.7 mg/dL, can develop in many acute and chronic conditions. Numerous drugs have been known to cause hypomagnesemia. These are listed in Table 7.2.

Low serum magnesium concentration is found in many clinical conditions, such as diabetes mellitus, hypertension, congestive heart failure (CHF), esophageal cancer, or chronic diarrheal disorders. In each of these conditions, hypomagnesemia is most likely the result of increased urinary excretion of magnesium caused by either spontaneous osmotic diuresis (as in untreated diabetes mellitus) or diuretic use (as in hypertension or CHF), by poor intake as in esophageal cancer, or by excessive intestinal loss.

Relationship of Hypomagnesemia to Diabetes Mellitus

Several studies have proposed an intricate relationship between hypomagnesemia and diabetes mellitus. The exact mechanism(s) of hypomagnesemia in diabetes is not yet clear but is most likely the result of increased urinary magnesium losses secondary to chronic glucosuria. The finding that short-term improvement in glycemic control does not increase the serum magnesium level to normal tends to refute a direct relationship

Factors Affecting Tubular Reabsorption of Magnesium	TABLE 7.1

Decrease tubular reabsorption, increase urinary excretion of magnesium
  Volume expansion
  Osmotic diuresis
  Diuretics
  Cardiac glycosides
  Alcohol ingestion
  High sodium intake
  High calcium intake
  Hormones: growth, thyroid, calcitonin, chronic mineralocorticoid therapy
  Drugs: gentamicin, cisplatin, cyclosporine

Enhance tubular reabsorption, decrease urinary excretion of magnesium
  Parathyroid hormone

between glucosuria and hypomagnesemia. However, hypomagnesemia accompanies many diabetic complications. For instance, acute hypomagnesemia may develop in diabetic ketoacidosis. Serum magnesium concentration may parallel changes in serum potassium concentration. Thus, after fluid and insulin therapy, magnesium levels may fall acutely, similar to serum potassium levels. A greater risk of severe diabetic retinopathy can be predicted when magnesium levels are lower than normal.

Relationship of Hypomagnesemia to Cardiovascular Disorders

Hypomagnesemia has been linked to multiple cardiovascular complications, including arrhythmia, hypertension, and decreased platelet activity. Magnesium facilitates cellular ion handling and maintains the cellular pumps necessary for peripheral vascular tone (Na-K-ATPase and calcium-activated potassium channels). Magnesium deficiency causes inhibition of NA-K pump activity. Numerous published reports imply hypomagnesemia in fatal and nonfatal cardiac arrhythmias. In all reports, however, a combination of hypokalemia and hypomagnesemia was considered the underlying etiology for these arrhythmias. From these reports it is difficult to ascertain whether hypomagnesemia itself gives rise to electrical abnormalities in the heart or whether it does so by merely potentiating the adverse effects of hypokalemia. Nonetheless, it is important to recall the implications of hypomagnesemia when treating patients with CHF, hypertension, and

TABLE 7.2   Causes of Hypomagnesemia

Physiologic
   Athletics
   Pregnancy and other hypermetabolic states
   Cold acclimatization

Nutritional
   Starvation
   Dietary deficiency
   Total parenteral nutrition
   Refeeding syndrome

Gastrointestinal tract losses
   Chronic diarrhea
   Malabsorption syndromes
   Laxative abuse
   Pancreatitis
   Specific magnesium malabsorption
   Prolonged nasogastric suctioning

Renal excretion
   Acute renal failure
   Renal tubular acidosis
   Postobstructive diuresis
   Primary renal tubular magnesium wasting
   Hypertension
   Drug-induced
      acetazolamide
      alcohol
      aminoglycosides
      amphotericin B
      capreomycin
      carbenicillin
      chlorthalidone
      cisplatin
      cyclosporine
      digoxin
      ethacrynic acid
      Furosemide

      mannitol
      methotrexate
      pentamidine
      theophylline
      thiazides

Nutritional deficiencies
   Malnutrition
   Magnesium-free parenteral feedings
   Esophageal cancer
   Long-term alcohol abuse

Endocrine disorders
   Hyperaldosteronism
   Hyperparathyroidism
   Hyperthyroidism
   Diabetes mellitus
   Ketoacidosis
      diabetic
      alcoholic
      vitamin D deficiency
   Hypoparathyroidism
   Syndrome of inappropriate secretion of
      antidiuretic hormone
   Bartter's syndrome
   Gitelman's syndrome
   Redistribution
   Insulin treatment for diabetic ketoacidosis
   High catecholamine states
   Major trauma or stress
   Hungry bone syndrome
   Multiple mechanisms
   Chronic alcoholism
   Alcohol withdrawal
   Major burns
   Liquid protein diet
   Congestive heart failure

Adapted from Tosiello L. Hypomagnesemia and diabetes mellitus. Arch Intern Med 1996;156:1143–1148, with permission, copyright 1996, American Medical Association.

other disorders in whom diuretics are used as therapy and in acutely ill and elderly patients in whom fluid and electrolyte disorders are common. The relationship of hypomagnesemia to cardiac arrhythmias, especially in association with acute myocardial infarction, must be emphasized because of the seriousness of these complications in the setting of myocardial infarction.

Both magnesium and potassium deficiencies are associated with increased ventricular ectopy, and magnesium and potassium repletion effectively decreases the frequency of ventricular ectopic beats. Both potassium and magnesium deficiencies occur during diuretic therapy and are particularly more prone to cause serious cardiac complications, such as arrhythmias in elderly persons. A magnesium deficit may coexist with hypokalemia in the absence of hypomagnesemia. Therefore, treatment in hypokalemic patients must take into account magnesium repletion even in the absence of overt hypomagnesemia.

Magnesium depletion is highly probable in patients with severe CHF and in those requiring hospitalization, aggressive diuretic therapy, or hemofiltration, along with having persistent hypokalemia. Digitalis toxicity, angina, and acute myocardial infarction add to a patient's susceptibility to the adverse effects of magnesium deficiency.

Arrhythmias

A close correlation between lymphocyte potassium and lymphocyte magnesium concentrations with the incidence of acute, potentially lethal arrhythmias in patients with acute myocardial infarction has been reported. High lymphocyte potassium concentrations were associated with a high incidence of fatal arrhythmias, whereas high lymphocyte magnesium concentrations were associated with a protective effect. Increasing the serum and lymphocyte magnesium concentrations in patients with acute myocardial infarction by a single intravenous dose of magnesium causes not only an absolute decrease in the incidence of serious arrhythmias but also the postponement by a few hours of arrhythmias that do occur. Several studies show that supplementation of magnesium may reduce the incidence of fatal and nonfatal arrhythmias after acute myocardial infarction.

Anesthesia and Magnesium Levels

Total or ionized magnesium levels can be low in patients after induction of anesthesia. Patients who receive diuretics preoperatively are more likely to develop hypomagnesemia after the induction of anesthesia than are patients with preexisting hypomagnesemia who are not on diuretics. Patients who were receiving digoxin preoperatively had significantly lower serum magnesium levels than did patients not taking digoxin. Cardiac arrhythmias (supraventricular or ventricular) are the most common postoperative complications. Multivariate analysis shows that patients treated with placebo had a significantly greater frequency of postoperative ventricular arrhythmias than did patients treated with magnesium. Thus, magnesium therapy is effective in reducing the frequency of clinically significant postoperative ventricular arrhythmias and in increasing cardiac index in the early postoperative period.

Evidence for the role of magnesium salts in decreasing the frequency of ischemia-induced cardiac arrhythmias originates from placebo-controlled trials of magnesium therapy in patients with acute myocardial infarction. Magnesium or placebo was administered to 130 patients with documented acute myocardial infarction. In the magnesium-treated group, the incidence of cardiac arrhythmias was 21%, compared with 42% in the placebo-treated group. The difference was highly significant. Mortality rates in the first 4 weeks after treatment were significantly lower in the magnesium treatment group than in the placebo group. Electrophysiologic studies in normal human subjects show that intravenous administration of magnesium prolongs the following:

- Sinoatrial node conduction time
- Atrioventricular nodal refractory period
- P-R intervals

It is not clear, however, whether the ability of magnesium to reduce the frequency of cardiac arrhythmias is related directly to the electrophysiologic, antiarrhythmic properties of magnesium or can be ascribed to its anti-ischemic properties.

Hypomagnesemia in Acutely Ill Patients

The presence of hypomagnesemia in acutely ill patients increases mortality rate independent of APACHE (acute physiology and chronic health evaluation) II scores. This increased mortality rate is seen in severely ill patients in medical intensive care units and in moderately ill ward patients. Other electrolyte abnormalities, consisting of hyponatremia, hypokalemia, and hypochloremia, and abnormalities in renal function and acid-base frequently accompany hypomagnesemia. However, in a previous study, azotemia and hypokalemia were found more frequently among the hypomagnesemic patients in both ward and medical intensive care unit settings.

Relationship of Magnesium to Hypertension

Intravenous magnesium is still widely used by obstetricians for treating eclampsia. The goal of this therapy is to prevent convulsions. However, blood pressures are reduced to the level of symptomatic hypotension. It is evident that, after years of magnesium therapy in eclampsia, intravenous administration of magnesium can result in a rapid and profound reduction of blood pressure. Because eclampsia is a specific condition, questions remain: Can this finding be applied to other types of hypertension? Can hypomagnesemia be related to elevated blood pressures? One study showed that hypomagnesemic patients with essential hypertension require more antihypertensive medications than do their counterparts with a normal level of serum magnesium, suggesting a causal relationship between serum magnesium concentration and blood pressure levels.

Controlled clinical trials were conducted to examine the validity of the aforementioned hypothesis. Results of the clinical trials neither proved nor refuted the hypothesis that oral magnesium supplementation provides an effective means of reducing blood pressure.

Signs and Symptoms

The signs and symptoms of hypomagnesemia are generally attributable to the primary disorders or drugs that have caused hypomagnesemia as well as associated fluid, electrolyte, and acid-base abnormalities. Most commonly, hypokalemia accompanies hypomagnesemia; therefore, signs and symptoms in hypomagnesemic patients are similar to those observed in hypokalemic patients. These features include:

- Neuromuscular irritability
- Cardiac arrhythmias
- Respiratory depression

Respiratory failure can be a common postoperative complication associated with hypomagnesemia. Skeletal and respiratory muscle weakness has been commonly described in hypomagnesemic critically ill neonates and adults.

Hypocalcemia can also accompany hypomagnesemia. Hence, signs and symptoms of hypocalcemia, including paraesthesia, tetany, and convulsions, that resemble those of hypomagnesemia may predominate or mask those of hypomagnesemia.

Diagnosis

Serum magnesium level is the only guide for treatment of magnesium abnormalities in clinical practice. However, it is not the best method for assessment of total body store of magnesium. For instance, the serum magnesium level may be elevated—with total body magnesium depletion—in the presence of impaired renal function. The magnesium concentration in red blood cells, lymphocytes, or muscle has been measured to determine magnesium deficiency. Because these tests are not readily available and are invasive (muscle biopsy) and expensive, they are not recommended for clinical practice.

Treatment

Magnesium deficiency or hypomagnesemia can be treated in the following ways:

- Magnesium supplementation
- Potassium-sparing diuretic agents
- Angiotensin-converting enzyme (ACE) inhibitor drugs

Summary of Diagnosis: Hypomagnesemia

- Diabetes mellitus, chronic diuretic therapy (loop diuretics), alcoholism, chronic diarrhea, antibiotic (gentamicin) use, cancer chemotherapeutic agents (cisplatinum), and immunosuppressives (cyclosporine) may cause magnesium wasting and hypomagnesemia.
- Acute hypomagnesemia may develop in diabetic ketoacidosis.
- Hypomagnesemia often coexists with hypokalemia.
- Both magnesium and potassium deficiencies are associated with increased ventricular ectopy.
- Hypomagnesemia may be a cause of significant postoperative ventricular arrhythmias.
- Intravenous magnesium therapy is widely used by obstetricians for treatment of eclampsia.
- Signs and symptoms of hypomagnesemia are generally attributable to the primary disorders and similar to those observed in hypokalemic patients.
- Major signs and symptoms may be neuromuscular irritability, cardiac arrhythmias, and respiratory depression.
- Respiratory failure can be a common postoperative complication associated with hypomagnesemia.
- Symptomatic hypomagnesemia with a serum magnesium level less than 1 mg/dL should be treated with magnesium supplementation.
- Magnesium preparations that can be used include magnesium sulfate, magnesium chloride, and magnesium oxide.
- The preparation of choice is magnesium sulfate, and the recommended route is by intramuscular injection.

Mild Asymptomatic Hypomagnesemia

Mild asymptomatic hypomagnesemia with a serum magnesium level greater than 1.5 mg/dL requires no treatment, provided the patient can eat a normal diet.

Symptomatic Hypomagnesemia

Patients with symptomatic hypomagnesemia or with serum magnesium levels less than 1 mg/dL, or hypomagnesemic patients unable to eat should be treated with magnesium supplementation. Numerous magnesium preparations can be used, such as magnesium sulfate ($MgSO_4$), magnesium chloride ($MgCl_2$), and magnesium oxide (MgO). $MgSO_4$ is the preparation of choice, and the recommended route is by intramuscular injection. Intravenous administration of magnesium may cause severe hypotension and is not routinely recommended. The dosage regimen in adults, even with normal renal function, is variable. The authors recommend 50% solution, 1 g (1000 mg) intramuscularly, every 6 hours for 24 hours on day 1; every 8 hours for 24 hours on day 2; and every 12 hours for 24 hours on day 3. The frequency of administration may be adjusted upward or downward based on serum magnesium level and renal function, which should be monitored daily during the treatment.

Acute Hypomagnesemia

In acute hypomagnesemia associated with tetany or convulsions, 10% magnesium solution 10 to 20 mL can be infused over 5 to 10 minutes, usually followed by a 250 to 500 mL infusion of 2% solution over the subsequent 4 to 8 hours. Flushing and, rarely, sinus bradycardia may develop following rapid infusions.

Maintenance Therapy

For maintenance therapy, magnesium chloride 16 to 32 mEq/day in oral form is best absorbed and retained and more reliably sustains serum magnesium level. Alternatively, magnesium oxide 500 mg three times daily may be given. Potassium-sparing diuretic agents and ACE inhibitors enhance the attainment of normal serum magnesium concentrations and whole-body magnesium content primarily by reducing renal excretion of magnesium. Therefore, routine magnesium supplementation is probably not necessary for patients with mild to moderate CHF who are normokalemic and who are receiving a potassium-sparing agent or an ACE inhibitor drug.

Magnesium plays a fundamental role as a cofactor for many enzymatic reactions, notably those involved in the hydrolysis of adenosine triphosphate (ATP). The cellular pumps that maintain the homeostasis of sodium, potassium, and calcium are dependent on this reaction for a source of energy. Accordingly, it has been demonstrated in both experimental and clinical studies that a diuretic-induced cellular potassium depletion cannot be corrected by potassium supplementation alone when there is a concomitant magnesium deficiency. A normal body magnesium status is a prerequisite for correction of cellular potassium content.

Amiloride is a potent and specific inhibitor of sodium transport in many cellular and epithelial transport systems. A combination of amiloride (5 mg) and hydrochlorothiazide (50 mg) is capable of preserving the internal and external balance of potassium and magnesium on a long-term basis in patients with hypertension and/or CHF.

Spironolactone is also an appropriate therapy in CHF patients at risk for potassium and magnesium deficiencies. ACE inhibitors have a magnesium-conserving effect in CHF patients when they are given in conjunction with loop diuretics. This effect is dependent on glomerular filtration rate, which is also reduced by ACE inhibitors. A strong correlation between urinary magnesium excretion and creatinine clearance in CHF patients treated with ACE inhibitors suggests that magnesium conservation may largely be a result of the reduction in glomerular filtration rate.

Other Uses of Magnesium Therapy

Magnesium in cardiac arrhythmias   Several studies show that intravenous magnesium is a safe and effective method for reducing the frequency of arrhythmias and mortality in acute myocardial infarction. The benefit of magnesium therapy in myocardial infarction is summarized in Table 7.3. In a randomized, double-blind, placebo-controlled study in which magnesium chloride was administered to patients with acute myocardial

---

Benefits of Magnesium Therapy in Acute Myocardial Infarction   **TABLE 7.3**

Reduction of arrhythmias
Systemic vasodilation lowering myocardial oxygen demand
Coronary vasodilation
Decreased platelet aggregation
Improved myocardial metabolism
Protection against catecholamine-induced myocardial necrosis
Reduction of myocardial infarct size

Adapted and modified from Horner SM. Efficacy of intravenous magnesium in acute myocardial infarction in reducing arrhythmias and mortality. Circulation 1992;86:774–779.

infarction, patients received 50 mmol magnesium chloride (equivalent to 1215 mg of magnesium) in the first 24 hours after myocardial infarction and 12 mmol (292 mg of magnesium) in the second 24 hours. At 4 weeks, magnesium chloride supplementation had significantly reduced the incidence of arrhythmias (21% in the magnesium group versus 47% in the placebo group) and mortality (7% in the magnesium group versus 19% in the placebo group).

A single intravenous bolus of magnesium sulfate has also shown to significantly reduce cardiac arrhythmias in myocardial infarction. Note, however, that magnesium is not a standard antiarrhythmic agent. If serum magnesium is low, magnesium should be given as a supplement.

Postoperative cardiac arrhythmia Magnesium therapy is effective in reducing the frequency of clinically significant postoperative ventricular arrhythmias and increasing the cardiac index (stroke volume) in the early postoperative period. Although magnesium is not yet a standard antiarrhythmic agent, magnesium supplement should be given if serum magnesium level is low.

Magnesium therapy in refractory hypokalemia Hospitalized patients have a high incidence of concomitant potassium and magnesium depletion. When the deficiencies coexist, repletion of both potassium and magnesium is essential. However, in cases of hypokalemia, although overt hypomagnesemia may be lacking, cellular magnesium depletion may still exist, making hypokalemia refractory. Therefore, in cases of hypokalemia when potassium replacement alone does not increase serum potassium level in 48 to 72 hours, serum magnesium should be obtained. In case of low or low normal magnesium level, magnesium should be administered in the dosage stated previously: 50% solution, 1 g (1000 mg) intramuscularly, every 6 hours for 24 hours on day 1; every 8 hours for 24 hours on day 2; and every 12 hours for 24 hours on day 3. Alternatively, a potassium-sparing diuretic will increase both potassium and magnesium levels promptly.

REFERRAL

Patients with hypomagnesemia should be referred to a nephrologist when it is associated with:

- Other electrolytes and/or acid-base abnormalities such as hyponatremia, hypokalemia, and hypophosphatemia
- When the cause of hypomagnesemia is obscure and requires intensive investigation
- In the presence of azotemia

KEY POINTS: HYPOMAGNESEMIA

- Diabetes mellitus, chronic diarrhea, and debilitating disorders such as malignancy (particularly esophageal malignancy) and chronic loop diuretic therapy are important causes of hypomagnesemia.

- Serum magnesium may parallel changes in serum potassium. Thus, after fluid and insulin therapy as in diabetic ketoacidosis, the magnesium level may fall acutely, similar to serum potassium.

- Magnesium deficiency may be an important cause of postoperative cardiac arrhythmias.

- Hypomagnesemia in acutely ill patients may increase the mortality rate.

- Intravenous magnesium is still a conventional therapy to treat eclampsia.

- Intravenous magnesium can result in a rapid and profound reduction of blood pressure.

- In CHF, potassium sparing agents and/or ACE inhibitors enhance attainment of normal serum magnesium concentration and whole-body magnesium content at a faster rate than by magnesium replacement alone.

Patients should be referred to a cardiologist when hypomagnesemia is observed:

- In association with hypokalemia and digitalis toxicity
- In the setting of acute myocardial infarction
- Associated with cardiac arrhythmias

HYPERMAGNESEMIA

Causes

Magnesium is excreted mainly by the kidneys; therefore, renal retention of magnesium in acute and chronic renal failure is the most common cause of hypermagnesemia. However, in renal failure, hypermagnesemia is not common except in patients with excessive magnesium intake. Thus, the use of magnesium-containing products such as Maalox (Rhone-Poulenc Rorer, Collegeville, PA) (antacid) or Milk of Magnesia (Roxane, Columbus, OH) (laxative) is a frequent cause of hypermagnesemia in renal failure patients. Other causes of hypermagnesemia include:

- Hypothermia
- Hypothyroidism
- Adrenal insufficiency
- Iatrogenic
- Eclampsia
- Magnesium intake through laxatives—adults
- Accidental ingestion of epsom salt (magnesium salt)—young children

With oral intake of hypertonic (50%) magnesium for laxative purpose instead of hypotonic solution by error, severe fluid loss through diarrhea, resulting in hypotension, renal hypoperfusion, and hypermagnesemia, may occur.

Signs and Symptoms

The signs and symptoms of hypermagnesemia are ascribed to neuromuscular and cardiovascular function. As the serum magnesium increases above 4 mEq/L, deep tendon reflexes become sluggish. With serum magnesium level above 10 mEq/L, deep tendon reflexes are absent. Flaccid quadriplegia, respiratory failure, dilated pupils, hypotension, and bradycardia may develop. Rarely, complete heart block and cardiac arrest may occur.

KEY POINTS: HYPERMAGNESEMIA

- The most common cause of hypermagnesemia is the intake of magnesium-containing products such as Maalox or the use of a magnesium-containing enema in patients with renal failure.

- Sluggish deep reflexes, quadriparesis, or quadriplegia may be noted.

- Respiratory failure and complete heart block may develop.

- Calcium is the direct antagonist of magnesium. In respiratory failure or cardiac arrest caused by hypermagnesemia, calcium gluconate 10%, 10 to 20 mL intravenous bolus is the treatment of choice.

- With good renal function, an intravenous bolus of 40 mg furosemide will reduce blood level rapidly.

Treatment

Calcium is the direct antagonist of magnesium. In severe hypermagnesemia, calcium gluconate 10%, 10

to 20 mL, should be administered by intravenous bolus to prevent cardiac arrest. Because magnesium is excreted mainly by the kidneys with normal renal function, renal excretion should be enhanced by infusion of fluid (isotonic saline or 0.5 normal saline) and furosemide intravenous bolus (40 to 60 mg). With abnormal renal function or renal failure wherein hypermagnesemia is common, hemodialysis with magnesium-free dialysate is recommended. Exchange transfusion in infants with hypermagnesemia may be beneficial.

REFERRAL

All patients with hypermagnesemia should be referred to a nephrologist.

SUGGESTED READINGS

Alfrey AC. Disorders of magnesium metabolism. In: Mandal AK, Jennette JC, eds. Diagnosis and Management of Renal Disease and Hypertension. 2nd ed. Durham, North Carolina: Carolina Academic Press, 1994:103–109.

Abraham SA, Rosenmann D, Kramer M, et al. Magnesium in the prevention of lethal arrhythmias in acute myocardial infarction. Arch Intern Med 1987;147:753–755.

Dyckner T, Wesler PO, Widman L. Amiloride prevents thiazide-induced intracellular potassium and magnesium losses. Acta Med Scand 1988;224:25–30.

England MR, Gordon G, Salem M, et al. Magnesium administration and dysrhythmias after cardiac surgery. JAMA 1992;268:2395–2402.

Hollifield JW. Magnesium depletion, diuretics, and arrhythmias. Am J Med 1987;82(suppl 3A):30–37.

Horner SM. Efficacy of intravenous magnesium in acute myocardial infarction in reducing arrhythmias and mortality. Circulation 1992;86:774–779.

Leier CV, Cas LD, Metra M. Clinical relevance and management of the major electrolyte abnormalities in congestive heart failure: hyponatremia, hypokalemia, and hypomagnesemia. Am Heart J 1996;128:564–574.

Massry SG. Pharmacology of magnesium. Am Rev Pharmacol Toxicol 1977;17:67–82.

Quamme GA. Control of magnesium in the thick ascending limb. Am J Physiol 1989;256(25):F197–F210.

Rubeiz GJ, Thill-Baharozian M, Hardie D, et al. Association of hypomagnesemia and mortality in acutely ill medical patients. Crit Care Med 1993;21:203–209.

Stevenson RN, Keywood C, Amadi AA, et al. Angiotensin-converting enzyme inhibitors and magnesium conservation in patients with congestive cardiac failure. Br Heart J 1991;66:19–21.

Tosiello L. Hypomagnesemia and diabetes mellitus. Arch Intern Med 1996;156:1143–1148.

Whelton PK, Klag MJ. Magnesium and blood pressure: review of the epidemiologic and clinical trial experience. Am J Cardiol 1989;63:26G–30G.

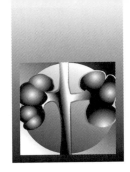

Polyuria and Diabetes Insipidus

Anil K. Mandal

POLYURIA

Background

Polyuria is the excretion of an excessive volume of urine per unit time; it is associated with increased frequency of urination to accommodate the large volume of urine produced. Polyuria is not to be confused with the frequency of urination caused by genitourinary tract infections such as urethritis, cystitis, and prostatism. This is accompanied by dysuria, a small volume of concentrated urine, and sometimes abnormal-appearing urine; the urinalysis is almost always abnormal. In contrast, polyuria caused by diabetes insipidus, diabetes mellitus, chronic renal disease, or compulsive water drinking is accompanied by polydipsia, elimination of very dilute urine, sleeplessness, and tiredness;

generally the urinalysis is normal. A thorough patient history, complete physical examination, and laboratory testing should establish the cause of polyuria in a given patient and help in formulating an appropriate plan for management.

Causes

The major causes of polyuria are listed in Table 8.1. The causes can be determined provided the mechanism of urinary concentration is well understood. Urinary concentration is determined by:

- Urinary flow rate
- Urinary solute load
- Medullary interstitial osmolality
- Plasma vasopressin level
- State of collecting tubule responsiveness to arginine vasopressin (AVP) or antidiuretic hormone (ADH)

Urinary Flow Rate

Pathophysiologically, expanded extracellular fluid volume increases the glomerular filtration rate (GFR), which increases urinary volume and frequency. Expan-sion of the extracellular fluid volume can occur as a result of excessive intake of free water or other types of fluids. Typical examples of excessive fluid intake include that by compulsive water drinkers and heavy beer drinkers.

Excessive Solute Load

An excessive solute load, such as glucose, sodium chloride, and urea, can give rise to polyuria and increased urinary frequency, as occurs in association with diabetes mellitus and chronic renal failure with impaired sodium conservation and enhanced urea excretion.

Medullary Interstitial Osmolality

Osmotic diuresis caused by excessive sodium and urea excretion may be associated with nephrostomy drainage, bladder decompression with a catheter in acute urinary retention, and the early stage of hypernatremia (before volume depletion occurs from natriuresis and water diuresis). Medullary interstitial hypertonicity is essential to provide the gradient for free water reabsorption under the influence of ADH. Therefore, if

Causes of Polyuria   **TABLE 8.1**

Causes	Examples
Expanded extracellular volume by free water intake	Compulsive water drinking
	Heavy beer drinking
Excessive urinary solute load	Glucose load: diabetes mellitus
	Mannitol load: mannitol infusion
	Sodium load: excessive ingestion (e.g., as occurs in drowning)
Profound natriuresis accompanied by urea diuresis	Polyuric phase of acute tubular necrosis
	Following relief of urinary tract obstruction
	Chronic renal failure
	Treatment with urea in SIADH
Impaired hypertonicity of medullary interstitium	Compulsive water drinking
	Loop diuretic therapy
	Acute and chronic tubulointerstitial nephritis
Reduced plasma vasopressin level	Partial and complete diabetes insipidus
Collecting tubule unresponsiveness to AVP (nephrogenic diabetes insipidus)	Congenital
	Acquired
	Drugs: demeclocycline, lithium
	Electrolyte and metabolic conditions: hypokalemia, hypercalcemia
	Parenchymal renal disease: acute and chronic tubulointerstitial nephritis

AVP, arginine vasopressin; SIADH, syndrome of inappropriate antidiuretic hormone.

the medullary interstitium is not adequately hypertonic, as may occur through renal parenchymal damage, the urine will not be fully concentrated regardless of the plasma vasopressin levels. Thus, polyuria, with elimination of dilute urine, may occur in acute and chronic tubulointerstitial nephritis as well as in other types of chronic renal diseases. The hypertonic medullary interstitium may be diluted by chronic water loading in compulsive water drinkers. Dilution may also occur by inhibition of sodium and chloride transport in the ascending thick limb of loop of Henle, which may account for the inability to concentrate urine in the water-deprived state induced by loop diuretics.

Plasma Vasopressin Level

Deficiency of AVP can result in a loss of 5 to 7% of filtered water, which is equivalent to 9 to 12 liters of urine per day (170 L of glomerular filtrate in 24 hours). A typical example of AVP deficiency occurs in patients with complete or partial central diabetes insipidus, the causes of which include idiopathic development, head trauma, and the posthypophysectomy state.

Collecting Tubule Responsiveness to AVP

In some individuals, even those with normal renal function, collecting tubule cells do not respond to ADH. This may be caused by defective receptor binding of ADH, as is seen in congenital nephrogenic diabetes insipidus. Acquired nephrogenic diabetes insipidus results from insensitivity of collecting tubule cells to ADH and can occur in a variety of renal diseases involving the medullary tubules and interstitium. Nephrogenic diabetes insipidus is also caused by a variety of drugs, including demeclocycline and lithium. Both agents inhibit adenylate cyclase and, hence, prevent production of cyclic adenosine monophosphate (cAMP), which is essential for the action of ADH.

DIABETES INSIPIDUS

Causes

Diabetes insipidus is a syndrome characterized by the elimination of abnormally large volumes of dilute urine (polyuria). It results from a deficiency in AVP release or in the action of AVP and can be caused by any of four fundamentally different defects of AVP. Thus, diabetes insipidus may be caused by the following:

- Impaired secretion of AVP, which is called neurohypophyseal diabetes insipidus
- Impaired renal response to AVP, which is called nephrogenic diabetes insipidus

- Excessive free water intake, causing impaired release of AVP, which is called primary polydipsia
- Increased metabolism of AVP by vasopressinase, as found in gestational diabetes insipidus

Neurohypophyseal, or Central, Diabetes Insipidus

Primary impairment in ADH secretion results from extensive destruction of the AVP-producing magnocellular neurons in the posterior pituitary (neurohypophysis). This destruction can be idiopathic or can be caused by a variety of acquired or genetic diseases.

Causes

Acquired   The acquired causes of neurohypophyseal, or central, diabetes insipidus include surgery in the hypothalamic area; head trauma; various primary, metastatic, and hematologic malignancies; granulomas; and infections of the meninges or brain.

Genetic   The only clearly defined genetic form of neurohypophyseal diabetes insipidus is transmitted in a completely penetrant autosomal dominant mode. It appears to result from selective postnatal degeneration of AVP-producing neurons and recently has been linked to mutations in the gene on chromosome 20 that codes for AVP—neurohypophysin II, the peptide precursor of AVP.

Idiopathic   The idiopathic form of neurohypophyseal diabetes insipidus resembles the genetic form in that the deficiency of AVP seems to be highly selective, occurs in the absence of any known cause, and, in some cases, appears to be caused by degeneration of magnocellular neurons in the neurohypophysis. The idiopathic form usually begins much later in life, however, and is not associated with a family history or with mutations in the coding region of the AVP-neurohypophysin II gene.

Pathophysiology

Destruction of the neurohypophysis causes a reduction in the amount of AVP secreted in response to the normal osmotic stimuli. This reduction in plasma AVP results in a decrease in urine osmolality and a reciprocal rise in the rate of urine flow. Along with increased urine flow, fluid intake rises to balance urine output, and dehydration is prevented. Thus, plasma AVP and urine concentration remain at levels that permit the development of symptomatic diabetes insipidus even though enough neurohypophysis remains to secrete adequate amounts of AVP in response to an abnormally intense stimulus, such as fluid deprivation. At this stage of response, the deficiency state can be classified as partial diabetes insipidus.

Partial diabetes insipidus may remain stable or may progress, with no AVP release in response to hypertonic dehydration. This state of complete unresponsiveness to release of AVP is called complete diabetes insipidus.

Patients with neurohypophyseal diabetes insipidus continue to exhibit usual diurnal variation in urine output. Thus, the rate of urine flow at night is approximately half that during the day, although both volumes are well above normal. Appreciable dehydration is rare in patients with neurohypophyseal diabetes insipidus so long as thirst perception is intact and there is access to free water. However, hypernatremic dehydration may develop if additional losses of fluid occur through vomiting, diarrhea, or inaccessibility to a water supply because of stroke or other impairments. The risk is highest for patients with complete diabetes insipidus because they cannot concentrate their urine regardless of the severity of their dehydration. Dehydration in diabetes insipidus is more likely to occur in young children and in patients with damage to the thirst center.

Nephrogenic Diabetes Insipidus

Nephrogenic diabetes insipidus is characterized by reduced renal sensitivity to the antidiuretic effect of AVP. Thus, decreased urinary concentration, a slight increase in urinary flow, and mild hypertonic dehydration may occur. If the renal insensitivity is minor, the rise in plasma AVP caused by dehydration may be adequate to overcome the defect and restore urinary concentration and flow toward normal. If the renal insensitivity to AVP is marked, the increase in AVP secretion needed to overcome the degree of insensitivity may not be achieved before hypertonic dehydration results in thirst and polydipsia. Patients with nephrogenic diabetes insipidus also exhibit the usual circadian variations in urine output and are subject to almost the same risks of hypertonic dehydration as those with neurohypophyseal diabetes insipidus. The main difference between neurohypophyseal and nephrogenic diabetes insipidus is that no damage to the thirst mechanism is evident in patients with nephrogenic diabetes insipidus.

Lithium-induced Diabetes Insipidus

Lithium is a commonly used drug for bipolar illness. Consequently, an increased number of renal consultations are obtained from psychiatric practitioners regarding a variety of renal problems observed in patients treated with lithium. The most common and probably most important adverse effect of lithium is polyuria. Total urine volume and osmolality in patients treated with lithium are similar to those in patients with hypophyseal or nephrogenic diabetes insipidus. Since AVP does not decrease urine volume or increase urine concentration, the defect is tubular unresponsiveness to ADH and is similar to other causes of nephrogenic diabetes insipidus. In patients treated with lithium, ADH levels are elevated compared with those in control subjects. This finding confirms that ADH production is normal but that the collecting tubule is unresponsive to ADH. The vasopressin-resistant diabetes insipidus caused by lithium may be caused by a circulating factor that either binds ADH and makes it inactive or that causes the secretion of an inactive form, which competes with active ADH for receptor sites in the collecting tubules. In addition to this functional defect, chronic tubulointerstitial nephritis may occur in chronic lithium users, which can result in further impaired urinary concentration and increase the polyuria caused by vasopressin-resistant diabetes insipidus.

Primary Polydipsia

Excessive water intake in patients with primary polydipsia decreases plasma osmolality and sodium concentration, which blunts release of AVP. This results in a water diuresis, which prevents the development of water intoxication. Patients with psychiatric disturbances may continue to have polyuria and polydipsia unless water intake is curtailed. Conversely, any attempt to reduce polyuria by administration of vasopressin will result in severe symptomatic hyponatremia because of water intoxication, which gives rise to central nervous system manifestations such as headache, confusion, coma, and even death. These patients can still concentrate their urine on water deprivation, although maximal concentrating capacity is frequently blunted.

Gestational Diabetes Insipidus

The signs and symptoms of gestational diabetes insipidus are associated with lower basal plasma osmolality and sodium levels than other types of diabetes insipidus. However, the symptoms remit soon after the placenta is delivered. Polyuria and polydipsia can appear in the third trimester or in the immediate postpartum period. Gestational diabetes insipidus is more common in the primigravida and may occur especially in women who develop preeclampsia or acute fatty liver of pregnancy. Thus, the association of transient diabetes insipidus with acute fatty liver of pregnancy appears more common than previously recognized.

Diabetes insipidus in pregnancy may be vasopressin-sensitive or vasopressin-resistant. The fundamental defect for gestational diabetes insipidus is excessive vasopressinase activity (produced in increasing amounts by placenta), causing inactivation of both endogenous and exogenous vasopressin. Histopathologic examination of the renal glomeruli from these patients may show glomerular lesions similar to those observed in women with preeclampsia.

POLYURIA OF HYPERCALCEMIA

There are several potential sites of action at which a drug or a physiologic disturbance such as elevated calcium levels may interfere with the urinary concentrating mechanism, causing polyuria. The impairment of urinary concentration in hypercalcemia could be caused by one or more abnormalities, including:

- A primary increase in water intake
- A reduced gradient for water permeability across the collecting tubules
- Decreased release of AVP
- Collect tubule lack of response to AVP

An important mechanism appears to be an increase in medullary blood flow as a result of increased prostaglandin associated with hypercalcemia.

DIAGNOSIS AND LABORATORY TESTING

Standard Clinical Tests

The standard clinical tests are:

- Water deprivation test
- Response to exogenous vasopressin

These two tests can help with the differentiation among the three major causes of polyuria: central (neurohypophyseal) diabetes insipidus, nephrogenic diabetes insipidus, and primary polydipsia.

Water Deprivation Test

Procedure The water deprivation test takes 12 hours and is done under strict medical supervision because some patients (e.g., compulsive water drinkers) with primary polydipsia may find access to water and continue to drink. The general procedure follows:

1. Body weight and urine osmolality and serum electrolyte measurements are obtained before the test begins, and plasma vasopressin levels are drawn.
2. Weight should be recorded hourly. The test is discontinued if a patient loses more than 5% of the baseline body weight at any time during the test.

3. At the end of the test, body weight is again recorded, urine osmolality and serum electrolytes are measured, and plasma vasopressin levels are obtained. Additional serum electrolyte measurements may be obtained during the test, especially in patients with rapid weight loss. Weight loss accompanied by hypernatremia suggests severe polyuria, which is most consistent with complete central diabetes insipidus.

Evaluating water deprivation test results In normal individuals, water deprivation increases urine osmolality to 800 to 900 Osm/kg. In patients with primary polydipsia (compulsive water drinkers), urine osmolality also increases substantially but may not reach the levels seen in controls. Urine osmolality may increase slightly or not at all from the baseline in patients with complete central and nephrogenic diabetes insipidus. However, in patients with partial central diabetes, AVP release may occur in response to plasma hypertonicity and permit some degree of urinary concentration to occur. Therefore, a slight or no increase in urinary osmolality from the baseline suggests either neurohypophyseal (complete central) or nephrogenic diabetes insipidus.

Therapeutic Vasopressin Test

The vasopressin test consists of subcutaneous injection of 5 U of aqueous Pitressin (Parke Davis, Morris Plains, NJ). In patients with central diabetes insipidus, urinary osmolality will promptly increase from 30 to 200%, depending on the severity of the deficiency. Less than a 10% increase in urinary osmolality will be noted in patients with nephrogenic diabetes insipidus or primary polydipsia.

Instead of conducting the cumbersome and protracted water deprivation test, a therapeutic test with vasopressin (or desmopressin) may be tried in the hospital setting, with the following outcomes:

- If desmopressin (or DDAVP; deamino-8-D-arginine vasopressin) at 2 to 4 μg subcutaneously every 12 hours for 2 days abolishes the polyuria and polydipsia without causing water intoxication, the odds are excellent that the patient has neurohypophyseal diabetes insipidus.

- If the polyuria is abolished, however, but causes a smaller or no reduction in polydipsia and results in the development of water intoxication (hyponatremia), the odds are great that the patient has primary polydipsia.
- No response is diagnostic of nephrogenic diabetes insipidus. Partial central diabetes insipidus at times can be difficult to distinguish from primary polydipsia because both entities variably respond to water depri-

vation with an increase of urinary osmolality, which further increases with administration of Pitressin.

Plasma AVP Measurement

Clinically, the cause of polyuria resulting from disorders of ADH release or ADH resistance (nephrogenic diabetes insipidus) can be identified by patient response to administration of exogenous vasopressin. Determining plasma vasopressin levels is helpful, but the results take several days to obtain. Furthermore, the test is expensive.

Single AVP levels are not helpful in distinguishing central diabetes insipidus from primary polydipsia because the AVP level can be low in both conditions, especially if the sample is drawn before the water deprivation test is initiated. However, a paired sample drawn before and at the end of the water deprivation test can help the clinician differentiate between the two conditions. In patients with central diabetes insipidus, a slight or no rise in the AVP levels may be seen in the second sample, depending on the severity of the deficiency, whereas an appreciable rise in AVP levels may be seen in compulsive water drinkers. In patients with nephrogenic diabetes insipidus, plasma AVP levels may not vary before and after the test.

Magnetic Resonance Imaging

Magnetic Resonance Imaging (MRI) of the brain may help to distinguish between partial central diabetes insipidus and primary polydipsia. A normal hyperintense signal is noted in almost 98% of patients without sellar disease; however, the signal is absent in those with sellar disease. Hyperintense signals are therefore likely to be found in the patient with primary polydipsia but absent in patients with central diabetes insipidus. The pitfall is that the signal may be absent in patients with nephrogenic diabetes insipidus. Thus, MRI can be useful in distinguishing central diabetes insipidus from primary polydipsia but may not be helpful in differentiating central from nephrogenic diabetes insipidus.

Cautions in Testing

- The water deprivation test should be done during the day and under strict medical and nursing supervision.
- The water deprivation test, even under vigilant supervision, may demonstrate less than optimal urinary concentration in patients with primary polydipsia. This is because of medullary "wash out" (interference with the medullary concentrating mech-anism) and a lack of hypertonicity. In these patients, the urinary concentration will increase

more if the patient is administered protein and salt before the water deprivation test.
- Any preparation of vasopressin, either aqueous vasopressin or desmopressin, should be administered with caution in a patient with suspected primary polydipsia. Continuous drinking of water after vasopressin therapy could lead to water intoxication and acute symptomatic hyponatremia (confusion, headache, convulsions, etc.).

Summary of Diagnosis

- Excessive free water intake (compulsive water drinking), solute overload (diabetes mellitus), and chronic renal disease are common causes of polyuria and nocturia.
- Deficiency of AVP (complete central diabetes insipidus) gives rise to massive polyuria.
- Nephrogenic diabetes insipidus is another cause of polyuria.
- Patients with central diabetes insipidus exhibit the usual diurnal variation in urine output; the rate of urine flow at night is approximately half that during the day, although both volumes are above normal.
- Patients with psychiatric disturbances may continue to have polyuria and polydipsia unless water intake is curtailed.
- Compulsive water drinkers can still concentrate their urine on water deprivation, although maximal concentrating capacity is frequently blunted.
- The water deprivation test and response to exogenous vasopressin can help with the differentiation among central diabetes insipidus, nephrogenic diabetes insipidus, and primary polydipsia.

TREATMENT

Therapeutic options are directed at the cause of polyuria. If polyuria is caused by excessive excretion of osmotically active substances such as glucose, urea, or mannitol, treatment is directed to reduce excretion of these substances in the urine. For instance, treatment of diabetes mellitus with insulin or an oral hypoglycemic agent is essential to reduce glucosuria and minimize polyuria. Similarly, a low protein diet prescribed to patients with chronic renal failure helps to reduce nitrogen load and urea excretion.

Primary Polydipsia

Patients with primary polydipsia frequently have underlying mental disorders. The first step should be the treatment of the underlying psychiatric disorder(s), which may help curtail the compulsive water drinking. With reduced water intake, urinary concentration will increase over time.

Neurohypophyseal Diabetes Insipidus

Vasopressin is the treatment of choice for neurohypophyseal diabetes insipidus. Although various treatment regimens for complete and partial central diabetes insipidus are presented in Table 8.2, desmopressin is the safest and most effective, albeit the most expensive, form of treatment. Development of significant hyponatremia is rare with desmopressin.

TABLE 8.2	Treatment of Diabetes Insipidus				
Medication	Dose	Route	Onset	Duration	Comments
Hormonal Therapy Vasopressin tannate (Pitressin in Oil) (arg & lys VP; 5 U/mL)	2–5 U	SC; IM	2–4 h	24–72 h	Emulsion must be shaken and warmed before use Vasoconstriction and smooth muscle contraction are common side effects
Synthetic vasopressin (lypressin; 50 U/mL)	5–10 U	Nasal spray	30–60 min	4–6 h	Replaced pituitary "snuff" because it is relatively nonallergenic and nonirritating
Desmopressin (DDAVP; 100 μg/mL)	5–20 μg	Nasal spray	30–60 min	12–24 h	Drug of choice for complete central diabetes insipidus
Desmopressin (DDAVP; 4 μg/mL)	1–4 μg	SC	30 min	8–12 h	Also a good choice for central diabetes insipidus Hyponatremia may occur
Desmopressin (DDAVP; 0.1-mg tablet)	0.1–0.4 mg	PO	30 min	8–12 h	Mild increase in liver enzymes may occur Contraindicated in patients with liver disease Gastrointestinal symptoms may occur
Adjunctive Therapy Chlorpropamide Diabinese (250-mg tablets)	100–500 mg/d	PO	2 h	24–36 h	May be given as single dose; start at 100 mg; increase 1 tablet every 3–4 days; expect hypoglycemia at doses over 500 mg/d; used only in partial central diabetes insipidus
Hydrochlorothiazide Hydro DIURIL (50-mg tablet)	50–100 mg/d	PO	2–4 h	12–24 h	Usual thiazide side effects; can be used in central or nephrogenic diabetes insipidus

Adapted with permission from Singer I. The management of diabetes insipidus in adults. Arch Intern Med 1997;157:1293–1301.
arg & lys VP, arginine and lypressin (8-lysine) vasopressin; DDAVP, deamino-8-D-arginine vasopressin; IM, intramuscular; SC, subcutaneous; PO, by mouth.

Pitressin in Oil is effective and long-acting, but causes increased blood pressure and hyponatremia.

Chlorpropamide is another safe and effective oral therapy. When used alone or in combination with hydrochlorothiazide, it usually reduces urine output to asymptomatic, if not normal, levels even in patients with severe AVP deficiency. The antidiuretic effect is usually rapid in previously untreated patients, but it may take longer (7–10 days) if the patient has been treated recently with Pitressin or desmopressin. The mechanism of action is unclear, but it does not involve increased release of AVP. Hypoglycemia (in particular prolonged hypoglycemia) may occur, especially if chlorpropamide is used alone. If the drug is used in conjunction with hydrochlorothiazide, the hypoglycemic effect may be minimized.

Nephrogenic Diabetes Insipidus

Nephrogenic diabetes insipidus may be treated by desmopressin or any of the oral hypoglycemic agents listed in Table 8.2. The dosage and administration of each agent is similar to those used in the treatment of central diabetes insipidus.

REFERRAL

Patients with polyuria, in whom the cause is not easily determined, should be referred to a nephrologist or an endocrinologist. If the cause of polyuria is determined and found to be central diabetes insipidus, an endocrinologist may be the appropriate consultant. A nephrologist may be the appropriate consultant for all other causes of polyuria.

COMMONLY ASKED QUESTIONS

Why do I need to go to the bathroom so often day and night?
Frequent urination could be caused by insulin deficiency, caused in turn by diabetes mellitus, or by vasopressin deficiency, caused in turn by diabetes insipidus. Insulin is released by the pancreas, whereas vasopressin is released by the pituitary gland, which is located at the base of the brain.

I am exhausted because I'm up all night going to the bathroom. Is there anything you can do to help me?
Yes. Once we determine why you must go so often, you can be treated effectively and the number of your visits to the bathroom will steadily decrease.

Do I have to continue the treatment for the rest of my life?
Yes. However, convenient treatment regimens are available. For instance, for diabetes mellitus, a variety of oral agents are available as a substitute for insulin injection, and pills or snuff can be used instead of injection for diabetes insipidus.

Are there side effects from these drugs?
Yes, there are side effects. You and a family member should be familiar with the side effects of the medications you are taking so that they can be recognized; when they occur, report to your physician or hospital in case of emergency.

(Male patient) I wake up a few times at night to go to the bathroom and have difficulty passing water. What should I do?
Most likely your prostate gland is enlarged, which is obstructing the urine flow. This condition can be treated medically or surgically.

SUGGESTED READINGS

Berl T, Schrier RW. Disorders of water metabolism. In: Sibnier RW, ed. Renal and Electrolyte Disorders. Boston, MA: Little, Brown & Company, 1992:1–87.

Moses AM, Clayton B, Hochhauser L. Use of T-1 weighted MR imaging to differentiate between primary polydipsia and central diabetes insipidus. AJNR 1992;13:1273–1277.

Myers JB, Morgan TO, Carney SL, et al. Effects of lithium on the kidney. Kidney Int 1980; 18:601–608.

Robertson GL. Diabetes insipidus. Endocrin Metab Clin North Am 1995; 24:549–572.

Singer I. Differential diagnosis of polyuria and diabetes insipidus. Med Clin North Am 1981; 65:303–320.

Singer, I, Oster JR, Fishman LM. The management of diabetes insipidus in adults. Arch Intern Med 1997;157:1293–1301.

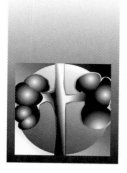

CHAPTER 9

Disorders of Urination

P. George John

NOCTURNAL ENURESIS

Background

Nocturnal enuresis is a common disorder, affecting 15 to 20% of 5-year-olds. By adolescence, the incidence drops to 1 to 2%. Nocturnal enuresis is defined as the involuntary voiding of urine beyond the age at which bladder control is obtained (4 to 6 years) in the absence of congenital or acquired defects of the urinary tract. Typically, involuntary voiding occurs at least two nights per month before it is classified as enuresis. Primary enuresis accounts for 75 to 80% of all cases and is defined as a child who has never gained nocturnal urinary control. Secondary enuresis is characterized by at least a six-month period of dryness that preceded the onset of wetting. Daytime incontinence is present in 15 to 20% of enuretic patients.

Epidemiologic studies suggest that 45% of 3-year-olds, 23% of 5-year-olds, 7 to 10% of 7-year-olds, and 1 to 2% of adolescents have nocturnal enuresis. Long-term follow-up suggests an annual spontaneous cure rate of 15%. There is a male to female ratio of 3:2. Enuresis is reported to occur more frequently in those individuals with lower socioeconomic status.

Nocturnal enuresis is a familial disorder. Incidence in identical twins is twice as likely as in fraternal twins. In 40% of children who are genetically predisposed to enuresis, one of the parents was enuretic. In 70% of these children, at least one family member was enuretic. In one survey, the incidence of enuresis was 77% when both parents were enuretic, 44% when one parent was enuretic, and 15% when neither had enuresis.

Causes

Central Nervous System (CNS)

The etiology of nocturnal enuresis is unclear. It is probably multifactorial, involving delay in the maturation of the CNS, the lack of normal daily rhythm for release of antidiuretic hormone (ADH), and insufficient wakening at night. The achievement of bowel and bladder control follows a common sequence: first, daytime bowel control; second, nocturnal bowel control; third, daytime bladder control; and last, nocturnal bladder control.

The most common, accepted theory of nocturnal enuresis is delayed functional maturation of the CNS, reducing the ability to inhibit bladder contractions at night. In normal children there is a circadian variation in secretion of ADH with an increase during the night. Enuretic children may not have this increase at night, and they may excrete significantly more dilute urine.

Sleep Disorders

Sleep disorders might also play a role in nocturnal enuresis. Studies of sleep patterns initially suggested that enuretic episodes occurred during slow-wave deep sleep, but current studies show that wetting can occur during different stages of sleep. Overall, it is unlikely that sleep anomalies have any effect on enuresis or that any particular correlation exists between the time of bed-wetting and the particular stage of sleep. However, insufficient wakening has been demonstrated in some patients with nocturnal enuresis.

Urodynamic studies show that functional capacity is reduced in enuretic children. Recent data suggest that there are no behavioral or psychological differences between enuretic and nonenuretic children. Nonetheless, distress or anxiety during the critical periods of development may have an effect on voiding and also on the development of enuresis secondary to psychological problems. Often, psychological effects are secondary to the enuresis. The incidence of underlying urinary tract abnormalities is very low.

Diagnosis

History

Patient history is the most important tool in diagnosing enuresis. The history should include:

- Frequency of bed-wetting
- Amount of bed-wetting

- Daytime voiding pattern (frequency, urgency, urinary stream)
- Previous urinary infections
- Bowel problems
- Family history

A positive family medical history of enuresis is common with uncomplicated enuresis. The psychosocial history is important to the diagnosis. Attitudes of the patients and their parents toward enuresis should be evaluated.

Physical examination should include:

- Abdominal examination
- Genital examination
- Screening neurologic evaluation

The neurologic evaluation should include:

- Checking the deep tendon reflexes
- Sensations (especially the perianal sensation)
- Tone of the anal sphincter

Gait should be evaluated for signs of neuromuscular disorder, and the back should be inspected and palpated for sacral dimpling to determine the presence of spinal congenital disorders.

Summary of Diagnosis: Nocturnal Enuresis

- Nocturnal enuresis is a common disorder affecting 15 to 20% of children aged 5 years.
- Nocturnal enuresis is a familial disorder. Incidence is very high if both parents were enuretic, whereas incidence is low if neither parent had enuresis.
- There are no behavioral or psychological differences between enuretic and nonenuretic children.
- Diabetes mellitus should be excluded by blood glucose studies.
- In intractable cases of nocturnal enuresis, plasma vasopressin should be obtained to rule out central diabetes insipidus.
- IVP, ultrasound of kidneys, and cystometric studies are rarely necessary to rule out urinary tract abnormalities.
- Identification and treatment of urinary tract infection (UTI) is an important therapeutic endeavor.

Laboratory Evaluation

Routine urinalysis is all that is required for uncomplicated enuresis. Urine should be tested for specific gravity and sugar. A urine culture is done if pyuria or bacteriuria is present. Other studies, including voiding cystourethrogram, intravenous pyelogram (IVP), ultrasound of kidneys, and cystometric studies, are usually unnecessary and indicated only when there is daytime wetting, poor urinary stream, other voiding problems, or a positive urine culture.

Treatment

Because the cure is spontaneous in most patients, drug treatment is not uniformly required. Reassurance and patient/parent education are extremely important. If the patients or family have no emotional or psychosocial problems, treatment may be postponed and the patient observed. When desired, treatment should be individualized depending on the patient's age, willingness, and motivation. Therapy should be offered to the child who is bothered by the symptoms. As a rule, patients with a strong family history of enuresis tend to delay therapy because they accept the temporary social inconvenience. The different therapeutic modalities and their advantages and disadvantages are presented in Tables 9.1 and 9.2.

Behavior Modification

Behavior modification requires considerable cooperation from both patient and parents. This therapy should be considered for children more than 6 years of age. Motivation therapy involves the use of positive reinforcement, including verbal praise and/or material rewards for a dry bed with cessation of punitive measures for continued wetting. The cure rate is reported at 25%. Behavior modification could be combined with other treatment modalities.

Therapy for Enuresis		**TABLE 9.1**
< 5 Years of Age	**5–7 Years of Age**	**> 7 Years of Age**
Education and reasoning	Education	Education
	Behavioral therapy	Behavioral therapy
	DDAVP on special occasions	DDAVP
	Alarm system	Imipramine hydrochloride
	Imipramine hydrochloride	Oxybutynin
	Oxybutynin	Cystoplasty[a]

[a]Rare, use only in patients not responding to other treatment
DDAVP, deamino-8-D-arginine vasopressin.

Enuresis Treatment: Advantages and Disadvantages		**TABLE 9.2**
Treatment Choice	**Advantages**	**Disadvantages**
DDAVP	Efficient	Expensive
	Easy to use	
	Minimal side effects	
Alarm system	No side effects	Difficult to use
		Initially expensive
		Efficacy not proven
Imipramine hydrochloride	Easy to use	Success rate low (10–50%)
	Relatively inexpensive	Side effects
Oxybutynin	Easy to use	Side effects
	Relatively inexpensive	

DDAVP, deamino-8-D-arginine vasopressin.

Bladder Exercises

Because many enuretics have reduced bladder capacity, bladder exercises sometimes help. Most regimens involve increasing the oral fluid intake and lengthening periods between daytime voiding.

Alarm Systems

Alarm systems consist of an alarm triggered when the electrodes become wet to wake the child and interrupt micturition. This is a conditioning therapy, and the cure rate is reported at 65 to 90%. The average duration of treatment to achieve overnight dryness is 18 days. This treatment works better alongside other measures such as motivation therapy, behavior modification, and exercise to increase bladder capacity. The relapse rate is 20 to 30% but is less if fluid intake is increased toward the end of treatment and if treatment is continued through a 4-week dry period. The alarm system is not acceptable for many patients.

Pharmacotherapy

Vasopressin or desmopressin   Patients and parents usually prefer drug treatment for enuresis. Common agents used are vasopressin, or deamino-8-D-arginine vasopressin (DDAVP), which reduces the urine output and gives good results with minimal morbidity.

DDAVP is available as either a nasal spray or an oral medication. An initial dose of 20 mg is given at bedtime, with a maximum dose of 80 mg. Optimal duration of DDAVP therapy is unknown. Therapy should be tapered and stopped intermittently to see if remission has occurred. Because the drug is effective immediately, it can be used intermittently for special occasions, such as school camps or sleep-overs, in children 5 to 7 years of age. Side effects are minimal. Hyponatremia is a theoretic possibility, but the nightly administration of DDAVP minimizes hyponatremia during the day because of increased urine volume (loss of free water).

Anticholinergics   Oxybutynin corrects good detrusor instability. It reduces the detrusor contractions and increases the bladder capacity. Recent studies suggest oxybutynin is of special benefit in patients shown to have small bladder and detrusor instability on urodynamic studies. The dose is 5 mg, two to three times per day. Occasionally one dose at night is sufficient. Therapeutic benefits occur in 30 to 50% of patients. Side effects include dry mouth, blurred vision, and flushing.

Tricyclic antidepressants   Imipramine hydrochloride is historically the most extensively used medicine. The exact mode of action is unclear. The antidepressant action, alteration of the sleep mechanism and arousal patterns, and anticholinergic effects are possible modes of action alone or in combination. Some clinicians have shown that imipramine may alter the secretion of ADH. The dose of imipramine in patients 6 to 8 years of age is 25 mg nightly. It is suggested to start with 10 mg and increase the dose slowly as needed. Older children may need 50 to 75 mg. Although the effect of imipramine therapy is immediate, it is best to continue the drug for 2 weeks before assessing its efficacy and a possible dose change. The optimal duration of therapy is unknown, although 3- to 6-month therapy has been beneficial. The dose should be tapered. The success rate of imipramine is 20 to 30%. Side effects include anxiety, insomnia, dry mouth, nausea, and personality changes. An overdose can be fatal from cardiac arrhythmia, hypotension, respiratory complications, and convulsions.

KEY POINTS: NOCTURNAL ENURESIS

- Most enuretic children are aged 3 and younger.

- Nocturnal enuresis is more common among children of lower socioeconomic status.

- No behavioral or psychological differences seem to exist between enuretic and nonenuretic children.

- The incidence of underlying urinary tract abnormalities is low, and investigations to find urinary tract abnormalities are not cost-effective.

- Therapeutic options consist of behavior modification, motivation therapy, bladder exercises, and pharmacologic interventions.

- Spontaneous cure occurs in most patients. Thus, drug treatment is not uniformly necessary.

- In pharmacologic intervention, DDAVP oral or nasal spray is a common choice.

URINARY INCONTINENCE

Background

Urinary incontinence is a common but underestimated problem in the geriatric population. The prevalence is underestimated because physicians rarely ask about it; patients consider it a part of the normal aging process and are often embarrassed to discuss the problem. Urinary incontinence affects approximately 15% of elderly people living in the community, 35% of elderly patients in acute care hospitals, and 60% of nursing home residents. Approximately 25% of incontinent patients in nursing homes are cognitively impaired. Urinary incontinence has social, economic, and medical impact. Urinary incontinence is often the main reason for institutionalization of elderly persons. By the time the patient is in a nursing home, the cost of care for incontinence increases more than that for patients living in the community.

Urinary incontinence can result in skin irritation and local pressure sores. Socially, an incontinent patient feels isolated and avoids social activities. Elderly persons should be asked about their attitudes toward incontinence and be assured that diagnosis and treatment options are usually noninvasive, inexpensive when done at a clinic, and effective.

The incidence of incontinence increases with age because of age-related physiologic changes. Bladder capacity decreases, involuntary bladder contractions are common, and mobility is more likely to be impaired. In females, there is a decline in bladder outlet and urethral resistance secondary to the relaxation of pelvic musculature. Women may also develop atrophic vaginitis, which in itself can cause dysuria, urgency, and UTIs. In males, prostate enlargement can cause decreased urinary flow rates, detrusor instability, and overflow incontinence.

Anatomy, Physiology, and Pathophysiology

The urinary bladder is a muscular reservoir. The wall of the bladder is composed of interlacing bundles of smooth muscle (detrusor). When the detrusor relaxes, urine storage results; when it contracts, micturition results.

Sensory stretch receptors located within the bladder wall function to assess the degree of fullness. That information is transmitted through the spinothalamic tracts to the CNS. The brain sends inhibitory signals when urine storage is required and excitatory signals when the bladder needs to be emptied. The information from the brain is transmitted through dorsal columns and the spinothalamic tracts.

The bladder has somatic, parasympathetic, and sympathetic innervations. The pudendal nerve somatic component innervates the external sphincter. The external sphincter has a limited role in maintaining continence because it is able to stay contracted for only a short period. It contracts during coughing, sneezing, and laughing, when intra-abdominal pressure rises for a short time. The parasympathetic nerve fibers arise from the second through the fourth segments of the sacral spinal cord and innervate the detrusor. When stimulated, the detrusor contracts. The internal sphincter is innervated by the sympathetic nervous system, the nerves of which originate from the lower thoracic and upper lumbar segments. When the sympathetic nerves are stimulated, the internal sphincter relaxes.

Micturition

The neurophysiology of micturition is complex. The brain recognizes bladder fullness when approximately 300 mL of urine accumulate in the bladder. When micturition is desired, the inhibitory signals are replaced by impulses that stimulate the parasympathetic system, resulting in detrusor contraction. This contraction is associated with relaxation of the internal sphincter. When the bladder is emptied, the brain sends impulses that result in parasympathetic inhibition and sympathetic stimulation, resulting in detrusor relaxation and internal sphincter contraction.

Causes

With advancing age, the size of the bladder decreases and detrusor contraction occurs more readily, resulting in higher frequency of urination. Fecal impaction, UTI, prolapse of the uterus, prostatism, pelvic floor relaxation, and immobility can also contribute to urinary incontinence.

Types of Incontinence

Urge incontinence or detrusor instability Urge incontinence is the most common type, accounting for approximately 70% of occurrences. The predominant symptom is urgency. In patients with detrusor overactivity, early, forceful detrusor contractions well before the bladder is full result in urinary urgency and frequency. These patients tend to pass small amounts of urine frequently. Detrusor overactivity can occur in conditions of defective CNS inhibition or increased afferent stimulation of the bladder. The CNS problems typically causing urge incontinence are:

- Strokes
- Masses (tumor, aneurysm, or hemorrhage)

- Demyelinating diseases (multiple sclerosis)
- Parkinson's disease

Increased stimulation of the bladder can result from:

- Lower UTIs
- Atrophic vaginitis
- Fecal impaction
- Uterine prolapse
- Benign prostatic hyperplasia

The diagnosis of detrusor overactivity is based on the patient's history. Physical examination may yield no specific finding. A careful pelvic, rectal, and neurologic examination may reveal any anatomic or neurologic lesion.

Overflow incontinence Overflow incontinence occurs in approximately 10% of patients with incontinence. Patients usually complain of continuous dribbling, difficulty in starting, and a weak urinary stream. Overflow incontinence can occur temporarily after regional or general anesthesia, after bladder instrumentation, or with the use of certain medications (such as narcotics). It can also occur with peripheral nerve disease, diabetic neuropathy, or spinal cord lesions. Bladder outlet obstruction resulting from an enlarged prostate can also cause overflow incontinence. Physical examination usually reveals a distended bladder. Neurologic examination may show signs of a spinal cord lesion or peripheral neuritis. Measurement of postvoid residual urine shows an increase in residual urine.

Stress incontinence Stress incontinence is usually the result of outlet incompetence and occurs mostly in women. In men it can occur as a result of surgical damage in urologic procedures. The patient usually complains of wetting during laughing, coughing, running, sneezing, and straining. This cause of incontinence is the result of pelvic floor relaxation caused by aging, multiple child births, or pelvic surgical procedures. The changes are more pronounced after menopause because of estrogen deficiency. Rarely, a neurologic lesion such as peripheral neuritis or a spinal cord lesion can cause stress incontinence. Patient history is most important for the diagnosis of stress incontinence. Physical examination may reveal cystocele, rectocele, or uterine prolapse.

Functional incontinence Functional incontinence is identified when the patient cannot reach the toilet in time because of physical or cognitive impairments or because of some medications. Functional incontinence may be caused by:

- Physical limitation as a result of severe arthritis, stroke, and use of restraints

- Dementia and delirium
- Diuretics, anticholinergic drugs, and sympathomimetic drugs

Generally, patients with functional incontinence have a normal functioning urinary system. Consequently, there is no typical finding on physical examination. Some medications can cause urinary incontinence either as a result of urine overproduction (diuretics) or by direct effect on detrusor muscle (anticholinergic) or internal sphincter (sympathetic agonists or antagonists).

In some patients, the cause of incontinence could be mixed. A patient may have both urge incontinence and stress incontinence, for example.

Diagnosis
History
To determine the type of incontinence, ask the patient about the frequency of incontinence and the amount of urine passed in each episode. Patients often more easily respond to direct questions about the use of absorbent undergarments and how frequently they need to change the undergarment. The frequency and severity of urine loss can be more accurately determined by having the patient keep a weekly diary or log.

The patient should be asked about the activities that cause incontinence and how the incontinence affects his or her social life. The patient's functional and cognitive status should be evaluated for signs of severe constipation, diarrhea, or fecal incontinence, which may suggest neurologic or autonomic dysfunction or fecal impaction.

Past medical history should be reviewed. The presence of the following may predispose to incontinence:

- Diabetes mellitus
- Benign prostatic hypertrophy
- Neurologic disease
- Recurrent UTIs
- Pelvic disease
- Postmenopausal genitourinary atrophy

Other information that could provide clues or further information include:

- Previous pelvic or abdominal operations
- Radiation treatment
- Hysterectomy, previous bladder suspension procedures, or prostate operations
- Previous surgery for modification of urinary incontinence
- In women, childbirth experiences, multiparity, large babies, and prolonged labor, all of which could predispose to sphincter incompetence or pelvic floor dysfunction

Physical Examination

A complete physical examination should be done:

- An abdominal examination is important to evaluate any bladder distension, which is common with overflow incontinence.
- A rectal examination should be done to detect any prostate abnormalities, fecal impaction, or pelvic pathology. Pelvic examination may reveal cystocele, uterine prolapse, rectocele, or atrophic urogenital tissues.
- The internal sphincter weakness can be assessed by having the patient cough while lying supine on the examination table. Urine leakage in this position is suggestive of outlet incompetence.
- A neurologic examination should include a CNS examination, mental status evaluation, and spinal cord and peripheral nerve function assessment.
- Reflexes and sensations of the lower extremities, anal wink reflex, and tone of the anal sphincter should be assessed.

Laboratory Tests

A urinanalysis may suggest a UTI. A urine culture should be done if the urinalysis suggests an infection. Blood tests should include a serum creatinine and blood urea nitrogen and electrolyte. If the history suggests polyuria, the patient should be tested for blood glucose, serum calcium, and phosphorus levels.

Urodynamic testing (radiologic) Urodynamic testing is not necessary in all patients. In patients with complicated incontinence, with more than one type of incontinence, and for those who do not respond to usual treatment, urodynamic testing is indicated. Testing should be done by a urologist or by an individual trained in radiologic evaluation. Some elderly persons with urinary incontinence may have normal urodynamic findings; others without incontinence may have abnormal urodynamic findings. Urodynamic studies are especially useful in patients with more than one type of incontinence. Urodynamic testing includes cystometry, urinary flow measurement, urethral pressure profile, and select imaging studies.

Cystometry. Cystometry measures the pressure of the bladder filling and can detect early detrusor contractions. A catheter is inserted into the bladder, the bladder is then filled with saline, and the intravesical pressure is measured as the volume within the bladder is increased. Of all the urodynamic studies, cystometry is probably the most useful for assessing patients with detrusor hyperactivity. Such patients will demonstrate detrusor contractions and characteristic pressure increases well before the bladder is filled. Multichannel urodynamic testing allows simultaneous measurements of intravesical, intra-abdominal, and urethral pressures

during resting, provocative maneuvers, and voiding, thereby distinguishing various types of incontinence.

Urinary Flow Measurement. Occasionally, urinary flow measurement is used to detect a urinary obstruction. The flow pattern may be abnormal in patients with a poorly contracting bladder. A normal urinary flow rate should be at least 10 mL per second.

Urethral Pressure Profile. The urethral pressure profile measures the pressure within the urethra and its functional length. This profile indicates whether the resistance is sufficient to prevent leakage of urine from the urinary bladder. This test may be useful for evaluating urinary stress incontinence.

Imaging Studies. Imaging studies commonly used are IVP and voiding cystourethrography. IVP is occasionally

Summary of Diagnosis: Urinary Incontinence

- The incidence of urinary incontinence increases with age because of age-related anatomic and physiologic changes.
- Urge incontinence is the most common type of incontinence, accounting for 70% of occurrences. Stroke, multiple sclerosis, and Parkinson's disease make up the majority of the occurrences.
- Urgency and frequency are the characteristic features of urge incontinence.
- Overflow incontinence occurs in approximately 10% of patients with urinary incontinence. Diabetic neuropathy and spinal cord lesions are examples of overflow incontinence.
- Stress incontinence is usually caused by outlet incompetence and occurs mostly in women.
- Diabetes mellitus, benign prostatic hypertrophy, neurologic disease, recurrent UTIs, pelvic disease, or postmenopausal genitourinary atrophy may predispose to urinary incontinence.
- Urodynamic studies, including cystometry, urinary flow measurement, urethral pressure profile, and select imaging studies, are available tests that may differentiate the type of incontinence.
- A detailed and thorough history is the most important diagnostic tool. A complete physical examination is also important. Elaborate testing, including urodynamic studies, are seldom needed.

useful if structural abnormalities are suspected. Voiding cystourethrography may detect bladder diverticula, pelvic floor relaxation, bladder outlet incompetence, uteteric reflux, or outlet obstruction. Genitourinary tract imaging by ultrasonography may be done to measure residual bladder volume when catheterization cannot be done.

Treatment

Medications used in the treatment of urinary incontinence and the dosage are given in Table 9.3. The side effects are presented in Table 9.4. Try to eliminate the cause of incontinence (e.g., enlarged prostate, uterine prolapse, fecal impaction).

Detrusor Instability

Detrusor instability is best treated with anticholinergic medications. Commonly used agents are:

- Oxybutynin, 5 mg, three times daily
- Imipramine, 25 to 50 mg, three times daily
- Flavoxate hydrochloride, 100 to 200 mg, three times daily
- Propantheline bromide, 25 to 50 mg, three times daily
- Dicyclomine, 10 mg, three times daily

Start with a small dose and increase slowly to minimize side effects. Calcium channel blockers are useful in the treatment of detrusor overactivity because of direct effect on smooth muscle relaxation.

Stress Incontinence

Pelvic floor exercises (Kegel's exercises) and biofeedback help stress incontinence. Adrenergic agents such as phenylpropanolamine hydrochloride and pseudoephedrine increase the tone of the internal sphincter and help stress incontinence. Intermittent use of medication for planned activities can be useful. Estrogen replacement therapy may help stress incontinence. Imipramine, a tricyclic antidepressant, has anticholinergic and direct relaxant effects on detrusor muscle and an α-adrenergic effect on bladder outlet. For this reason, imipramine is commonly used for stress incontinence or mixed urge and stress incontinence. Surgical treatment may be necessary in certain patients who do not respond to the medical treatment.

Overflow Incontinence

Overflow incontinence is caused by functional or anatomic obstruction. Obstructive problems could be surgically corrected. Pharmacologic treatment may be useful in the patient who does not want surgery or who is not a surgical candidate. α-Adrenergic antagonists reduce internal sphincter tone and can improve urine flow. Some α-adrenergic blocking agents are:

TABLE 9.3	Medications Used in the Treatment of Incontinence
Drug[a]	**Dosage**
Overflow incontinence	
Bethanechol	20–100 mg every 6 hr
	For underactive detrusor
Terazosin	1–10 mg once daily
	Increase as tolerated for outlet obstruction
Prazosin	3–12 mg in divided doses 2 or 3 times daily
Stress incontinence	
Phenylpropanolamine hydrochloride	Adult: 25–50 mg every 6–8 hr
	Child: 6.25–12.5 mg every 4–6 hr
Pseudoephedrine	60 mg every 6–8 hr
Imipramine hydrochloride	25–100 mg at bedtime
Estrogen intravaginal cream	2 g 2 times weekly
Urge incontinence	
Oxybutynin	2.5–5.0 mg 3 times daily
Flavoxate	100–200 mg 3 or 4 times daily
Imipramine hydrochloride	25–100 mg at bedtime
Estrogen intravaginal cream	2 g 2 times weekly
Oral estrogen	0.625 mg daily
Transdermal estrogen	0.05 mg every 24 hr
Nifedipine	10 mg 2 times daily

[a]Drugs listed in order of preference.

Side Effects of Drugs Commonly Used in the Treatment of Urinary Incontinence	TABLE 9.4

Anticholinergics	Tricyclic antidepressants
Dry mouth	Fatigue
Blurred vision	Tremor
Drowsiness	Cardiac arrhythmias
Constipation	Dry mouth
Occasional urinary retention	Blurred vision
Palpitations	Drowsiness
Orthostatic hypotension	Constipation
Smooth muscle relaxants	α-Adrenergic agonists
Dry mouth	Headache
Blurred vision	Sweating
Drowsiness	Tachycardia
Constipation	Hypertension
Calcium antagonists	Insomnia
Headaches	Estrogens
Dizziness	Hormonal side effects
Constipation	
Nausea	

- Prazosin hydrochloride
- Terazosin hydrochloride
- Doxazosin mesylate

These agents must be used cautiously in elderly patients because of the propensity to cause orthostatic hypotension. Doses should be started low initially and gradually increased as tolerated.

Patients with overflow incontinence resulting from a hypotonic or neurogenic bladder can benefit from cholinergic medications such as bethanechol. Most postoperative patients are likely to benefit from a short-term course of this medication.

Assistive voiding techniques, such as the abdominal strain or Credé's maneuvers, can help patients with overflow incontinence. Patients with overflow incontinence may be managed with intermittent self-catheterization or indwelling bladder catheterization. Intermittent self-catheterization is used for long-term management of patients with overflow incontinence who are cognitively intact and have adequate manual dexterity. Long-term indwelling urinary catheterization is indicated for patients unable to empty their bladders and unresponsive to treatment measures. External catheters for male patients can also be helpful, although their use may be limited by improper fit and skin irritation.

Functional Incontinence

Functional incontinence is treated first by trying to eliminate the contributing conditions. Environmental modification, such as reducing the distance to the toilet or using a bedside commode, can be useful in selected patients. Mobility may be improved and confusional states may be cleared by eliminating some of the patient's medications.

Patients with dementia benefit from prompted voiding, scheduled voids, and attention to behavioral signals that indicate a desire to void. Adjustment of medications that may cause incontinence should be considered.

Absorbent Undergarments

Several types of absorbent undergarments are often used by incontinent patients; some are disposable and others are reusable. These products can help elderly patients regain the freedom lost as a result of urinary incontinence. Conversely, they may also cause many patients to forego medical evaluation and merely accept the incontinence as another age-related inconvenience.

Prevention

Proper obstetric care and delivery may help avoid stress incontinence. Multiparity and difficult prolonged labor predispose women to incontinence. Pelvic floor exercises (Kegel's exercises) after deliveries may improve the tone of the pelvic muscles. Estrogen replacement in certain patients may reduce the incidence of incontinence.

In men who undergo urologic surgery, including transurethral resection or prostatectomy, proper technique may avoid incontinence.

REFERRAL

Most patients with incontinence can be effectively treated by the primary care physician. For certain patients, a urologist, gynecologist, or psychiatrist should be consulted. The indications for referral are given in Table 9.5. Assessment by a gynecologist knowledgeable in incontinence may be useful in women with previous genitourinary surgery, cystocele, rectocele, or uterine prolapse.

KEY POINTS: URINARY INCONTINENCE

- The incidence of urinary incontinence increases with age.

- Urinary incontinence has social, economic, and medical impact.

- A thorough history is essential. Elaborate testing, including urodynamic studies, is seldom necessary.

- The primary care physician can effectively treat most cases of incontinence. Elderly subjects should be asked about incontinence and assured that diagnosis and treatment options are usually non-invasive, inexpensive, and effective.

- In elderly women, estrogen therapy to treat atrophic vaginitis may reduce the incidence of incontinence.

- In elderly men, use of proper technique during prostate surgery could prevent incontinence.

- Therapeutic options consist of treatment of the cause, anticholinergic drugs, calcium channel blockers, antidepressants, and α-adrenergic blockers.

- α-Adrenergic blockers are useful in overflow incontinence caused by anatomic obstruction, such as benign prostatic hypertrophy.

- An α-adrenergic blocker, such as doxazosin, reduces internal sphincter tone and can improve urine flow.

TABLE 9.5	Indications for Urologic Consultation or Referral in Patients with Urinary Incontinence

Diagnosis is unclear (e.g., patient describes more than 1 type of incontinence)
Overflow incontinence is documented
Patient does not respond to treatment
Gross or microscopic hematuria is present
Findings on prostate examination suggest a malignant lesion

COMMONLY ASKED QUESTIONS

Enuresis

Is enuresis a sign of kidney or bladder disease?
Enuresis is not caused by any bladder or kidney abnormality. It stems from a delay in the child gaining bladder control.

Is enuresis a symptom of any psychological problems?
Most authorities believe that enuresis is not caused by psychological problems, although enuresis may occur temporarily when the child is growing and subject to psychological stress. Psychological problems are usually the result of rather than the cause for enuresis.

My husband said he had a bed-wetting problem when he was small. I did not. Is my son predisposed to bed-wetting because his father did? Is my son more likely than my daughter to have this problem?
There is a small chance that son or daughter may have this problem.

What is the best way I can train my child to avoid this problem?
Enuresis rarely has anything to do with toilet training. However, do not force the issue of toilet training.

My child goes to the bathroom right before he goes to bed. Should I stop liquids earlier in the day? How much before bedtime?
In a child with enuresis, stop liquids approximately 3 hours before bedtime.

Are children with enuresis more prone to kidney disease or UTIs?
There is no chance of any bladder or kidney disease resulting from enuresis, and children with enuresis are not more prone to UTIs.

How long does the enuresis last?
There is a 30% chance that the enuresis will clear each year. It is unusual to have enuresis after age 10, although, rarely, it can continue until adulthood.

What if I do not want to give my child medications?
No harm, except that it is a nuisance to wash the bed clothes every night. If the child is not upset and you are not upset, you may elect not to treat the problem with medication.

Incontinence

Is incontinence a normal consequence of aging?
Incontinence could be caused by the relaxation of the pelvic floor muscles resulting from estrogen deficiency. More often, the weakness is caused by repeated child births or surgery.

Will I need surgery? Will surgery "cure" the incontinence permanently?
It depends on the cause of the incontinence. Many patients can be managed medically. In most patients, incontinence is easily treatable and the workup is simple, painless, and inexpensive.

Are there pills I can take to stop incontinence when I am in public or out at social events?
Depending on the cause of incontinence, many people can control incontinence when out for social activities. Medication has to be decided by the physician after evaluating the type of incontinence.

My mother had this problem. Does this mean I'm likely to have it too?
Incontinence is not necessarily genetic.

Does it get worse as I get older? What can I do to prevent it from getting worse?
Bed-wetting may get worse gradually as you grow older because nerve and pelvic floor functioning become less effective. Pelvic floor

exercises could ameliorate the incontinence. Estrogen replacement may be beneficial in certain cases.

SUGGESTED READINGS

Nocturnal Enuresis
Apon US. Nocturnal enuresis. Pediatr Nephrol 1995;9:94–103.
Mark SD, Frank JD. Nocturnal enuresis. Br J Urol 1995; 75:427–434.
Rushton HG. Evaluation of the enuretic child. Clin Pediatr 1993:14–18. [Special edition]
Rushton HG. Older pharmacologic therapy for enuresis. Clin Pediatr 1993. [Special Edition]

Urinary Incontinence
Bard DM, Wein AJ, Steers WJ, et al. Voiding dysfunction: diagnosis, classification and management. In: Adult Pediatric Urology. 3rd ed. St Louis: Mosby, 1996:1222–1325.
Burns PA, Pranikoff K, Nochajsk T, et al. Treatment of stress incontinence with pelvic floor exercises and biofeedback. J Geriatr Soc 1990;38:341–344.
Chutka DS, Flemming KC. Urinary incontinence in elderly population. Mayo Clin Proc 1996;71:93–101.
Peggs JF. Urinary incontinence in elderly: pharmacological therapies. Am Fam Phys 1992;46:1763–1769.
Resnick NM. Urinary incontinence in older adults. Hosp Pract 1992;27:139–142.
Rosenthal AJ, McMarty CT. Urinary incontinence in the elderly. Postgrad Med 1995;97:109–116.
Wein AJ. Pharmacology of urinary incontinence. Urol Clin North Am 1995;22:557–577.
Clinical Practice Guidelines. Urinary Incontinence in Adults. US Dept of Health and Human Services, 1992, 1996.

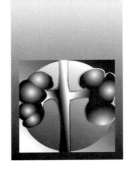

An Outpatient Approach to Proteinuria

Brad H. Rovin

BACKGROUND

Although a large amount of protein passes through the kidneys daily, adults with normal functioning kidneys do not usually excrete more than 150 mg of urinary protein per day. This norm of 150 mg is because of the glomerular permeability barrier, which effectively prevents proteins larger than albumin (66,000 daltons) from passing into the urinary space. Lower molecular weight proteins (e.g., beta$_2$ microglobulin, molecular weight of 11,600) are filtered at the glomerulus and reabsorbed by the proximal tubules; they do not appear in urine unless filtered in high concentration. Elevated protein levels in the urine thus imply a problem with tubular protein reabsorption, a breach in the glomerular filtration barrier, or abnormally high levels of low molecular weight proteins in the plasma.

Proteinuria As a Marker of Primary Renal Disease

Proteinuria is not an uncommon finding in adults and is often asymptomatic. Proteinuria is frequently detected during routine office testing by the primary care physician. Because proteinuria may be a marker of serious primary renal disease or of kidney involvement by a systemic process, the initial diagnostic evaluation of abnormal proteinuria is crucial for determining further workup and potential therapy. An approach to proteinuria that is easily undertaken in the outpatient setting follows.

CAUSES

Glomerular Proteinuria versus Tubular Proteinuria

Perhaps the most important, and confusing, aspect of the evaluation of proteinuria is the diagnosis of glomerular and tubulointerstitial diseases. Abnormal proteinuria may occur as the result of intrinsic renal disease that involves the glomerulus or tubulointerstitial space. Alternatively, the kidney may be involved secondarily in a systemic process that affects glomeruli or tubules. Table 10.1 presents common diagnostic possibilities that should be considered when evaluating a patient with proteinuria. This list, although not exhaustive, covers many of the conditions one is likely to encounter in general practice. Several of these diseases deserve further comment.

Glomerular diseases are generally associated with heavy proteinuria and may have nephrotic-range proteinuria.

Minimal change disease has a high incidence in children but is also seen in older adults. It is characterized by heavy proteinuria, an unremarkable urinary sediment, and normal renal function.

Focal segmental glomerulosclerosis and **membranous nephropathy** are common forms of primary glomerular disease that cause proteinuria or nephrotic syndrome in adults. These diseases may present with benign urinary sediments. Depending on when the disease is discovered, patients may have normal renal function or may have renal insufficiency.

IgA nephropathy and **membranoproliferative glomerulonephritis** feature active urinary sediments with glomerular bleeding or casts. Renal function is frequently abnormal in these conditions.

Ablative nephropathy occurs long after the resolution of a process that caused a greater than 50% reduction in nephron mass. The initiating processes can be diverse and are not restricted to old glomerular diseases. Typical examples are vesicoureteral reflux in young children and chronic urinary tract obstruction in older adults. The resulting glomerular hypertrophy and

	Differential Diagnosis of Proteinuria	**TABLE 10.1**
Primary Glomerulopathies	**Secondary Glomerulopathies**	**Tubulointerstitial Disease**
Membranous glomerulonephritis	Diabetes mellitus	Heavy metal toxicity
Minimal change disease	Immune-mediated diseases (e.g., SLE)	Drugs
Focal-segmental glomerulosclerosis	Neoplasia	Allergic interstitial nephritis
IgA nephropathy	Infection	Immune interstitial nephritis (e.g., Sjögren's syndrome)
Membranoproliferative glomerulonephritis	Amyloidosis	Fanconi's syndrome
	Drugs	Pyelonephritis
	Toxemia of pregnancy	
	Hereditary (e.g., Alport's syndrome)	
	Ablative nephropathy	

glomerular hypertension cause glomerular damage and the appearance of sometimes heavy proteinuria.

Proteinuria Caused by Drugs

Drugs are a common cause of proteinuria, hence a thorough history of medication use is important. Gold, penicillamine, and nonsteroidal anti-inflammatory drugs (NSAIDs) may cause glomerular lesions. Antibiotics are a frequent cause of allergic interstitial nephritis.

Proteinuria Associated with Systemic Diseases

Proteinuria may be a clue to serious systemic diseases, such as:

- Vasculitis
- Systemic lupus erythematosus (SLE)
- Systemic infections (e.g., endocarditis, visceral abscess)
- Initial manifestation of a malignancy (lymphoma or adenocarcinoma of the colon or breast, squamous cell carcinoma of the lung)

These possibilities should be evaluated in proteinuric patients with appropriate risk factors or physical findings.

SIGNS AND SYMPTOMS

Mild to moderate levels of urinary protein usually do not result in specific signs or symptoms. If severe, proteinuria may lead to the nephrotic syndrome (see "Urine Protein Immunoelectrophoresis" later in this chapter), and the patient may report swelling. Most often, swelling will manifest as dependent edema. Occasionally a patient may present with sacral edema, ascites, or anasarca. Patients may also become aware of a "foamy" quality to their urine if proteinuria is significant. Foam in the urine results from urinary protein becoming denatured.

DIAGNOSIS AND TESTING

Dipstick Test

Proteinuria is most often initially detected using commercially available dipsticks. These dipsticks are sensitive to albumin in concentrations as low as 10 to 20 mg/dL but are insensitive to globulins (e.g., immunoglobulin light chains). Dipsticks may yield false-positive results. For example, the interpretation of dipstick-positive proteinuria may be difficult if the urine is very concentrated, if the patient has gross hematuria, or if the patient's urine is excessively alkaline (pH greater than 8).

Combining dipstick results with an acid precipitation test may improve the sensitivity for detecting urine protein. The addition of 5 to 10 drops of 5% sulfosalicylic acid (SSA) to 2-3 mL of urine will cause proteins (including globulins) to precipitate, resulting in turbid urine. The degree of turbidity reflects protein concentration. SSA will detect immunoglobulin light chains excreted in the urine in patients with multiple myeloma and is not affected by urine pH.

SSA can give a false-positive result if the urine contains high concentrations of the following:

- X-ray contrast media
- Tolbutamide
- Sulfisoxazole
- Penicillin
- Nafcillin
- Methicillin sodium

In general, detection of any level of protein on urine dipstick merits follow-up urinalysis. Moderate to high levels of proteinuria (i.e., dipstick values of 100 to 500 mg/dL, or "++ to +++") require the physician to promptly begin the evaluation outlined below.

Microscopic Analysis of the Urine

When proteinuria is detected, microscopic analysis of the urine should be done (see Chapter 1). Although proteinuria may be an isolated finding, urinary abnormalities are often found when significant structural changes are present. A urinary sediment containing dysmorphic red blood cells or red blood cell casts is strongly suggestive of a glomerular lesion. White blood cell casts may be indicative of glomerular or interstitial inflammation, or pyelonephritis. The presence of oval fat bodies indicates heavy (nephrotic range) proteinuria.

Characterizing Proteinuria

Once protein is detected in the urine, it is useful to characterize the urinary protein by using the classification scheme shown in Table 10.2. These categories

TABLE 10.2	Classification of Proteinuria
Temporal Pattern	**Pathophysiologic Mechanism**
Transient proteinuria	Plasma proteins in urine
Persistent proteinuria	Overflow proteinuria
Orthostatic	Glomerular proteinuria
Constant	Tubular proteinuria
	Tissue protein in urine
	Postglomerular proteinuria

will help the physician focus the differential diagnosis according to the mechanism of proteinuria. The temporal pattern and magnitude of proteinuria have prognostic implications. Moderate to heavy proteinuria that is persistent and nonorthostatic is usually seen in significant renal disease, whereas proteinuria that is transient or orthostatic carries a more favorable outlook.

The condition or clinical circumstances of the patient at the time the urine sample is obtained should be taken into consideration to avoid aggressive evaluation of transient proteinuria in an otherwise normal person.

The following factors may cause a transient increase in protein excretion, usually of less than 1 gram per day, in patients with normal kidneys:

- Fever
- Heavy exercise
- Vasopressor agents
- Albumin infusion

The physician should retest for proteinuria when the aforementioned conditions are no longer present to determine if the proteinuria has resolved or is persistent.

Persistent Orthostatic Proteinuria

One must determine whether persistent proteinuria is orthostatic. Orthostatic proteinuria occurs when the patient is in an upright position but resolves in the recumbent position.

The mechanism of orthostatic proteinuria is unknown but is likely associated with subtle abnormalities of the glomerular capillary wall. Characteristics of orthostatic proteinuria include the following:

- Often occurs in young adults ($<$ 40 years of age)
- Usually causes less than 1 to 2 grams of urinary protein per day
- Is associated with an otherwise normal urinary sediment
- Tends to remit with time
- Renal insufficiency, generally, does not develop even if proteinuria persists for years

The protocol used to establish the diagnosis is outlined in Figure 10.1. No further workup is indicated once the diagnosis is established. These patients should be followed at least yearly to make sure the proteinuria remains orthostatic.

Nonorthostatic or Constant Proteinuria

Nonorthostatic or constant proteinuria refers to the presence of abnormal urinary proteins regardless of a patient's posture. This type of proteinuria may worsen with upright posture but is present throughout the day. Generally, persistent proteinuria that is constant indicates the presence of a significant renal disease or kidney involvement in a systemic process.

Overflow Proteinuria

Overflow proteinuria is caused by an abnormally high level of low molecular weight protein in the plasma that is filtered at the glomerulus and exceeds the capacity of tubular reabsorption. Overflow proteinuria includes excretion of:

- Monoclonal light chains in patients with multiple myeloma
- Excessive hemoglobin released from massive hemolysis of red blood cells
- Myoglobin released as a result of rhabdomyolysis

As discussed in the following section, urine protein immunoelectrophoresis (UPIEP) will identify monoclonal light chains in the urine. The presence of hemoglobin or myoglobulin in the urine should be suspected if the urine is red or brown in the absence of urinary red blood cells. The history and physical examination will also help to distinguish the cause of the red or brown urine. Both hemoglobin and myoglobulin are nephrotoxic and can cause acute renal failure.

Urine Protein Immunoelectrophoresis

Obtaining a UPIEP to characterize proteinuria can often be helpful. This will distinguish between glomerular proteinuria, tubular proteinuria, and monoclonal light chains.

Because glomerular proteinuria reflects the loss of larger molecular weight proteins in the urine, the UPIEP will show a prominent albumin peak. The diagnostic possibilities of glomerular proteinuria are shown in Table 10.1. If glomerular proteinuria is severe, it may result in the nephrotic syndrome.

Nephrotic proteinuria exceeds 3.5 grams per 24-hour period. This degree of proteinuria may be accompanied by systemic complications that collectively constitute the nephrotic syndrome. These complications are presented in Table 10.3; treatment options are outlined below. Tubular proteinuria is characterized by excessive excretion of protein that is smaller than albumin; UPIEP will show a broad, heterogenous peak in the gamma region. Albumin is not a prominent component of tubular proteinuria. A finding of tubular proteinuria should focus the physician's attention on a tubulointerstitial process (Table 10.1). Monoclonal

ALGORITHM TO ESTABLISH A
DIAGNOSIS OF PROTEINURIA

PATIENT INSTRUCTIONS

5:00 pm   EVENING MEAL. Take only 1 glass of fluid with evening meal.

8:00 pm   BEDTIME. Lie in bed in any position. Do not sit up in bed. A pillow may be used.

10:00 pm   VOID into urinal without getting out of bed. Discard this specimen.

6:00 am   VOID into clean urinal without getting out of bed. SAVE this specimen in bottle marked #1.

8:00 am   VOID into clean urinal without getting out of bed. SAVE this specimen in bottle marked #2.

8:15 am   OUT OF BED. REMAIN AMBULATORY FOR DURATION OF TEST. BREAKFAST.
           Take only 1 glass of fluid with breakfast, no liquids between meals, no coffee.

11:00 am   VOID. Save this specimen in bottle marked #3.

12:00 pm   VOID. Save this specimen in bottle marked #4.

12:15 pm   LUNCH. Take only 1 glass of fluid with lunch.

1:00 pm   VOID. Save this specimen in the bottle marked #5.

ANALYSIS OF DATA

Specific gravity and urine protein (measured with dipstick or sulfosalicylic acid) are determined for each specimen, #1 through #5.

INTERPRETATION OF DATA

1. Specific gravity >1.020
   A. Negative protein = no abnormal proteinuria
   B. Positive protein = abnormal proteinuria

2. Specific gravity <1.020
   A. Negative protein = test indeterminate. (Repeat test—does patient have concentrating defect indicating tubular disease?)
   B. Positive protein = abnormal proteinuria

Orthostatic proteinuria = Abnormal proteinuria (as defined above) only in the urines obtained
                          while the patient is upright (Specimen #3, #4, #5).
Constant proteinuria   = Abnormal proteinuria in all specimens.

FIGURE 10.1.

Testing for orthostatic proteinuria. This protocol has instructions for patients and indicates how to analyze and interpret the data. Note that the urine must be appropriately concentrated for a valid test.

TABLE 10.3	Systemic Complications of Nephrotic Syndrome

Protein malnutrition
Predisposition to infection
Hypercoagulable state
Hyperlipidemia
Edema

light chains will be apparent as a narrow spike in the gamma region of the UPIEP. Glomerular or tubular proteinuria that is constant indicates significant renal disease.

Protein may be secreted by other structures of the upper and lower urinary tract in response to infection, tumor, or calculi, resulting in postglomerular proteinuria. Total protein secreted is usually no more than a few hundred milligrams of protein per day. A urinalysis to look for pyuria and bacteria, and/or radiographic imaging of the urinary tract (e.g., renal ultrasound, CAT scan, or intravenous pyelography), is useful in establishing a diagnosis.

Quantifying Proteinuria

In the presence of persistent proteinuria that is moderate to heavy by dipstick measurement, the physician should determine the amount of protein excreted per day. Typically, a 24-hour urine collection is used for this purpose. When obtaining a 24-hour urine collection, in addition to measuring protein, the amount of creatinine in the urine should be measured to gauge the "completeness" of the collection (see Chapter 1).

Twenty-four hour protein collections are inconvenient to do and often done improperly, thus imparting a moderate degree of inaccuracy to the measurement. An alternative to the 24-hour urine collection that is especially useful for following proteinuria serially in the outpatient setting is a random, mid-day urine sample for measuring protein and creatinine. The numeric ratio of protein to creatinine in a mid-day sample, multiplied by the expected 24-hour urine creatinine excretion (see Chapter 1), correlates well with an individual's 24-hour urinary protein excretion. For example, if a 70-kg patient's spot urine protein to creatinine ratio is 3.0, and the patient is expected to excrete 20 mg/kg of creatinine per day, that patient is excreting approximately 4.2 grams of protein per 24 hours. A protein to creatinine ratio of less than 0.2 would be considered normal.

The magnitude of urinary protein has prognostic value, may help determine the source of the protein (glomerular versus tubular), and will alert the physician to potential extrarenal complications of proteinuria (e.g., nephrotic complications). Nephrotic range proteinuria almost always indicates significant damage to the glomerular filtration barrier (especially if overflow proteinuria is excluded). Proteinuria that is less than 2 grams per day may be glomerular in origin, or may be secondary to tubulointerstitial disease. Persistent proteinuria greater than 1 gram per day is a risk factor for progressive renal insufficiency; thus, therapy should be tailored to reduce proteinuria below this level.

An approach to the patient with persistent proteinuria in whom postglomerular proteinuria, hemoglobinuria, and myoglobulinuria have been excluded is illustrated in Figure 10.2.

Additional Testing

Serum Creatinine Test

During the evaluation of proteinuria, a measurement of renal function should be taken. This is most conveniently done with a serum creatinine measurement and a 24-hour urine excretion test for creatinine, so that creatinine clearance can be calculated (see Chapter 1). Other blood tests should include serum chemistries and a complete blood count. Serologies, such as antinuclear antibody, serum complement levels, and antineutrophilic cytoplasmic antibodies (C-ANCA, P-ANCA), should be obtained as needed when evaluating for specific diseases.

Radiographic Evaluation

Radiographic evaluation of the anatomy of the urinary tract should also be done in patients being considered for renal biopsy or in patients suspected of having a urinary tract abnormality. Renal ultrasound provides information on renal size, cortical scarring, and the presence of renal stones or tumors. Small, atrophic kidneys suggest the presence of a chronic, irreversible process. A renal biopsy of atrophic kidneys would probably not yield much information. Small kidneys with cortical scarring, especially with a history of recurrent urinary tract infections, suggest old reflux nephropathy, and proteinuria is possibly secondary to ablative nephropathy. Renal calculi or tumors may contribute to postglomerular proteinuria. Renal ultrasound will not help in evaluating the bladder or ureters, hence other imaging procedures may be required if problems with the lower urinary tract are suspected.

Renal Biopsy

In many situations, the cause of glomerular proteinuria can only be determined by a renal biopsy (Fig. 10.3). This is true for all primary glomerulopathies and many systemic processes involving the kidney.

In general, a biopsy is indicated for all patients with nephrotic range proteinuria unless a cause can be identified by clinical evaluation, the proteinuria is expected as part of the natural history of the disease, and renal histology would not dictate a specific treatment. Examples of these are drug-induced proteinuria that resolves on discontinuing the suspected drug and diabetic nephropathy.

In other cases, although an obvious cause of proteinuria may be found (e.g., SLE), a biopsy would still be indicated because the pattern and severity of renal involvement will influence therapy.

Patients with glomerular proteinuria below 1 gram per day and who have an unremarkable urinary sediment, normal renal function, normal renal anatomy, and who are normotensive do not immediately need a renal biopsy but must be followed closely for a change in the level of proteinuria or renal function.

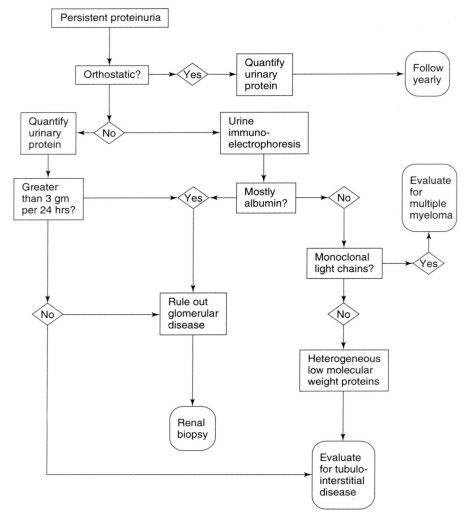

FIGURE 10.2.

Evaluation of persistent proteinuria. This algorithm provides an approach for evaluating persistent proteinuria. For the purpose of this algorithm, it is assumed that patients do not have hemolysis, rhabdomyolysis, or a postglomerular source as the cause of their proteinuria because these diagnoses are usually suggested by history, physical examination, or clinical course.

If proteinuria increases or renal function decreases, renal biopsy is essential to assess the severity of the pathologic process. Information from the biopsy will be useful in deciding the most appropriate therapy.

Patients who have unexplained glomerular proteinuria between 1 and 3 grams per day often will require a biopsy because of the prognostic implications of this degree of proteinuria (see "Treatment"). If the etiology of moderate glomerular proteinuria can be readily identified (e.g., reflux nephropathy, hypertensive neph-

rosclerosis), biopsy usually can be avoided. Biopsy is usually not required for overflow proteinuria or postglomerular proteinuria.

If the diagnostic workup suggests a tubular origin for urinary protein (i.e., low molecular weight urinary proteins usually excreted at less than 2 g/day), diagnostic testing based on the possibilities outlined in Table 10.1 should be undertaken. Occasionally, a biopsy will be necessary if the etiology cannot otherwise be determined or if the patient has renal failure.

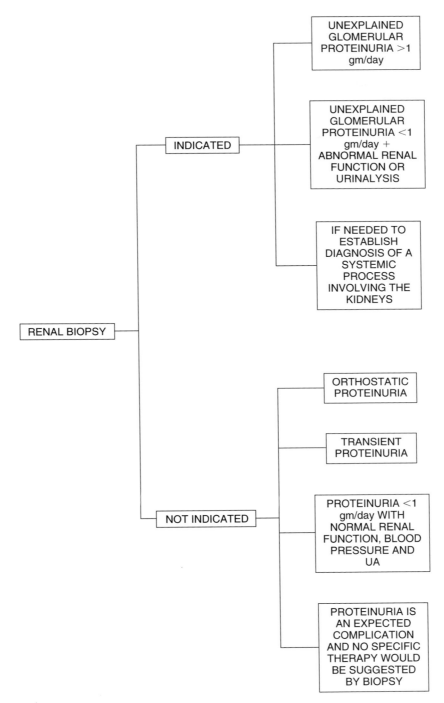

FIGURE 10.3.

Indications for renal biopsy in patients with glomerular proteinuria. These indications are not absolute but are guidelines that a nephrologist may use in determining whether to do a renal biopsy. Other factors often enter the biopsy decision, such as patient suitability, complicating medical conditions, and whether a patient would be a candidate for aggressive immunosuppressive therapy based on a biopsy. UA, urinalysis.

In addition to providing a diagnosis and a direction for treatment, the biopsy will be useful in predicting the response to therapy and the likelihood of recovery or progression to renal failure. Useful information obtained from the biopsy in this regard will be the amount of glomerular or interstitial scarring and the presence and severity of inflammatory cell infiltrates.

Summary of Diagnosis

- Proteinuria is not an uncommon finding in the adult population and is often asymptomatic.
- Mild to moderate levels of urinary protein (< 1 g/24 hr) generally do not result in signs or symptoms.
- Severe proteinuria (≥ 3.5 g/24-hr) gives rise to edema, hypoalbuminemia, and hyperlipidemia.
- It is important to determine whether persistent proteinuria is orthostatic. Orthostatic proteinuria occurs when the patient is in the upright position but resolves in the recumbent position.
- Nephrotic range proteinuria almost always indicates significant damage to the glomerular filtration barrier.
- Proteinuria that is less than 2 grams per day could be glomerular in origin or may be secondary to tubulointerstitial disease.
- Persistent proteinuria greater than 1 gram per day is a risk factor for progressive renal insufficiency.
- In hypertensive patients, tight blood pressure control is essential to reduce proteinuria.
- ACE inhibitors or angiotensin receptor blockers should be part of the antihypertensive regimen if there are no contraindications.

TREATMENT

Treatment of proteinuria may be divided into nonspecific and specific therapy. Nonspecific therapy is aimed at reducing proteinuria of any cause. Specific therapy is tailored to the disease causing proteinuria. Specific and nonspecific approaches are often used together to achieve a reduction in proteinuria. The rationale for reducing the amount of urinary protein is that proteinuria (particularly glomerular proteinuria) is more than simply a marker of renal disease. It is also an independent risk factor for progressive renal dysfunction.

Twenty-four hour urinary protein values greater than 1 gram are associated with an increased tendency for progressive decline in renal function. Reducing glomerular proteinuria below this level is thus an important therapeutic goal.

Nonspecific Therapy

Angiotensin-converting Enzyme Inhibitors (ACEi) and Angiotensin Receptor Blockers

At present, angiotensin-converting enzyme inhibitors are the main tools for decreasing proteinuria. Although ACEi lowers systemic blood pressure, the beneficial effect on the magnitude of proteinuria beyond other antihypertensive medications may be secondary to a decrease in intraglomerular pressure through effects on efferent arteriolar tone. Some evidence also suggests that ACEi can directly affect glomerular cell biology. Angiotensin receptor blockers are expected to confer the same benefit as ACEi.

This information should not diminish the importance of other antihypertensive agents in treating proteinuric patients, because the combination of hypertension and glomerular proteinuria significantly increases the risk for progressive renal failure. Furthermore, uncontrolled hypertension will worsen the degree of proteinuria. Excellent blood pressure control thus is mandatory for patients with proteinuria. An ACEi or angiotensin receptor blocker should be part of the antihypertensive regimen if no contraindications are present (e.g., renal insufficiency with the possibility of worsening renal function or hyperkalemia). Additional antihypertensive agents also should be added to the patient's regimen to achieve a target blood pressure of 120–130 systolic and 70–80 diastolic.

Moderate Reduction of Dietary Protein

Another nonspecific measure that may be beneficial to proteinuric patients with renal insufficiency is a moderate reduction of dietary protein intake to 0.7-0.8 g/kg ideal body weight per day. (This may need to be modified if the patient is severely nephrotic, as discussed later in this chapter.) Dietary protein reduction may slow progression of renal failure and may also result in smaller increases in urinary protein excretion, which proteinuric patients tend to experience with time. Although the issue of dietary protein restriction in proteinuric patients with normal renal function is still controversial, it is a relatively benign therapy that may be useful and is probably worth trying.

Specific Therapy

Immunosuppressive Therapy

Specific therapy for proteinuria is directed at removing the underlying cause of the abnormal protein excretion. Certain forms of primary glomerulonephritis respond to immunosuppressive therapy. The therapy usually consists of a combination of steroids and cytotoxic agents. Because this type of therapy is potentially toxic, it should be guided by renal biopsy findings. Similarly, if the kidney is involved in a systemic process, the therapy of proteinuria is the therapy of that disease. Depending on the systemic disease, this may involve steroids and cytotoxic agents for vasculitis, antibiotics for infection-associated glomerulopathy, or antineoplastic drugs for malignancy.

Complications of Nephrotic Syndrome

Protein Malnutrition

The complications of the nephrotic syndrome deserve special consideration. In the nephrotic syndrome, massive protein loss in the urine can occur and may lead to protein malnutrition. To avoid this complication, the natural inclination would be to place a patient on a high protein diet. Unfortunately, high protein intake may actually increase proteinuria and decrease a patient's serum albumin level. A normal dietary protein intake of 0.8 to 1 g/kg/day is appropriate for such nephrotic patients.

Infection

Patients with severe nephrotic syndrome may lose a large quantity of immunoglobulins in the urine, predisposing to infection with encapsulated bacteria. Nephrotic patients with ascites are at risk for developing spontaneous bacterial peritonitis. Thus, nephrotic patients must be carefully monitored for infection.

Elevated Cholesterol Levels

Cholesterol levels can be elevated in nephrotic patients. Because some glomerular diseases can persist for years with nephrotic proteinuria, it is not unreasonable to speculate that the associated hyperlipidemia may predispose patients to atherosclerotic cardiovascular disease. Furthermore, recent studies suggest a correlation between hyperlipidemia and progressive renal injury. Unfortunately, definitive data on the risks associated with nephrotic hyperlipidemia are lacking. Thus the benefits of treatment remain controversial. Nonetheless, it may be prudent to consider a low cholesterol diet and possibly an hepatic hydroxymethylglutaryl coenzyme A (HMG-CoA) reductase inhibitor in patients with unremitting proteinuria.

Edema

Hypoalbuminemia may cause edema in patients with nephrotic syndrome by decreasing plasma oncotic pressure or through a direct intrarenal effect to enhance salt and water reabsorption. Such patients are both fluid and sodium overloaded, and may be hyponatremic. Moderate edema is generally only of cosmetic significance, unless the patient has heart disease. In these patients, reabsorption of edema during recumbency may lead to pulmonary congestion. Edema can also be harmful if it is severe enough to cause skin breakdown. Edema is treated by restricting fluid intake, placing the patient on a 2-gram sodium diet, and administering loop diuretics (e.g., furosemide).

Hypercoagulable State

Nephrotic patients can develop a hypercoagulable state that results from numerous factors, including the loss of antithrombin III into the urine. The thrombotic tendency may result in arterial and venous clotting, especially renal vein thrombosis and deep venous thrombosis. Pulmonary embolism can also occur. Thrombosis is most commonly seen in patients with severe nephrotic syndrome (serum albumin < 3 g/dL and > 10 gram urinary protein/day), resulting from processes causing nonselective proteinuria (e.g., membranous nephropathy).

Renal vein thrombosis should be suspected in nephrotic patients who:

- Develop sudden onset of flank pain
- Develop a varicocele of the left testicle (caused by occlusion of the gonadal vein, which empties into the left renal vein)
- Have an unexplained increase in serum creatinine and/or proteinuria
- Have large or asymmetric kidneys

Renal vein thrombosis may be definitively diagnosed with a renal vein angiogram or an MRI. If a thrombotic event is discovered in a patient with nephrotic syndrome, maintain the patient on anticoagulant therapy until proteinuria falls below nephrotic range. Acute onset of a serious thrombotic event may require thrombolytic therapy. A daily dose of adult low-strength aspirin (81 mg) may be considered for prophylaxis in patients at risk for thrombosis.

KEY POINTS

- Orthostatic proteinuria often occurs in young adults, tends to remit in time, and, generally, renal insufficiency does not develop even if proteinuria persists for years.

- Nonorthostatic proteinuria may worsen with upright posture but is present throughout the day.

- Hemoglobin or myoglobin should be suspected if the urine is red wine-colored but shows no red blood cells on microscopic examination.

- The magnitude of urinary protein has prognostic value, may help determine the source of the protein (glomerular versus tubular), and will alert the physician to potential extrarenal complications (thromboembolism) or associated conditions (cancer or lymphoma).

- To provide exact diagnosis and determine appropriate therapy and prognosis, proteinuric patients should be referred to a nephrologist.

REFERRAL

A nephrologist should evaluate all patients with nephrotic range proteinuria or nephrotic syndrome. Additionally, patients with any level of proteinuria and renal insufficiency or an abnormal urinary sediment should be referred to a nephrologist. If a biopsy is being considered to establish a diagnosis in a proteinuric patient, consult a nephrologist.

SUMMARY

The workup and diagnosis of proteinuria can be initiated as an outpatient. This evaluation should rapidly identify patients with persistent, nonorthostatic proteinuria and provide the physician with an idea of whether the proteinuria is glomerular or tubular in origin. In many cases, renal biopsy will be necessary to definitively identify the cause of glomerular proteinuria and to direct specific therapy. Nonspecific therapy may be started before a tissue diagnosis of the cause of the proteinuria.

COMMONLY ASKED QUESTIONS

If I have protein in my urine, do I need to eat more protein?
Eating more protein will not necessarily compensate for the loss of protein in the urine. In fact, high levels of protein consumption may actually worsen proteinuria and lower serum protein levels further. Additionally, a high protein intake may accelerate the decline in renal function in patients with renal insufficiency. Thus, we recommend a moderate reduction in dietary protein intake.

Why is my urine foamy?
The bubbles in the urine are an indication of a significant amount of protein in the urine.

Can my proteinuria be treated?
Various measures may be used to reduce proteinuria. These include a reduction in dietary protein intake, good blood pressure control, and the use of an ACEi. Specific therapies are aimed at the disease causing the proteinuria, and often a renal biopsy is required to guide therapy.

Does the protein in my urine hurt my kidneys
Many laboratory studies suggest that urinary protein is not only a marker of kidney disease but may also directly injure the kidney.

SUGGESTED READINGS

Burton C, Harris KPG. The role of proteinuria in the progression of chronic renal failure. Am J Kidney Dis 1996; 27:765–775.
Ginsberg JM, Chang BS, Matarese RA, et al. Use of single voided urine samples to estimate quantitative proteinuria. New Engl J Med 1983;309:1543–1546.
Hebert LA, Bain RP, Verme D, et al. Remission of nephrotic range proteinuria in type I diabetes. Kidney Int 1994; 46:1688–1693.
Madais MP, Harrington JT. The diagnosis of acute glomerulonephritis. New Engl J Med 1983;309:1299–1302.
Petersen JC, Adler S, Burhart JM, et al. Blood pressure control, proteinuria, and the progression of renal disease. Ann Intern Med 1995;123:754–762.

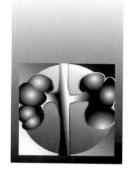

CHAPTER 11

Hypertension:
Management Strategies

Stephanie E. Ladson-Wofford
Patrick J. Fahey

BASICS

Hypertension is one of the most common indications for visits to a physician. Hypertension therapy is instituted to avert the morbidity and mortality associated with uncontrolled blood pressure.

Predisposing Factors

The prognosis of an individual patient is worsened when hypertension is associated with certain disorders. Therefore, in addition to obtaining a patient's medical history and determining any family history of hypertension, it is important to ascertain if the patient has one of the following disorders:

- Premature coronary heart disease
- Stroke
- Cardiovascular disease
- Diabetes mellitus
- Dyslipidemia

Technique for Blood Pressure Measurement

Typically, the diagnosis of hypertension is based on elevated blood pressure measurements recorded during at least two subsequent office visits over a period of one to several weeks. An average measured systolic blood pressure of 140 mm Hg or greater, or a diastolic blood pressure of 90 mm Hg or greater, or both, is required for diagnosis. If a blood pressure measurement of 140/90 mm Hg or higher is confirmed consecutively within a 2-month period, appropriate therapeutic interventions to control blood pressure should be implemented.

Blood pressure must be measured properly. The technique recommended by the Fifth Report of the Joint National Committee on Detection, Evaluation, and Treatment of High Blood Pressure (JNC V; 1993) is as follows:

1. Patients must refrain from smoking or ingesting caffeine at least 30 minutes prior to measurement.
2. Patients should be allowed to rest 5 minutes prior to measurement.
3. Patients should be seated with the arm bared, supported, and at heart level.
4. A cuff with a bladder that nearly (at least 80%) or completely encircles the arm should be used. Alternatively, the width of the cuff should equal approximately two-thirds of the distance from the axilla to the antecubital space.
5. Both systolic and diastolic pressures should be recorded. Diastolic pressure should be defined as the disappearance of sound (Korotkoff sounds).
6. Two measurements should be done 2 minutes apart and then averaged. There should be a difference of no more than 5 mm Hg between the two measurements, and, if so, additional measurements should be made until two readings are within 5 mm Hg.
7. Measurements should be done with a mercury sphygmomanometer, a recently calibrated aneroid manometer, or a calibrated electronic device.

Blood pressure and pulse should also be measured while the patient is both sitting and standing, with a 2-minute wait between measurements. A rapid heart rate may indicate anxiety or autonomic neuropathy; if the patient is orthostatic, it may be a sign of pheochromocytoma.

On the initial visit, the blood pressure should be measured in both arms. If the pressure is higher in one arm than the other, all subsequent measurements should be done in the former. If the arm pressure is elevated, the pressure should be measured in one leg, particularly if the patient is less than 30 years of age and the femoral pulse is delayed or diminished compared with the radial pulse.

White Coat Hypertension

It is well known that blood pressure measurements in the office may not be the same as those obtained at home. This phenomenon is referred to as "white coat" hypertension. Another well-documented phenomenon is one in which blood pressure is higher when taken by a physician compared with one taken by a nurse.

If white coat hypertension is suspected, it is important to review home blood pressure measurements. If the patient has an aneroid or electronic manometer, it should be calibrated against a mercury sphygmomanometer. The patient should then measure the blood pressure at home, and the measurements should be recorded and brought in on the next appointment.

Ambulatory blood pressure monitoring is another tool that can identify white coat hypertension. Evidence of target organ damage rules out white coat hypertension, and thus should be sought on physical examination.

TABLE 11.1   Poor Prognostic Factors Associated with Hypertension

Dyslipidemia
Diabetes mellitus
Cardiovascular disease
Cerebrovascular disease
Renal disease

Pseudohypertension

A falsely elevated blood pressure measurement is defined as pseudohypertension. This phenomenon can occur in elderly and obese patients. In the elderly, it is the result of stiff, calcified arteries that are not compressible by the blood pressure cuff. Pseudohypertension should be suspected if the vessels feel rigid and, in some cases, if the radial artery remains palpable despite occlusion of the brachial artery by the blood pressure cuff (defined as a positive Osler's maneuver). Korotkoff sounds over the brachial artery are absent when the maneuver is done. Osler's maneuver, however, is not 100% accurate.

Other clues of increased vascular rigidity include minimal or completely absent target organ damage despite the degree of blood pressure elevation, treatment-resistant hypertension, and significant postural symptoms with minimal therapeutic intervention. Intra-arterial blood pressure can be measured to confirm the diagnosis of pseudohypertension.

Pseudohypertension in an obese patient occurs when an inappropriately small cuff is used. This can be avoided by using a large (thigh) cuff or, if one is not available, by placing a regular cuff around the forearm and measuring the pressure in the radial artery.

DIAGNOSIS

History

Patient History

During the initial office visit, a careful history geared toward identifying any risk factors associated with a poor prognosis for hypertensive patients should be taken (Table 11.1). Table 11.2 lists all pertinent historical factors to identify in the hypertensive patient.

A history of diabetes, dyslipidemia, kidney disease, or hypertension is pertinent. If the patient has a history of hypertension, determine how it was previously managed and how well it had been controlled. Psychosocial factors pertaining to work status, family situation, and educational level should be reviewed. Sexual function is also important because impotence can be indicative of vascular disease, and fear of impotence from antihypertensive agents can affect patient compliance.

Family History

The patient's family history should be reviewed, with particular attention paid to identifying the following:

- Hypertension
- Premature cardiovascular morbidity and mortality
- Diabetes mellitus
- Kidney disease
- Dyslipidemia
- Pheochromocytoma

Review of Medications

During the initial workup of the patient, carefully review any medications the patient is taking, including those that are not prescribed. Medications may be responsible for an increased blood pressure or may interfere with therapy (Table 11.3).

Excessive sodium intake can elevate the blood pressure. Chronic alcohol ingestion of more than 2 ounces of ethanol per day can have adverse effects. Illicit drug use, particularly cocaine and amphetamines, is also important to know.

Physical Examination

As previously noted, the blood pressure must be measured properly. The physical examination should focus on identifying evidence of end organ damage, the symptoms of which may have been elicited in the history. Table 11.4 outlines pertinent body features to assess during the physical examination.

History Needed in Hypertensive Patients — **TABLE 11.2**

Medications (prescribed and over-the-counter)
Tobacco use
Alcohol consumption
Illicit drug use
Dietary habits (sodium, cholesterol, fat intake)
Physical activity
Recent weight changes
Obesity
Family history (hypertension, premature cardiovascular disease, diabetes mellitus, kidney disease, dyslipidemia, pheochromocytoma)
Environmental stresses (family, work, employment status, education)
Sexual dysfunction

Medications That Worsen Hypertension and Interfere with Therapy — **TABLE 11.3**

Sympathomimetics	Psychotropic agents
Anabolic steroids	Cyclosporine
Corticosteroids	Erythropoietin
Oral contraceptives	Yohimbine
Anorectics	Nonsteroidal antiinflammatory drugs (NSAIDs)

TABLE 11.4	Physical Examination
Body Region	**Finding**
General	Facial roundness
	Truncal obesity
	Discrepant arm and leg muscle development
Fundi	Hemorrhages, exudates, or papilledema
	Arteriolar narrowing, arteriovenous nicking or silver wiring
Neck	Carotid artery distension bruits
	Jugular venous distension
	Thyroid size
Lungs	Rales or rhonchi
Heart	Size, rate, rhythm
	Murmurs, gallops, rubs
	Precordial lift
Abdomen	Masses
	Bruits
Extremities	Pulses
	Edema
	Femoral bruits
Nervous system	Focal sensory or motor deficits
Integument	Striae, bruises

General assessment of the patient should include the following:

- Note facial roundness.
- Truncal obesity and a discrepancy in muscle development in the arms compared with the legs should be noted.
- The fundi should be examined to determine if there are changes consistent with hypertensive retinopathy (hemorrhages, exudates, and papilledema) or arteriosclerotic retinopathy (arteriolar narrowing, arteriovenous nicking, or silver wiring).
- The carotid artery should be palpated and auscultated for bruits.
- Jugular venous distension should be noted.
- The thyroid should be examined for evidence of goiter or bruits.
- Determine if the patient has rhonchi or rales (asthma, chronic bronchitis, or chronic obstructive pulmonary disease [COPD]).

The cardiac examination should focus on the size of the heart, rhythm, and evidence of murmurs, gallops, rubs, or precordial lift.

The abdomen should be palpated for masses and auscultated for abdominal and renal arterial bruits. If an abdominal or renal bruit is present, determine if it has a diastolic component because isolated systolic bruits tend to have less significance. Abdominal bruits are best heard just to the right or left of the midline, above the umbilicus or in the flanks. The peripheral pulses should be palpated, and edema in the extremities should be noted if present. Determine if the femoral pulse is decreased or delayed compared with the radial pulse; it is necessary to listen for bruits. Evaluate the patient for focal sensory or motor neurologic deficits, and examine the skin for striae or bruises.

Signs and symptoms of target organ damage should be sought, including:

- Headache
- Transient blindness
- Weakness
- Dyspnea
- Chest pain
- Claudication

Laboratory Evaluation

Unless the history and physical examination are suggestive of a secondary form of hypertension, the initial laboratory data to be obtained is listed in Table 11.5.

Once the diagnosis of hypertension is established, the following tests may be performed:

- Electrocardiography for a baseline reading and to assess cardiac status, particularly identifying evidence of left ventricular hypertrophy
- Possibly a chest radiograph if the patient is 40 years of age or older
- A 24-hour urine collection for sodium, microalbumin, and creatinine (the latter to ensure an adequate urine collection)
- Possibly other tests, such as echocardiography and plasma renin/urinary sodium determination

SECONDARY HYPERTENSION

Secondary hypertension should be suspected if there is abrupt onset, significant elevation in a person under age 20 or over age 50, or pertinent clinical clues are elicited in the history or on physical examination. Some forms of secondary hypertension are potentially curable and therefore should not be overlooked. Table 11.6 provides an overall guide for the workup of secondary causes of hypertension.

Causes of Secondary Hypertension

Chronic Renal Disease

Chronic renal disease is the most common cause of secondary hypertension. Although symptoms of early renal disease are frequently absent, the patient may have symptoms of nocturia, lower extremity edema, or hematuria. When taking the history, determine if the patient has had multiple episodes of pyelonephritis or kidney stones. There may be a family history of polycystic

Initial Laboratory Tests in the Newly Diagnosed Hypertensive Patient	**TABLE 11.5**

Complete blood count
Electrolytes
Blood urea nitrogen (BUN)
Creatinine
Glucose levels
Calcium
Uric acid
Lipid profile (total cholesterol, high-density lipoprotein cholesterol, triglycerides)
Urinalysis with microscopy
Electrocardiogram

Diagnostic Workup of Secondary Hypertension		**TABLE 11.6**
Diagnosis	**Initial Diagnostics**	**Additional Procedures**
Chronic renal disease	Urinalysis, serum creatinine, renal ultrasound	Isotopic renogram, renal biopsy
Renovascular disease	Plasma renin before and 1 hr after captopril	Isotopic renogram 1 hr after captopril, aortogram
Coarctation	Blood pressure in legs	Aortogram
Primary aldosteronism	Plasma potassium, plasma renin and aldosterone ratio	Urinary potassium, plasma, or urinary aldosterone after saline load Adrenal CT and scintiscans
Cushing's syndrome	Morning plasma cortisol after 1 mg dexamethasone at bedtime	Urinary cortisol after variable doses of dexamethasone Adrenal CT and scintiscans
Pheochromocytoma	24-hour urine for metanephrine, normetanephrine, VMA	Plasma catechols, basal and after 0.3 mg clonidine Adrenal CT and scintiscans

VMA, vanilylmandelic acid.

kidney disease, kidney stones, hematuria, deafness, or immunoglobulin A (IgA) nephropathy. The patient may have palpable kidneys on abdominal examination. Proteinuria seen on urinalysis can also be indicative of renal disease.

Renal Artery Stenosis (RAS)

Renovascular hypertension, or high blood pressure secondary to RAS, should be suspected if the patient has a history of abrupt onset of hypertension, worsening blood pressure that was previously controlled, or severe hypertension. There may be a negative family history of hypertension. In the older patient, the history may be significant for widespread vascular disease or tobacco use. A history of flash (abrupt-onset) pulmonary edema coupled with renal insufficiency is particularly suggestive of RAS. Use of an angiotensin-converting enzyme (ACE) inhibitor that caused acutely worsening renal function is another clue. Abdominal bruits should be sought on physical examination.

Coarctation of the Aorta

Coarctation of the aorta usually presents with hypertension in the arms coupled with a diminished or delayed femoral pulse. Physical examination may be remarkable for decreased muscle tone in the lower extremities.

Pheochromocytoma

In patients with pheochromocytoma, paroxysmal hypertension may occur, but sustained high blood pressure is the rule. Other symptoms include headache, sweating, palpitations, and pallor. Fifty to seventy percent of patients may have orthostatic hypotension. Flushing, although a symptom, is not commonly seen. There may be a family history.

Hypokalemia

Hypokalemia in a hypertensive patient who is not on diuretic therapy may be a sign of primary hyperaldosteronism. The patient may have symptoms of polydipsia, polyuria, and muscle weakness. Laboratory data may demonstrate hypernatremia, metabolic alkalosis, and excessive urinary loss of potassium. Unlike other causes of secondary hypertension, suspected when the age of onset is atypical, this disease is usually seen in patients between ages 30 and 50. Another clue is resistant hypokalemia despite the administration of potassium-sparing diuretics, ACE inhibitors, or potassium supplements.

Cushing's Syndrome

Hypertension occurs in the majority of patients with Cushing's syndrome, but it is rarely accompanied by hypokalemia. Most patients are obese, typically with a central distribution, and have cushingoid features such as moon facies, facial plethora, red to purple deep striae, and easy bruisability. The patient may also have carbohydrate intolerance, myopathy or muscle weakness, hirsutism, menstrual disturbances, poor wound healing, or osteoporosis.

Sleep Apnea

Although not frequently considered, sleep apnea is another cause of secondary hypertension. Therefore, the patient should be evaluated for early morning headaches, excessive daytime sleepiness, loud snoring, and poor sleep quality, particularly if obese. Laboratory clues include polycythemia and an elevated arterial carbon dioxide (PCO_2) tension.

Summary of Diagnosis

- It is well known that measurement of blood pressure in the physician's office may not be the same as that obtained at home, a phenomenon referred to as "white coat" hypertension.
- Evidence of target end organ damage, such as left ventricular hypertrophy and renal insufficiency, rules out white coat hypertension.
- A review of medications (prescription, over-the-counter, nonprescription, and illicit) is essential in the management of hypertension. Numerous prescription drugs can elevate blood pressure (Table 11.3).
- Chronic renal disease is the most common cause of secondary hypertension. Proteinuria and elevated blood urea nitrogen (BUN) and serum creatinine levels are supportive.
- Renovascular hypertension should be suspected if the patient has a history of abrupt onset of hypertension, worsening blood pressure that was previously controlled, or hypertension associated with headache.
- Hypokalemia in a hypertensive patient who is not on diuretic therapy may be a sign of primary hyperaldosteronism.
- Nonpharmacologic measures for mild to moderate hypertension include weight reduction and physical exercise.
- Moderation of sodium intake should help to lower blood pressure in patients with excessive intake.

TREATMENT

The purpose of treating hypertension is to prevent the morbidity and mortality associated with high blood pressure. The recommendations of the JNC V are that the systolic blood pressure be below 140 mm Hg and the diastolic blood pressure be below 90 mm Hg. However, if the patient is diabetic, the goal should be 130/85 mm Hg or less.

Nonpharmacologic Approaches

Weight Reduction

Weight reduction is well established as one method of lowering blood pressure in obese patients. Patients with central, or upper body, obesity have an increased incidence of insulin resistance and hyperinsulinemia. Obesity, particularly when predominantly abdominal, correlates not only with hypertension but also with other coronary risk factors, such as hyperlipidemia and diabetes, as well as with an increased mortality rate from coronary artery disease in general. Blood pressure is usually lowered relatively early in a weight loss program. Obese patients should be enrolled in a weight reduction program with a recommended therapy of regular physical activity and a balanced low-sodium, calorie-restricted diet. Weight reduction without antihypertensive medication may be tried initially to lower blood pressure in patients with modest blood pressure elevation.

Tobacco Cessation

Tobacco cessation is extremely important for hypertensive patients who smoke. Nicotine use is not a risk factor for hypertension; however, both cigarette smoking and hypertension are risk factors for coronary artery disease. Smoking cessation may involve not only individual counseling by the physician but also perhaps appropriate medication and referral to an effective smoking cessation program.

Reduction of Excessive Alcohol Intake

Excessive alcohol use can elevate blood pressure in some patients and prevent medicinal control of blood pressure with the usual dosages. Patients with hypertension who drink alcoholic beverages should be advised to limit their daily intake to no more than 1 ounce of ethanol (equivalent to 24 ounces of beer, 8 ounces of wine, or 2 ounces of 100-proof whiskey). Furthermore, a medical problem such as the development of high blood pressure may present the physician with a significant opportunity to deal with the primary problem of alcohol abuse.

Regular Physical Activity

Regular physical activity is an important aspect in treating hypertension. Sedentary people are at a higher risk for developing hypertension, and studies show that exercise can reduce the systolic blood pressure in hypertensive patients by as much as 10 mm Hg. For sedentary patients, moderate activity such as 30 to 45 minutes of walking four to five times each week can prove beneficial. Patients with known cardiac disease likely merit a full examination (including an exercise stress test) before starting an exercise program, but most patients can safely begin a program of gradually increasing levels of physical activity.

Moderation of Sodium Intake

Moderation of sodium intake should help to lower blood pressure in patients with excessive intake. Multiple studies have demonstrated that the systolic blood pressure may drop 5 to 10 mm Hg with sodium restriction. Certain populations, such as African-Americans, diabetic patients, and the elderly, appear to be more sensitive to a reduction in dietary sodium. The average American diet has more than 150 mmol of sodium per day; recommendations are that sodium intake be reduced to less than 100 mmol per day, which is less than 6 grams of sodium chloride—an achievable goal.

Potassium and Calcium Intake

Although some reports claim that lower than average intake of potassium and calcium causes elevated blood pressure, many hypertensive patients with low potassium or calcium intake do not have high blood pressure. If a patient has a low potassium or calcium intake, the necessary dietary changes to correct the deficiency should be recommended; however, it is unlikely that a significant blood pressure response will occur in most patients. It is not recommended that a high potassium or calcium intake be instituted as basic antihypertensive therapy.

Relaxation Therapy

Relaxation therapy does not appear to be reliable as a definitive mode of therapy for most hypertensive patients (Trials of Hypertension Prevention, 1992).

However, relaxation techniques may be beneficial for other reasons in some patients, and if there is an antihypertensive effect, it is an added benefit.

Medication Selection Based On Populations

Younger Patients

Younger patients (defined as those under age 45) with hypertension may respond better to some medications than do other populations. Before initiating antihypertensive agents, the nonpharmacologic approaches discussed above should be implemented. Younger patients often eat fast foods, which can be high in fat and salt, or use excessive amounts of alcohol. Thus, recommending appropriate dietary changes is particularly important. Remember also that birth control pills are risky in women with hypertension.

Generally, any class of antihypertensive agent may be used in a younger patient, but there are selected issues to consider.

- Migraine headaches is a problem seen relatively frequently in the younger population. For patients with frequent migraines, a beta blocker should be considered to treat two problems with one medication.
- Beta blockers also work well in younger patients, who typically have hyperdynamic cardiovascular systems. However, for physically active patients, many of the beta blockers cause diminished exercise tolerance and create a sense of general fatigue.
- Beta blockers may also cause impotence, an unacceptable consequence for younger males, as well as decreased libido. This no doubt accounts for the large increase in the use of ACE inhibitors and calcium channel blockers in recent years, although the antihypertensive effectiveness of beta blockers tends to be better in the younger population than in the elderly.
- The younger population may also have fewer problems than the elderly with constipation secondary to medication with calcium channel blockers, and thus may tolerate them better.
- In general, the younger population tends not to tolerate agents that work through the central nervous system (CNS) because the potential side effects may interfere with work and family responsibilities.
- Given the lifestyle of younger patients, it is advisable to prescribe medications that are taken once daily to improve compliance.
- With the major efforts to identify and treat hypercholesterolemia in younger adults, a medication that does not raise cholesterol levels is desirable.

Elderly Patients

The incidence of isolated systolic hypertension increases in elderly (older than age 60) patients. The Systolic Hypertension in the Elderly Program (1993) demonstrated the danger of isolated systolic hypertension in older patients and the marked benefit of reducing the systolic blood pressure. The initial goal of therapy is to reduce systolic blood pressure to less than 160 mm Hg in those patients whose systolic blood pressure is greater than 180 mm Hg, and to decrease the systolic blood pressure by 20 mm Hg in those patients whose blood pressure measurements are between 160 and 179 mm Hg. If the change in blood pressure is well tolerated, it is appropriate to attempt to slowly lower the systolic blood pressure further, to a goal of 140 or less. Because elderly patients have diminished baroreceptor and sympathetic nervous system responsiveness and impaired cerebral autoregulation, therapy should be instituted at lower dosages and with a more gradual dose increase than is appropriate for younger patients.

- Elderly patients tend to respond better to diuretics, calcium channel blockers, and ACE inhibitors, and less to beta blockers, than does the younger population.
- Isolated systolic hypertension may respond to a diuretic alone.
- Although there can be a good response to agents that work through the CNS (e.g., clonidine, reserpine), the elderly are more prone than younger patients to adverse effects.
- Postural hypotension is a particular risk, and therefore agents that are associated with this problem may need to be avoided.

The elderly often have numerous coexisting conditions. Some antihypertensive agents may adversely affect the patient with a coexisting disease or interact unfavorably with a medication. Conversely, many beneficial effects are associated with some drugs, which can treat more than one disease process (e.g., the symptoms of benign prostatic hypertrophy in an older man can be reduced by using selective α_1-blockers).

Because the elderly may have an increased prevalence of either identified or yet-to-be identified cardiac conduction abnormalities, the dihydropyridine calcium channel blockers are probably a better choice than the nondihydropyridine calcium channel blockers (verapamil and diltiazem), which depress sino-atrial and atrioventricular nodal functions.

Many elderly people live on fixed incomes and their medical expenses perhaps are covered only by Medicare.

It is important that consideration be given to lower-priced medications, such as the generic thiazides and beta blockers and certain ACE inhibitors and calcium channel blockers, which are available generically.

African-Americans

The high prevalence of hypertension in the African-American population is well identified. In the Multiple Risk Factor Intervention Trial (1982), African-American men with blood pressure control comparable to their white cohorts experienced a greater increase in serum creatinine levels during follow-up. Presently, the National Institutes of Health (NIH) is sponsoring a national multicenter study of African-Americans with hypertension and kidney disease to determine how hypertensive nephrosclerosis is affected by blood pressure controlled at two different levels, with either a beta blocker, a calcium channel blocker, or an ACE inhibitor. The findings of this study may demonstrate whether Africans-Americans better benefit from a blood pressure goal of 130/80 mm Hg versus a lower blood pressure of 120/75 mm Hg.

Studies over the years have suggested that African-Americans tend to respond better to calcium channel blockers and diuretics than they do to ACE inhibitors and beta blockers. However, there still may be some response to the latter two drug families. Even if there is only a 14-mm Hg drop in systolic blood pressure with a beta blocker, compared with an 18-mm Hg drop with another agent, the selection of a beta blocker makes sense for the patient with modest hypertension who has had a myocardial infarction (MI) or angina.

Similarly, the ACE inhibitors are reasonable choices for the patient with congestive heart failure (CHF). Because of the increased prevalence of volume-mediated hypertension, many African-Americans respond well to diuretic therapy, the effectiveness of which is improved by restricted dietary sodium intake.

Patients with Diabetes

Diabetic patients on antihypertensive medications pose a special challenge. Particular concerns include:

- Thiazide diuretics can increase insulin resistance and, in some patients, worsen diabetic control. However, many diabetic patients tolerate low doses of a thiazide diuretic without such complications.
- Diabetic patients tend to have volume-mediated hypertension, which is another indication for diuretic therapy. However, careful follow-up is required to avoid hypokalemia, which is considered a cause of increased mortality seen in diabetic patients using diuretics.

- Another concern is that diabetic patients who use beta blockers, particularly those who take insulin, are at increased risk for asymptomatic hypoglycemic reactions, which can be prolonged and result in seizures. Initial antihypertensive choices should include ACE inhibitors and calcium channel blockers.
- ACE inhibitors offer a particular advantage for patients with diabetic nephropathy. Recent published reports suggest that these products may slow the progression of renal failure.
- α_1-receptor blockers are now classified as first-line agents for hypertension by the JNC V and therefore should be considered for diabetic patients because of their ability to improve lipid levels and insulin sensitivity. These agents must be used cautiously, however, because they may aggravate orthostatic hypotension.

Patients with COPD or Asthma

Patients with COPD or asthma typically are not good candidates for beta blockers because of the risk of bronchospasm. Even cardioselective agents become less selective at higher doses. Many patients who have COPD also have coronary artery disease, and if these patients are able to tolerate modest doses, a cardioselective beta blocker (atenolol 25–50 mg/day or metoprolol 50–100 mg/day) should be tried.

If a beta blocker is necessary, warn the patient about the potential adverse effects to the respiratory system and initiate medications at low doses with close supervision.

Some patients with COPD do not experience wheezing but instead have a chronic cough. The cough may become worse with ACE inhibitors, although it tends to originate from the throat. Regardless the cough's origin, it may not be well tolerated by the patient. If an alternative to ACE inhibitors is required, particularly if the patient has concomitant CHF, angiotensin II receptor blockers may be considered. Calcium channel blockers may be the best tolerated.

Patients with Chronic Renal Failure (CRF)

The hypertensive patient with CRF poses another special challenge for the primary care physician. Hypertension in patients with CRF is worsened or caused solely by sodium and water retention. In general, if the serum creatinine level is above 2 mg/dL, thiazide diuretics are less effective than are loop diuretics. A loop diuretic such as furosemide, bumetanide, or indapamide, should be used for adequate diuresis.

If the patient does not respond well to a loop diuretic, an additive effect may be obtained with a distal diuretic, particularly metolazone. The thiazide diuretic may enhance the diuretic effect of its action in the distal nephron.

Nearly all other classes of antihypertensive agents can be used in patients with CRF. However, some medications may cause hyperkalemia, particularly if the patient is diabetic or has interstitial renal disease. These medications include ACE inhibitors, beta blockers, and potassium-sparing diuretics. Angiotensin II receptor blockers are thought to be less likely to cause hyperkalemia, but this has not yet been established.

When ACE inhibitors or angiotensin II receptor blockers are started, check the patient's renal function within 24 to 72 hours of initiating therapy. If CRF is the result of unilateral arterial obstruction to a solitary kidney or of bilateral RAS, ACE inhibitors and angiotensin II receptor blockers can cause a marked hypotensive response and acutely worsen renal function, and thus should not be used in this setting. Typically, renal function is restored after stopping the medication, and it is therefore best to consider initiating therapy with a shorter-acting agent, such as captopril.

The physician must keep in mind that as renal function deteriorates, the dose of most ACE inhibitors, with the exception of fosinopril, should be reduced. The dose of diuretics typically needs to be increased to effect a diuresis.

Resistant hypertension is frequently the setting in which minoxidil is initiated. Before starting minoxidil, it is prudent to consult a nephrologist. It is important to maintain tight blood pressure control in patients with resistant hypertension because studies suggest that lowering the blood pressure to 130/85 mm Hg or less can significantly slow the progression of renal failure.

Patients with Cardiovascular Disease

Angina   Beta blockers can be used to treat angina as well as hypertension. The same may be said for calcium channel blockers.

Myocardial infarction   If the hypertensive patient has suffered an MI, a beta blocker is a good choice if left ventricular function is preserved. If left ventricular function is not preserved, an ACE inhibitor can be used.

Congestive heart failure   A wealth of data demonstrates the value of ACE inhibitors in treating CHF. Because CHF is also a salt- and water-retentive condition, diuretics together with ACE inhibitors can be used to control blood pressure. However, an exagger-

ated hypotensive response may occur in patients with diastolic dysfunction, particularly in the elderly. Also, the combination of ACE inhibitors and diuretics carries with it a high risk of acute renal failure (ARF) when used in patients with CHF.

If the patient has diastolic dysfunction, he or she might better benefit from a beta blocker or calcium channel blocker. Although historically beta blockers have been avoided in treating most forms of CHF, new beta blockers such as carvedilol demonstrate marked improvement in morbidity in patients with certain types of CHF. For patients with a compromised ejection fraction, however, the older beta blockers may markedly worsen CHF because of the decreased inotropic and chronotropic effects.

Arrythmias   There are special considerations for patients with arrhythmias. Patients who take diuretics are at increased risk of developing arrhythmias if hypokalemia or hypomagnesemia, or both, occurs. The physician may wish to add a potassium supplement or use a potassium-sparing diuretic. For those hypertensive patients with tachyarrhythmias, beta blockers and nondihydropyridine calcium channel blockers are appropriate medications to consider.

Classes of Antihypertensive Medication

Diuretics

Diuretics are the most frequently prescribed drugs used to treat hypertension. Diuretics work by decreasing plasma volume and cardiac output and, over time, by decreasing total peripheral resistance. The most widely used diuretics since the 1950s are the thiazides. Loop diuretics such as furosemide and bumetanide are less effective than the thiazides, except in individuals with chronic renal impairment.

Thiazides have the advantage of once-daily dosing and are typically inexpensive. Thiazides are identified by the JNC V as one of two preferred agents (the other is the beta blocker) recommended for initial hypertension therapy.

Metolazone is a thiazide diuretic that is effective in renal failure. However, like other thiazides, it is contraindicated in patients with anuria and in patients allergic to sulfa.

The potassium-sparing diuretics such as triamterene are actually weak diuretics and are typically used in combination with other diuretics to reduce hypokalemia.

Indapamide decreases not only blood pressure but also vascular reactivity and resistance. It has less effect on lipid metabolism than do thiazides.

Side effects and contraindications The most common side effects of diuretics include:

- Hypokalemia
- Hypomagnesemia (with loop diuretics)
- Hyperuricemia
- Hyperglycemia (less of a problem with loop diuretics)
- Hyperlipidemia (occurs more frequently with thiazides)

Hyponatremia may also occur, but usually it is in the elderly female patient on a thiazide diuretic.

With the exception of ethacrynic acid, thiazides and loop diuretics are contraindicated in those patients with sulfa allergies. After a few decades of thiazide use, physicians recognized that potential adverse effects could be reduced significantly by decreasing the dosage and that approximately 80 to 90% of the blood pressure lowering effect would occur. As an example, hydrochlorothiazide was historically given in doses of 50 or 100 mg daily, whereas currently a 25-mg daily dose is usual. A large patient may require 50 mg but the small or older patient may respond well to 12.5 mg. Despite there being fewer adverse effects associated with a lower dose, periodically take the patient's electrolyte, uric acid, glucose, and lipid measurements.

Beta Blockers

Beta blockers have long been used as antihypertensive agents. These agents may lower blood pressure by decreasing cardiac output and sympathetic outflow and by blocking plasma renin release and postsynaptic peripheral β-receptors.

Some beta blockers are cardioselective agents, including:

- Atenolol
- Betaxolol
- Bisoprolol
- Metoprolol

As with diuretics, many beta blockers are available generically. As a group, the JNC V recommends their use for initial therapy. These agents can be used in patients with coexisting diseases such as migraine headaches and coronary artery disease. There are numerous generic beta blockers, but it may be best to consistently use one or two instead of trying them all.

Side effects and complications Some of the older beta blocking agents, such as propranolol, are used less frequently than newer agents because they cause more CNS side effects as a result of increased lipid solu-

bility and bronchoconstriction. Other beta blocker side effects include:

- Bradycardia
- Heart block
- Bronchoconstriction
- Abnormal glucose metabolism
- Hyperglycemia

α_1-Receptor Blockers

The α_1-receptor blocker family includes prazosin, terazosin, and doxazosin, which can be considered for step I therapy. These agents work by blocking the postsynaptic α_1-receptors and causing vasodilation. Rarely, they may cause first-dose syncope or hypotension; however, this is more likely to occur in patients who are volume depleted, on diuretics, are elderly, or who have diabetes. Thus, each of the three agents should be initiated at a low dose of 1 mg at bedtime, and then carefully titrated to an effective level that the patient can tolerate.

Because these drugs improve symptoms of benign prostatic hypertrophy, they should be considered for the older, hypertensive male patient with this problem. They are also notable for their lipid-lowering effect and enhanced insulin sensitivity, making them particularly attractive for those patients with hyperlipidemia or diabetes.

Side effects The most common side effects, which are most likely the result of decreased blood pressure, include:

- Headache
- Drowsiness
- Fatigue
- Weakness

ACE Inhibitors

The ACE inhibitors (the "prils") have played an increased role in antihypertensive therapy. The original agent, captopril, is now available generically, which may lead to lower prices for this family of drugs.

The ACE inhibitors block the formation of angiotensin II, which results in direct vasodilation and decreased aldosterone secretion. It is advisable to reduce the dose in the patient already on diuretics before starting the ACE inhibitor to prevent excessive hypotension.

Side effects and complications As noted earlier, hyperkalemia may become a problem in some patients, and thus patients who have other risk factors for hyperkalemia, such as renal failure or diabetes, need to be observed closely. ACE inhibitors have been shown to cause ARF in patients with severe bilateral RAS or stenosis in an artery leading to a solitary kidney (from renal transplantation or a nonfunctional contralateral kidney).

The side effects include:

- Dry cough
- Skin rash
- Taste alteration
- Angioedema

The effectiveness of these agents is increased when the patient maintains low sodium intake and avoids the concomitant use of nonsteroidal antiinflammatory drugs (NSAIDs). NSAIDs also increase the risk of developing ARF, particularly when the patient is volume depleted, typically because of concomitant diuretic therapy.

Angiotensin II Receptor Blockers

The angiotensin II receptor blockers represent a relatively new family of antihypertensive drugs. The drugs act by blocking one of two identified receptors for angiotensin. Unlike ACE inhibitors, they are not associated with a dry cough, a side effect believed to result from the accumulation of bradykinin. However, like the ACE inhibitors, they can cause ARF in patients with RAS. Hyperkalemia is less likely to develop with angiotensin II receptor blocking agents.

Calcium Channel Blockers

Calcium channel blockers are widely used for antihypertensive therapy. They are also recommended as first-line therapy by the JNC V. These drugs gained broad use in the 1980s. Calcium channel blockers act by inhibiting the influx of calcium ions through slow channels in vascular smooth muscle tissue, resulting in the relaxation of arterioles. They have a mild natriuretic effect and a neutral or favorable effect on lipids. They have been shown to reduce left ventricular hypertrophy.

The calcium channel blockers include:

- Verapamil
- Diltiazem
- Dihydropyridines (e.g., nifedipine, amlodipine, felodipine, and isradipine)

Side effects and complications　Conduction disorders are seen with verapamil and, to a lesser degree, diltiazem. Verapamil and diltiazem block the slow calcium channels in the heart and thus generally should be avoided in patients with sick sinus syndrome, second- or third-degree heart block, or CHF.

The dihydropyridines are more potent peripheral vasodilators and hence more effective in lowering blood pressure. Vasodilatory side effects, such as headaches, flushing, and local ankle edema, are more common with dihydropyridines but less common with the second generation of slower-release and longer-acting preparations.

Because calcium channel blockers are also approved for angina management, these agents are often used in patients having both hypertension and angina. Controversy developed in the mid-1990s when a study linked calcium channel blockers to an increased rate of MIs. This was a case-controlled, retrospective study in which shorter-acting formulations of calcium channel blockers were used. The current recommendation is to use longer-acting agents approved for use in hypertension and to avoid shorter-acting agents.

Centrally Acting α_2 Agonists

Centrally acting α_2 agonists are not considered a step I option but are often used as supplements. This family includes:

- Clonidine
- Guanabenz
- Guanfacine
- Methyldopa

These drugs act by stimulating the central postsynaptic α_2-adrenergic receptors, thereby reducing the sympathetic nervous system activity, which also results in decreased plasma renin activity.

Side effects and complications　Because of the drugs' mode of action, side effects are related to the CNS and include sedation, dry mouth, fatigue, and dizziness. With the exception of guanfacine, these agents must be taken two to three times daily, which can affect compliance. Although the risk of an abrupt withdrawal syndrome can be seen with almost any antihypertensive agent, it occurs most frequently with clonidine. The risk of rebound hypertension, however, is less with a daily dose of less than 1.2 mg. These agents are available in generic forms.

Peripheral-acting Adrenergic Agents

Peripheral-acting adrenergic agents include guanadrel and guanethidine. They are not often used in primary care settings because they are potent agents that may cause significant orthostatic hypotension and are poorly tolerated by most patients. The physician may want to seek a nephrology consultation if considering one of these agents.

The Rauwolfia alkaloid group includes primarily reserpine. Reserpine is an older agent that is occasionally used today. It is taken once daily and is better tolerated in low doses. Its major drawback is CNS depression.

Direct Vasodilators

Another family of drugs used less often in the primary care setting is the direct vasodilators. These products include hydralazine and minoxidil. They enter vascular smooth muscle and cause vasodilation.

With the development of more effective agents such as the calcium channel blockers and ACE inhibitors, hydralazine is used less often today for hypotension. When hydralazine is used, it can serve as a third agent for individuals with severe hypertension.

Minoxidil is more potent than hydralazine and is typically reserved for those individuals with severe hypertension. It is seldom used in the primary care setting, and the assistance of a nephrologist should be considered before starting this medication.

Side effects and complications Hirsutism is the most common side effect of direct vasodilators, typically beginning on the face, which is unacceptable to most women. Development of a pericardial effusion is considered a risk associated with taking minoxidil; however, it typically develops in patients with chronic renal failure and may be secondary to uremia. Vasodilators are notorious for causing fluid retention and reflex tachycardia; therefore, diuretics and either a beta blocker or clonidine are often required to reduce the heart rate.

Step Therapy

Given the multitude of antihypertensive drugs, it is fair to say that step therapy has changed from the original presentation of this concept in the 1970s. However, it may not be useful to conclude that step therapy is obsolete. It still conveys the concept that medications should be tried for most patients one at a time.

If the initial medication is not adequately controlling the blood pressure, it should not be increased to the maximum recommended dose because it may cause undesirable side effects. A second agent should be added instead, preferably one of a different class. However, if there is minimal blood pressure response to a particular medication, consider discontinuing the drug and trying another agent, unless the two medications act synergistically. If the patient has a moderate blood pressure elevation, it should not be necessary to start two medications at the same time. With the exception

of the hospitalized patient in a hypertensive crisis, the goal should be to control the blood pressure gradually.

Compliance Issues

Simplifying Complicated Regimens

Hypertension is a chronic condition and typically asymptomatic. As a result, patient compliance can be an issue.

The noncompliant patient may miss several appointments or may not have physiologic or laboratory evidence of taking certain medications (e.g., bradycardia from a beta blocker or mild hypokalemia or hyperuricemia from a diuretic). Knowledge of a patient's educational level, attitude toward the disease, and perception of the importance of hypertension may help offer solutions for getting the patient to take a more active role in controlling his or her disease.

Compliance can be improved by educating the patient about hypertension, its sequelae, and the goal of therapy. Compliance is also improved by giving the patient careful, written instructions on how to take the medication and how to make appropriate lifestyle changes. If possible, prescribe medications that can be taken once daily, simplifying complicated regimens.

Side Effects and Complications

Side effects are a major source of noncompliance. The physician must determine how well a patient is tolerating medication. If a patient has difficulty with excessive fatigue, weakness, impotence, edema, or polyuria, he or she often will discontinue the medication. Fortunately, there are many agents with different side effect profiles to choose from.

Cost

The cost of medications can be a problem for many patients. Because many hypertensive patients are elderly and live on fixed incomes, with only Medicare for insurance coverage, the cost of antihypertensive medications can be significant. The minimum effective dosage should be used, as well as generic forms of the drugs. Combination drugs, when applicable, can be considered, and the use of tablets that can be broken in half can be economic.

REFRACTORY HYPERTENSION

Patients with blood pressure measurements that are consistently higher than 140/90 mm Hg (or higher than 160/90 mm Hg in patients older than age 60), despite use of two or more antihypertensive agents, adequate duration of therapy, and lack of evidence suggestive of secondary hypertension, are considered to have refractory, or resistant, hypertension. When considering this diagnosis, it is important to:

- Determine whether the blood pressure was measured properly and rule out pseudohypertension.
- For those patients in whom white-coat hypertension is suspected, obtain a record of measurements done outside the office (preferably from home) or order 24-hour ambulatory blood pressure monitoring.
- Make certain that the patient is compliant with dietary restrictions and medications.
- Review all medications taken by the patient and make certain that the doses are adequate. If more than one agent is required, make certain that they are complementary and not of the same drug family.
- Evaluate drug resistance by 24-hour ambulatory blood pressure monitoring.
- Encourage weight loss, because obesity can cause poor blood pressure control (perhaps in some patients because of associated insulin resistance and glucose intolerance).

Measuring Sodium Intake

Often, resistant hypertension is the result of volume overload, which is caused by either excessive sodium intake or inadequate diuresis. A 24-hour urine collection to measure sodium (together with creatinine measurement to ensure an adequate collection) can be ordered to determine if the patient is compliant with a low-sodium diet.

A urine sodium concentration greater than 120 mEq/24 hr is indicative of poor dietary compliance. Blood pressure is particularly sensitive to excessive sodium intake in African-Americans, in elderly patients, and in individuals with diabetes or renal insufficiency. With the possible exception of calcium channel blockers, most antihypertensive agents are more effective if the patient follows a low-sodium diet.

To assure adequate diuresis, the appropriate diuretic must be selected. Thiazide diuretics should be used in individuals with normal renal function because they are better antihypertensive agents than are loop diuretics. If the creatinine clearance rate is less than 30 mL/min, a loop diuretic must be used.

DISABILITY DETERMINATION AND REFERRAL

Patients may seek disability because they believe that job-related stress is causing or worsening their hypertension. Although each case is different, hypertension in and of itself is not a reason for a patient to be declared disabled. Decisions should be based on evidence of significant end organ damage, such as strokes or severe heart failure.

If the patient is having adverse sequelae related to stress, this would be an excellent opportunity to enlist the ancillary services of a social worker, psychologist, or psychiatrist. If the patient insists on using hypertension as a disability, it may be appropriate to consult a nephrologist or cardiologist who has a special interest in hypertension. Of course, a patient may simply skip the medication on the day of the office visit and claim to have refractory hypertension.

KEY POINTS

- A beta blocker, such as propranolol or atenolol, is a good choice for medication for a young hypertensive patient, in particular one with a history of migraines.

- Impotence, as well as decreased libido, may be an unacceptable side effect of beta blockers and may require switching to ACE inhibitors or calcium channel blockers.

- α_1 blockers, such as doxazosin, may be a good choice of medication to treat an elderly hypertensive patient, especially if nocturnal urinary frequency is associated.

- Beta blockers and thiazide diuretics are the least expensive of the drugs to treat hypertension and are as effective as other antihypertensive agents, but with three side effects: impotence, decreased insulin sensitivity with elevated glucose levels, and hyperlipidemia.

- The fewer the number of drugs prescribed, the more easily compliance is achieved.

- Compliance is key to successfully treating hypertension.

COMMONLY ASKED QUESTIONS

How do I know if my blood pressure is not just high because of stress?

To avoid misdiagnosing someone with hypertension, the blood pressure is measured on more than one occasion. Furthermore, the blood pressure can be checked at home and by 24-hour monitoring to confirm or refute a solitary blood pressure measurement.

Will I always have hypertension?

This depends on several factors, such as the cause of the high blood pressure, dietary habits, weight, age, race, and family history. Nonpharmacologic treatment measures such as weight loss and decreased sodium intake may improve blood pressure control. However, these are not the only factors that contribute to hypertension, and therefore continued blood pressure monitoring is necessary. Although hypertension may be resolved if it is the result of a secondary process, essential hypertension must be followed, especially since the prevalence of hypertension increases with advancing age.

Will over-the-counter medications such as decongestants be safe for me to use?

Generally, over-the-counter agents such as decongestants can be taken as directed by patients whose blood pressure is under control. Patients may wish to check their blood pressure one hour after taking an over-the-counter medication to be sure it is not rising. If blood pressure is poorly controlled, the use of such agents is not recommended unless under medical supervision. Patients should inform their physicians about any medications with warnings pertaining to hypertension, particularly if they will be taken for more than 48 hours.

How did I get hypertension if my parents did not have it?

Other factors besides genetics can play a role in development of hypertension. These include age, obesity, excessive salt intake, and stress, with great individual variation regarding how blood pressure responds to certain factors. Most patients with hypertension have no identifiable reasons for being hypertensive.

Are the medications that I am taking for hypertension safe?

Medications used to treat hypertension are usually "safe," although any medication has the potential for side effects and allergic reactions.

If a medication is associated with unacceptable side effects, the patient should inform the physician because there are many alternative drugs that can be prescribed.

SUGGESTED READINGS

Joint National Committee. The Joint National Committee on detection, evaluation, and treatment of high blood pressure (JNC V). Arch Intern Med 1993;153:156–183.

Mancia G, Parati G, Pomidossi G, et al. Alerting reaction and rise in blood pressure during measurement by physician and nurse. Hypertension 1987b;9:209–215.

Mandal AK, Markert RJ, Saklayen MG, et al. Diuretics potentiate angiotensin-converting enzyme inhibitor–induced acute renal failure. Clin Nephrol 1994;42:170–174.

Multiple Risk Factor Intervention Trial Research Group. Multiple risk factor intervention trial. JAMA 1982;248:1465–1477.

Peiris AN, Stagner JI, Vogel RL, et al. Body fat distribution and peripheral insulin sensitivity in healthy men: role of insulin pulsatility. J Clin Endocrinol Metab 1992;75:290–294.

Systolic Hypertension in the Elderly Program Cooperative Research Group. Implications of the systolic hypertension in the elderly program. Hypertension 1993;21:335–343.

Trials of Hypertension Prevention Collaborative Research Group. The effects of nonpharmacologic interventions of blood pressure in persons with high normal levels: results of the Trials of Hypertension Prevention Phase I. JAMA 1992;267:1213–1220.

World Hypertension League. Physical exercise in the management of hypertension: a consensus statement by the World Hypertension League. Hypertension 1991;9:283–287.

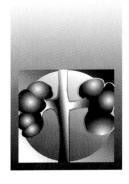

12
CHAPTER

Renovascular Hypertension

Shelly M. Heidelbaugh
N. Stanley Nahman, Jr.

BACKGROUND

Renovascular hypertension is a secondary form of hypertension resulting from renal artery stenosis (RAS). It is important that the clinician identify the disease because it is a potentially curable form of hypertension, as are other forms of secondary hypertension (Table 12.1). Most forms of RAS result from atherosclerosis or fibromuscular dysplasia of the renal artery. RAS resulting from atherosclerotic vascular disease is the most common form of renovascular hypertension.

CAUSES

In general, the patient tends to be older and may have a history of large-vessel vascular disease (coronary artery

disease or peripheral vascular disease). Other risk factors include those associated typically with atherosclerotic vascular disease (obesity, smoking, hyperlipidemia). Pathologically, the disease is characterized by accumulation of atherosclerotic plaque with subsequent luminal narrowing leading to renal ischemia and resulting in hypertension and/or renal insufficiency.

Fibromuscular Dysplasia

Fibromuscular dysplasia is a less common form of RAS affecting primarily young, Caucasian females. Pathologically, fibromuscular dysplasia results from dysplasia of the intima, media, or periarterial vessel wall. The most common type of lesion in fibromuscular dysplasia is

Secondary Forms of Hypertension	**TABLE 12.1**

Renal hypertension
  Renal parenchymal disease
  Renovascular hypertension
    Atherosclerotic RAS
    Renal artery fibromuscular dysplasia
    Coarctation of the aorta with renal ischemia
    Aortoarteritis
Endocrine hypertension
  Primary hyperaldosteronism
  Cushing's syndrome
  Pheochromocytoma
Miscellaneous causes
  Decongestant ingestion
  Appetite suppressants
  Excessive ethanol
  Oral contraceptives
  Licorice, mineralocorticoids, or corticosteroids

medial hyperplasia, which produces a characteristic "string of beads" appearance on renal angiography. Fibromuscular dysplasia presents as hypertension and, in contrast to atherosclerotic RAS, rarely gives rise to chronic renal failure. However, the diagnostic approach and therapy for fibromuscular dysplasia are similar to those for atherosclerotic renovascular hypertension.

Increased Renal Renin Release

Generally, hypertension resulting from RAS is secondary to renal ischemia with increased renal renin release (Fig. 12.1). Renin is an enzyme that catalyzes the conversion of angiotensinogen to angiotensin I. Angiotensin I is, in turn, converted to angiotensin II by angiotensin-converting enzyme (ACE). Angiotensin II is a potent vasoconstrictor and increases the release of aldosterone from the adrenal glands. Aldosterone increases distal tubular sodium reabsorption and potassium excretion. The combination of increased vascular tone from

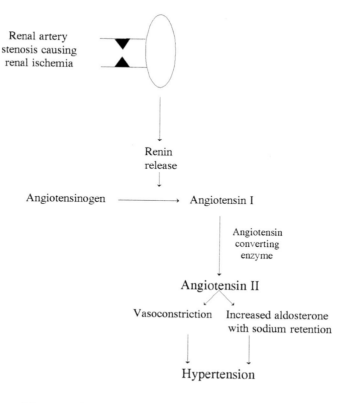

FIGURE 12.1.
Pathophysiology of hypertension resulting from renal ischemia and activation of the renin angiotensin system.

angiotensin II and volume expansion from aldosterone results clinically in hypertension. Reversing RAS with either angioplasty or surgery improves renal perfusion and thus inactivates the series of responses delineated previously. This may result in a decrease in blood pressure and, in some cases, improvement in renal function.

DIAGNOSIS

RAS may result in hypertension and/or chronic renal insufficiency. Clues to the diagnosis are based on the history and physical examination.

History

Renovascular hypertension should be suspected when the onset of hypertension is abrupt in patients younger than 20 (fibromuscular dysplasia with RAS) or older than 50 (atherosclerotic RAS) years of age. The development of labile or resistant hypertension in a patient with previously stable blood pressure control may also signal the onset of RAS. Finally, any patient with a history of malignant hypertension is a candidate for renovascular disease.

Patients with hypertension and known large-vessel atherosclerosis should also be considered at higher risk for development of RAS. This includes patients with the following characteristics:

- Documented peripheral vascular disease or claudication
- Status postcerebral vascular accident or carotid endarterectomy
- Known coronary artery disease or angina
- Postcoronary artery bypass grafting

Patients who have any of the aforementioned characteristics, who are heavy smokers, as well as others at risk for large-vessel peripheral vascular atherosclerosis should also be considered at risk for development of renovascular hypertension. Finally, hypertension with an unexplained history of acute pulmonary edema (flash pulmonary edema) is also associated with bilateral RAS.

Physical Examination

The classic presentation of renovascular hypertension is the presence of hypertension and a systolic-diastolic abdominal or flank bruit. Systolic bruits without a diastolic component may still represent RAS but can also be confused with loud cardiac murmurs, aortic coarctation or aneurysms, and vascular bruits associated with the celiac or mesenteric circulations. **Hypertension and the presence of bruits, whether specific for RAS or consistent with generalized peripheral vascular disease, should heighten one's suspicion for the presence of renovascular hypertension.**

Index of Clinical Suspicion and Confirmation of Diagnosis

The diagnosis of atherosclerotic RAS is usually considered in patients with difficult-to-control hypertension or in hypertensive patients with unexplained azotemia. The prevalence of renovascular hypertension in patients with hypertension is low (1–5%); thus, suspicion of the disease must be based on specific clinical clues. The presence of such clues allows the clinician to define an index of clinical suspicion that can guide the evaluation (Table 12.2).

TABLE 12.2 Criteria for Developing an Index of Clinical Suspicion in Patients with Suspected RAS

Index of Clinical Suspicion	Clinical Criteria
Low	Borderline or mild hypertension
Moderate	Diastolic blood pressure ≥ 120 mm Hg
	Hypertension refractory to therapy
	Abrupt onset of hypertension in the young or elderly
	Hypertension with abdominal bruit
	Moderate hypertension plus: smoking history, large-vessel atherosclerosis, unexplained increase in serum creatinine
	Prompt blood pressure reduction response to ACE inhibitor or beta-blockers
High	Severe hypertension (diastolic blood pressure > 120 mm Hg with unexplained azotemia or refractory to antihypertensive therapy)
	Accelerated hypertension
	Malignant hypertension
	Renal asymmetry
	Ischemic nephropathy (see Table 12.3)

Modified from Mann S, Pickering T. Detection of renovascular hypertension, state of the art. Ann Intern Med 1992;177:845-853.

| Conditions Associated with Ischemic Nephropathy | TABLE 12.3 |

Acute renal failure associated with ACE inhibitors or control of blood pressure
Renal insufficiency with renal asymmetry
Unexplained, progressive azotemia ($<$ 1 gm proteinuria) with refractory hypertension
Unexplained, progressive azotemia in the elderly
Hypertension and azotemia in any patient with a solitary functioning kidney (including renal transplant patients)
Progressive azotemia following medical therapy of known RAS
Flash pulmonary edema in azotemic, hypertensive patients

Modified from Jacobson H. Ischemic renal disease: an overlooked clinical entity? Kidney Int 1988;34:729-743.

Low Index of Clinical Suspicion

Patients for whom there is a low index of clinical suspicion include those with borderline or mild hypertension. These patients need no further evaluation and only require medical therapy for the hypertension.

Moderate Index of Clinical Suspicion

Patients for whom there is a moderate index of clinical suspicion would be expected to have a 5 to 15% likelihood of having renovascular hypertension.

Clinical clues include:

- Diastolic hypertension ($\geq$120 mm Hg) refractory to therapy
- Abrupt onset of severe hypertension in the young or elderly
- Hypertension with appropriate abdominal bruit
- Moderate hypertension in patients with the following features: smoking history, documented large-vessel atherosclerosis, unexplained serum creatinine elevation, or prompt blood pressure reduction by an ACE inhibitor or beta-blocking drug.

A "middle of the road" diagnostic approach to patients with a moderate index of clinical suspicion is taken by Mann and Pickering; they suggest that these patients should undergo noninvasive testing. The authors' group is more aggressive and, in general, would proceed straight to angiography (intra-arterial digital subtraction angiography) in these patients. However, the role of angiography needs to be tailored to its availability, the technical expertise of angiographic support, and the ease of obtaining and interpreting noninvasive studies.

Noninvasive studies are used to identify patients requiring angiography. Thus, a noninvasive test with a positive result implies the presence of renovascular disease and necessitates further evaluation by diagnostic arteriography. In contrast, a negative or normal result from a noninvasive test should terminate the clinical evaluation. Currently, the common noninvasive tests

(discussed later, under "Testing") used to screen for renovascular disease include:

- Captopril stimulation test
- Captopril renography
- Duplex ultrasonography
- Magnetic resonance angiography

Both intravenous pyelography ("hypertensive IVP") and routine renal scintigraphy lack sensitivity and specificity and have been largely abandoned as screening tests for the detection of renovascular disease.

High Index of Clinical Suspicion

The incidence of RAS in patients with a high index of clinical suspicion may be as high as 25% or more. Patients in whom there is a high index of clinical suspicion require diagnostic angiography to assess renovascular anatomy. Syndromes in which the index of clinical suspicion is high include severe hypertension (diastolic blood pressure greater than 120 mm Hg) with unexplained azotemia or hypertension unresponsive to aggressive antihypertensive therapy, accelerated or malignant hypertension, renal asymmetry without significant proteinuria, and any form of ischemic nephropathy.

Ischemic nephropathy (Table 12.3) refers to azotemia resulting from renal hypoperfusion and may be associated with numerous clinical syndromes. These syndromes include:

- Acute renal failure (ARF)-associated angiotensin converting enzyme (ACE) inhibitor therapy
- ARF associated with control of blood pressure
- Renal insufficiency with renal asymmetry
- Progressive azotemia (with less than 1 gm proteinuria/ 24 hr) with refractory hypertension
- Unexplained progressive azotemia in the elderly
- Hypertension and azotemia in any patient with a solitary kidney (including transplant kidneys)
- Progressive azotemia following medical therapy of known RAS

- Flash pulmonary edema in azotemic and hypertensive patients

Hypertensive patients who present with unexplained renal insufficiency and any of the aforementioned findings should be strongly considered for diagnostic angiography.

Testing

The diagnostic evaluation of patients with suspected renovascular disease includes assessment of renal function by measurement of serum creatinine as well as physiologic and radiographic tests that may give clues to the presence of RAS.

Noninvasive studies include:

- Determination of peripheral plasma renin activity (PRA)
- Captopril stimulation test
- Captopril renography
- Duplex ultrasonography
- Magnetic resonance angiography

Invasive testing, discussed in the following section, includes:

- Digital subtraction arteriography or venography
- Conventional renal arteriography

Noninvasive testing

BLOOD SAMPLE STUDIES   On routine laboratory screening, an elevated serum creatinine in a hypertensive patient is the most important finding to suggest the presence of renovascular hypertension. It also signals the most advanced form of the disease because it implies a loss of kidney function of sufficient magnitude to raise serum creatinine. This almost always occurs in patients with bilateral RAS. Another clinical clue may include the presence of mild hypokalemia (caused by elevated aldosterone levels). Elevated peripheral PRA found on random studies may be associated with RAS stimulation, but normal or low PRA does not exclude the diagnosis.

CAPTOPRIL STIMULATION TEST   The captopril stimulation test in renovascular disease is based on increased renal renin release from the ischemic kidney following an oral dose of captopril. The test is optimally used in patients who have normal salt intake, are not taking diuretics and, when possible, have stopped taking all antihypertensive medications for at least three weeks.

The test is done in an outpatient clinic or in a doctor's office according to the following steps:

1. The patient arrives in the clinic or office at a scheduled time and rests for 30 minutes.

2. Blood pressure is recorded three times and the average of three readings is noted.
3. A sample of blood is drawn for basal PRA.
4. Captopril, 25 mg, is crushed and mixed with water and given to the patient.
5. Forty-five minutes later, blood pressure is recorded.
6. Ninety minutes later, blood pressure is recorded and a second sample of blood is drawn for PRA. This sample is labeled as #2 PRA.

A positive test result is implied when the following criteria are met:

- Stimulated PRA is greater than 12 ng/mL/hr
- Absolute increase in PRA is at least 10 ng/mL/hr
- Increase in PRA is 150% or greater over baseline, or 400% or greater if the baseline PRA is less than 3 ng/mL/hr
- Sensitivity and specificity ranges from 34 to 100% and 72 to 95%, respectively

The test is relatively inexpensive and, when appropriate patients for testing can be identified, may be a useful screening tool.

CAPTOPRIL RENOGRAPHY   The use of captopril renography in the diagnosis of RAS has the same physiologic rationale as the captopril stimulation test; in the presence of significant renal artery occlusion, ACE inhibition will induce transient renal ischemia in the affected kidney. In contrast to the captopril test, captopril renography uses scintigraphy to localize the stenotic renal artery by demonstrating decreased renal uptake of the marker and/or delayed excretion. The test has a sensitivity and specificity range of 44 to 96% and 42 to 100%, respectively.

One advantage over the captopril stimulation test is that antihypertensive medication, other than ACE inhibitors, need not be discontinued before the test. A major disadvantage, however, is that captopril renography is much more expensive than the captopril stimulation test. In a prospective comparison of the two tests, Elliot et al. showed the tests to be comparable, with a slight advantage to captopril renography. A comparison of the two tests is included in Table 12.4.

PERIPHERAL PLASMA RENIN ACTIVITY   Low peripheral PRA has been suggested to exclude the presence of RAS. The test requires that peripheral PRA be interpreted in the context of dietary sodium intake. After stopping antihypertensive medication for at least 2 weeks, 24-hour urinary sodium excretion is assessed, followed by determination of peripheral PRA. The renin-sodium profile is used to determine the significance of the PRA. When practical to stop a patient's antihypertensive medication, the test may allow for

Comparison of Noninvasive Methods for the Detection of RAS			**TABLE 12.4**
Method	Sensitivity (%)	Specificity (%)	Comments
Peripheral PRA	56–80	up to 80	Simple blood test, requires sodium profiling and withholding all antihypertensive drugs
Captopril test	34–100	72–95	Simple blood test, relatively specific; requires stopping antihypertensive drugs for 3 weeks
Captopril renography	44–96	42–100	Relatively specific; expensive
Duplex sonography	up to 89	up to 99	Operator-dependent; interpretation complicated by obesity, bowel gas
Magnetic resonance angiography	53–100	92–97	Operator-dependent; moderately expensive; may only detect lesions in the proximal one-third of main renal artery; may overestimate severity of lesion

Compiled from Vaughan E. Nephrology forum: renovascular hypertension. Kidney Int 1985;27:811-827. Elliot W, Martin W, Murphy M. Comparison of two non-invasive screening tests for renovascular hypertension. Arch Intern Med 1993;153:755-764. Wilcox C. Use of angiotensin-converting enzyme inhibitors for diagnosing renovascular hypertension. Kidney Int 1993;44:1379-1390. Pickering T, Sos T, Vaughan E, et al. Predictive value and changes of renin secretion in hypertensive patients with unilateral renovascular disease undergoing successful renal angioplasty. Am J Med 1984;76:398-404.

screening of patients not requiring angiography. Random PRA (without sodium profiling and adherence to the study protocol) is not a useful screening test. In the authors' study of renal angioplasty in patients with RAS, up to one-third may have normal or low random PRA, despite high-grade renovascular lesions.

DUPLEX ULTRASONOGRAPHY   Duplex ultrasonography may be used to diagnose significant RAS by identifying decrements in blood flow velocity between the aorta and the renal artery. The test is limited by the technical difficulties associated with imaging deep vessels such as the renal arteries, and the diagnostic utility of the test is strongly dependent on the expertise of the technician doing the test. Furthermore, interpretation of the test may be confounded by the presence of bowel gas, obesity, aortic aneurysm, or history of recent abdominal surgery.

MAGNETIC RESONANCE ANGIOGRAPHY   Magnetic resonance angiography may prove to be a useful noninvasive test for detecting RAS. After an intravenous injection of gadolinium (a nontoxic contrast agent), magnetic resonance scanning is done and the renal arteries are imaged and reconstructed in appropriate planes. The technique has a reported sensitivity and specificity of 53 to 100% and 92 to 97%, respectively. As imaging technology improves, magnetic resonance angiography may become a useful test for identifying patients that require diagnostic angiography.

In summary, a moderate index of suspicion for the presence of renovascular disease may exist in hypertensive patients with normal renal function. Patients with a moderate index of clinical suspicion may be identified as requiring renal angiography using noninvasive testing. If test results are suggestive of RAS, angiography is indicated. When the test results are normal (or negative), they can be used to terminate the work-up. A strong angiography team may allow for more aggressive diagnostic evaluation of hypertensive patients combined with normal renal function and thus alleviate the ambiguities associated with each noninvasive test.

Invasive testing

INTRA-ARTERIAL DIGITAL SUBTRACTION RENAL ARTERIOGRAPHY (IADSA)   IADSA provides acceptable imaging of the main renal arteries and proximal branches. It typically requires femoral arterial cannulation and uses 10 mL or less of ionic or nonionic contrast. IADSA is the screening procedure of choice for high-risk patients at the authors' institution because it provides adequate imaging, is an outpatient procedure, and, given the small volume of contrast, there is a decreased risk of contrast-induced ARF.

CONVENTIONAL RENAL ARTERIOGRAPHY   Conventional renal arteriography is the diagnostic procedure of choice for imaging the renal arterial tree to the level of the arterioles. It is more accurate than IADSA and provides more angiographic detail.

The major disadvantage of conventional renal arteriography is the large volume of contrast (100–200 mL) used in the study. Whether ionic or nonionic contrast is used, these volumes of contrast material increase the incidence of contrast-induced ARF, particularly in patients with impaired renal function.

INTRAVENOUS DIGITAL SUBTRACTION ANGIOGRAPHY (IVDSA) IVDSA can be used to get an image of the renal arteries. IVDSA has the major advantage of being an outpatient procedure and requires only peripheral venous cannulation. However, there are major disadvantages associated with the procedure, including:

- Necessity of using a large-bore venous catheter in the basilic vein
- Large volumes of contrast needed (up to 200 mL) and the inherent risk of contrast-induced ARF
- Poor resolution of the images generated, as the venous contrast load must traverse the right heart and the pulmonary circulation before delivery to the arterial system. This results in dilution of the contrast load and less clear images of the renal arterial tree than can be seen with direct arteriography.

Given the relative advantages of IADSA, IVDSA is not commonly recommended for imaging the renal arteries.

Summary: testing In summary, the diagnostic approach to RAS is based on the clinical index of suspicion, which is an attempt to classify patients according to the expected prevalence of RAS for given clinical findings (Fig. 12.2). Patients with a low index of suspicion do not require further evaluation, whereas patients with a high index of suspicion require arteriography (which for the authors' would be IADSA). Diagnostic dilemmas occur with patients in whom a moderate index of clinical suspicion exists. In the authors' practice, most of these patients would receive IADSA, but the captopril test provides a reasonable alternative in appropriate patients.

TREATMENT

The goal of therapy in RAS is to alleviate the hydrostatic pressure gradient between the aorta and renal circulation distal to the stenotic region. Thus, clinical criteria are used to define renovascular lesions that might be responsive to angioplasty or surgery. Clinically significant renovascular lesions are defined by visual inspection of the angiogram for estimation of magnitude of stenosis or direct measurement of the systolic pressure gradient between prestenotic and

Summary of Diagnosis

- Most forms of RAS result from atherosclerosis or fibromuscular dysplasia of the renal artery.
- RAS resulting from atherosclerotic vascular disease is the most common form of renovascular hypertension.
- Fibromuscular dysplasia is a less common form of RAS affecting primarily young, Caucasian females.
- Renovascular hypertension should be suspected when hypertension is rapid in onset, particularly in patients younger than 20 or older than 50 years of age.
- The development of resistant hypertension in a patient with previously stable blood pressure control may also signal the development of RAS and superimposed renovascular hypertension.
- Patients with documented coronary artery disease or stroke have a higher risk for renovascular hypertension.
- Hypertension with an unexplained history of acute pulmonary edema is likely to be caused by bilateral RAS.
- The common noninvasive tests to screen for renovascular disease include captopril stimulation test, captopril scintigraphy, duplex ultrasonography, and magnetic resonance angiography. If the test results are suggestive of RAS, contrast angiography is indicated.
- Contrast angiogram is done when angioplasty or surgery is contemplated.

poststenotic lesions. By direct inspection, a 50 to 60% reduction in luminal cross-sectional area is generally used to define a significant occlusion. In animal models, a 50% reduction in cross-sectional area corresponds to a 70% reduction in flow. When the systolic pressure gradient is used to grade the severity of luminal compromise, the authors use a gradient of greater than 50 mm Hg as an indication for angioplasty.

Surgical and medical therapy can be used to treat RAS. Surgical options include renal artery angioplasty and vascular bypass surgery and carry the potential advantage of obliterating the renal artery hydrostatic pressure gradient between the aorta and the renal artery, thus curing the condition. In contrast, medical therapy of RAS includes medical management of hypertension and the institution of dialysis when indicated.

Renal Artery Angioplasty

Renal artery angioplasty reverses the systolic pressure gradient associated with RAS. In the authors' series of 171 patients with atherosclerotic RAS, renal artery angioplasty resulted in a significant reduction of the systolic pressure gradient between the aorta and the renal artery from 109 ± 50 mm Hg to 12 ± 16 mm Hg. The majority of patients (72%) had a postangioplasty systolic pressure gradient of 20 mm Hg or less, and 98% of patients had a postangioplasty gradient of less than 60 mm Hg. The procedure was well tolerated and helped to preserve or improve renal function in patients with serum creatinine levels as high as 9 mg/dL. This series was unique in that the authors documented the effect of angioplasty on the renal artery systolic pressure gradient before and after angioplasty. Many other series have demonstrated the therapeutic efficacy of renal artery angioplasty in this disease, but most did not report the effect of the procedure on the gradient.

Renal artery angioplasty is currently first-line therapy in patients with atherosclerotic RAS and is frequently the only option in patients who are not surgical candidates. Complications include those associated with angiography; in the authors' series, there were 12 incidences of groin hematoma and 2 episodes of ARF (increase of serum creatinine by more than 50%). No deaths were associated with the procedure. Two patients (1.1%) required acute surgical intervention because of renal artery rupture at the time of angioplasty (both events occurred early in our experience). Thus, the risk of arterial rupture must be weighed against the benefit of the procedure and/or alternate surgical or medical options. An obvious advantage is that the procedure can be done on an outpatient basis.

Surgical Bypass Procedures

Operative correction of RAS represents the historical standard of therapy. Surgical correction of RAS may be accomplished using aortorenal bypass or other arteriorenal bypass approaches using saphenous vein graft, or renal artery endarterectomy with resection of the stenotic segment and end-to-end or end-to-side anastomosis.

In experienced hands, patients can be cured or demonstrate clinical improvement in up to 80% of cases, with response rates as high as 95% when stringent preoperative selection criteria are applied. Mortality rates following surgical bypass range from 3 to 10%, depending on the extent of atherosclerosis and the patient's general health.

Medical Management of Documented Renal Artery Stenosis

Medical management of RAS is directed at attaining good blood pressure control, mitigating progression of renal failure, and retarding progression of atherosclerosis, including cessation of smoking and control of serum lipid levels.

Medical management of RAS implies that the reno-vascular lesion will not be repaired and thus compromised renal blood flow should be anticipated. On this basis, ACE inhibitors should be avoided or used with great caution in the therapy of hypertension in these patients. ACE inhibitors may further impair renal blood flow and worsen or precipitate azotemia. In patients with bilateral disease and renal failure, the risks of worsening renal failure or the development of significant hyperkalemia are substantial.

Despite optimal blood pressure control, many patients medically managed for RAS develop progressive renal insufficiency and require renal replacement therapy. When this occurs, dialysis is indicated for uremia, volume overload, or refractory hypertension.

KEY POINTS

- The presence of an abdominal bruit in a hypertensive patient heightens the suspicion of renovascular hypertension.

- The diagnosis of atherosclerotic RAS is usually considered in patients with difficult-to-control hypertension or in hypertensive patients with unexplained azotemia.

- Positive results for a captopril stimulation test and captopril scintigraphy test have high predictive values.

- If both tests have normal (or negative) results, the results can be used to terminate the work-up.

- Renal artery angioplasty is first-line therapy in patients with atherosclerotic RAS, in the authors' opinion.

- Medical management consists of good blood pressure control, preferably with antihypertensive drugs other than ACE inhibitors.

- ACE inhibitors should be avoided or used with great caution, as converting-enzyme drugs may further impair blood flow and worsen or precipitate azotemia.

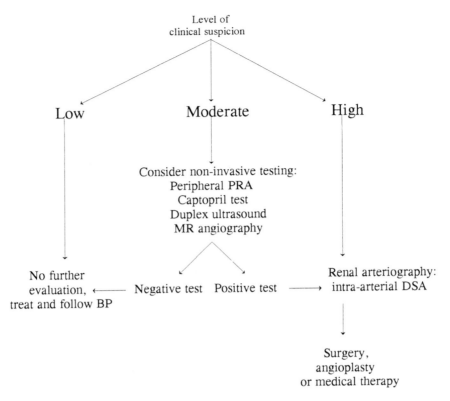

FIGURE 12.2.
Approach to the evaluation of renal artery stenosis in hypertensive patients. (Adapted from Mann S, Pickering T. Detection of renovascular hypertension, state of the art. Ann Intern Med 1992;177:845–853.)

REFERRAL

Referral of patients in whom there is a moderate level of clinical suspicion for RAS should be considered if outpatient support for conducting the appropriate test is unavailable or ill-defined. Those patients in whom there is a high level of clinical suspicion for RAS may be more easily managed in consultation with a nephrologist. The nephrologist may have in-depth experience with the local availability of angiographic support, can help manage acute changes in renal function that may occur in conjunction with diagnostic or therapeutic maneuvers, and can assist in decisions regarding angioplasty, surgery, or medical management.

It is the authors' practice to refer patients back to their primary care physician following surgical or angioplastic correction of RAS or if medical management is elected. At the discretion of the referring physician, the patient may be followed by the consultant once or twice a year for reassessment of blood pressure control, cardiopulmonary status, urinalysis, renal function, and antihypertensive drug regimen.

COMMONLY ASKED QUESTIONS

Can renal artery stenosis lead to kidney failure?
Yes. Renal artery stenosis may lead to end-stage kidney disease. When this occurs, dialysis is instituted.

Can renal arteries re-occlude following angioplasty?
Yes. The restenosis rate is probably not as high as the 20% associated with coronary angioplasty, but restenosis does occur. For this reason, any significant change in blood pressure control or serum creatinine level in patients with corrected renal artery stenosis necessitates re-arteriography (intra-arterial DSA, in the authors' practice).

What is the role of ACE inhibitor therapy in renovascular hypertension?
ACE inhibitors will reduce circulating angiotensin II levels and may improve blood pressure. However, the reduction in angiotensin II concentrations may reduce glomerular filtration of the kidney served by the stenotic renal artery. Rarely, renal artery thrombosis

has been reported in conjunction with ACE inhibitor therapy of renal artery stenosis. It is the authors' practice to not use ACE inhibitors for renovascular hypertension until the anatomy has been defined and, if possible, the stenotic lesion corrected (i.e., after angiography and angioplasty or surgery). Any patient treated with ACE inhibitors who exhibits a rise in serum creatinine meets one of the criteria for ischemic nephropathy (Table 12.3) and should be considered for angiography.

SUGGESTED READING

Elliot W, Martin W, Murphy M. Comparison of two non-invasive screening tests for renovascular hypertension. Arch Intern Med 1993;153:755–764.

Jacobson H. Ischemic renal disease: an overlooked clinical entity? Kidney Int 1988;34:729–743.

Mann S, Pickering T. Detection of renovascular hypertension, state of the art. Ann Intern Med 1992;177:845–853.

Pickering T, Sos T, Vaughan E, et al. Predictive value and changes of renin secretion in hypertensive patients with unilateral renovascular disease undergoing successful renal angioplasty. Am J Med 1984;76:398–404.

Vaughan E. Nephrology forum: renovascular hypertension. Kidney Int 1985;27:811–827.

Wilcox C. Use of angiotensin-converting enzyme inhibitors for diagnosing renovascular hypertension. Kidney Int 1993;44:1379–1390.

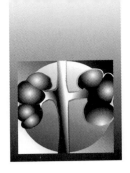

Congestive Heart Failure

John A. Larry

James L. Knepler, Jr

Bruce T. Vandehoff

BACKGROUND

Congestive heart failure (CHF) affects nearly 5 million Americans. Approximately 400,000 new cases are diagnosed each year. As the population ages, the incidence will continue increasing. One of every 100 people older than 65 years in the United States has CHF; it is the number one reason for hospitalization of patients in this age group. The condition results in a high mortality rate; the majority of patients who manifest overt CHF symptoms die within six years.

In patients with renal disease, CHF is relatively common. Although impaired renal function is a significant contributing factor in the development of CHF, it is not the sole cause. Patients with renal disease also have a high incidence of cardiac disease.

Pathophysiology

CHF is a clinical syndrome signaling the inability of the heart to maintain sufficient output to satisfy the metabolic requirements of the body. Because patients with ventricular dysfunction have limited cardiac function, the body attempts to compensate through a variety of mechanisms. These compensatory changes include ventricular remodeling with left ventricular dilatation, and hypertrophy and activation of neurohormonal systems. The neurohormonal systems best studied include the renin-angiotensin-aldosterone axis and the catecholamine-adrenergic system. Although these systems strive to maintain systemic pressure and renal perfusion, ultimately they become maladaptive by causing increased systemic vascular resistance, further compromising cardiac output. Impairment of left ventricular function and the compensatory changes that result characterize the pathophysiology of CHF (Fig. 13.1).

The Renin-Angiotensin System

The most significant neurohormonal system is the renin-angiotensin system. Angiotensin II is a potent systemic vasoconstrictor and also causes vasoconstriction of the efferent arteriole of the glomerulus, thus maintaining glomerular perfusion. Angiotensin II has two additional important systemic effects: stimulation of release of aldosterone from the adrenal gland and the release of antidiuretic hormone (ADH) from the posterior pituitary. Thus, aldosterone causes increased sodium resorption from the distal nephron, while ADH results in increased thirst and increased free water resorption from the distal and collecting system of the nephron.

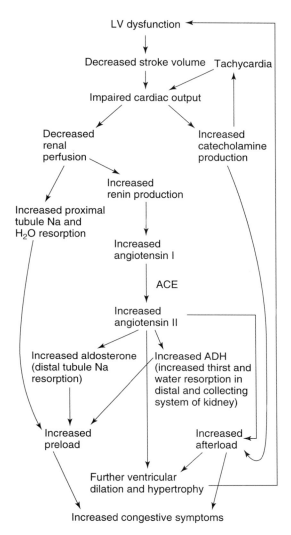

FIGURE 13.1.

Neurohormonal alterations in LV systolic dysfunction. *LV,* left ventricular; *ACE,* angiotensin-converting enzyme; *ADH,* antidiuretic hormone.

The Adrenergic System

The adrenergic system is also activated in patients with ventricular dysfunction. Increased levels of epinephrine and norepinephrine can be measured in patients with CHF. Although catecholamines can increase cardiac output by increasing heart rate and contractility of the ventricle, they can also cause an increase in systemic vascular resistance and a decrease in diastolic filling time, which may compromise coronary perfusion in patients with significant coronary artery disease.

Although serum norepinephrine is not routinely measured in clinical practice, it carries some prognostic information and suggests a negative correlation with survival.

Role of the Kidneys

The kidneys play a pivotal role in the body's adaptation to impaired pump function. As cardiac output declines, the kidneys take over the function of maintaining adequate perfusion of vital organs by expanding plasma volume through increased proximal tubular sodium reabsorption. Distal sodium resorption increases as a result of elevated aldosterone levels. This increase in renal sodium resorption is counterbalanced to some extent by increases in atrial natriuretic peptide (ANP) produced in response to distension of the cardiac atria. Thus, a new steady state of extracellular fluid volume is reached. With chronic atrial distension and further cardiac compromise, however, the effect of ANP becomes attenuated or overwhelmed and this balance is lost. Further renal sodium retention and extracellular fluid volume expansion ensue, and overt edema formation develops.

Cardiac Function

The cardiac function of a patient can be expressed as a relationship among three parameters: contractility, preload, and afterload. Contractility reflects the inherent ability of the cardiac myocytes to perform work. This can be altered by changes in catecholamine levels. Preload reflects the volume or pressure at end diastole. Increase in preload will result in increased cardiac output. In the impaired ventricle, maintaining cardiac output may require increased preload, which can exceed the threshold above which pulmonary edema develops. Afterload reflects systemic vascular resistance and ventricular wall tension;

it is increased via activation of the renin-angiotensin and adrenergic systems, further compromising cardiac output.

CAUSES

CHF is ultimately the result of a variety of underlying cardiac conditions, including coronary artery disease, cardiomyopathy, hypertensive heart disease, valvular heart disease, pericardial disease, cor pulmonale, congenital heart disease, and postviral myocarditis (Table 13.1).

In the United States, heart failure is most often related to coronary artery disease or cardiomyopathy, the latter often the result of long-standing untreated hypertension. The decompensation that produces frank CHF is, however, typically precipitated by other, more acute conditions (Table 13.2). Common precipitating factors of frank CHF include myocardial ischemia or infarction, cardiac arrhythmia, noncompliance with medical therapy, increased sodium intake, drugs such as nonsteroidal anti-inflammatory drugs (NSAIDs), infection and fever, pulmonary embolism, acute exacerbations of chronic hypertension, anemia, thyrotoxicosis, and pregnancy.

Diastolic Dysfunction

Most clinicians associate CHF with impaired systolic function of the left ventricle. It is important to realize that a significant number of patients with CHF or renal disease have diastolic dysfunction of the left ventricle and normal or near normal systolic function.

Diastolic dysfunction results from abnormal relaxation or increased stiffness of the ventricle during diastole, and occurs in conditions such as:

TABLE 13.1	Underlying Cardiac Conditions Predisposing to Congestive Heart Failure
	Coronary artery disease
	Hypertensive heart disease
	Cardiomyopathy
	Valvular heart disease
	Pericardial disease
	Congenital heart disease
	Myocarditis
	Cor pulmonale

TABLE 13.2	Precipitating Factors of Congestive Heart Failure
	Noncompliance with medical therapy
	Increased dietary sodium intake
	Myocardial ischemia or infarction
	Cardiac arrhythmias
	Infection
	Fever
	Pulmonary embolism
	Acute exacerbations of chronic hypertension
	Anemia
	Thyrotoxicosis
	NSAIDs
	Pregnancy

- Ischemia
- Hypertensive heart disease
- Aortic stenosis
- Infiltrative diseases of the heart (e.g., amyloidosis)

Patients with diastolic dysfunction exhibit an altered compliance curve, accepting a given volume into the ventricle at a higher filling pressure. This pressure is transmitted back to the left atrium, pulmonary venous bed, and pulmonary capillary bed, producing dyspnea and, sometimes, frank pulmonary edema. One must distinguish between the entities of systolic and diastolic dysfunction because therapy differs.

DIAGNOSIS

CHF is characterized by symptoms of volume overload, such as dyspnea, and edema. It is also characterized by manifestations of inadequate tissue perfusion, such as fatigue or decreased exercise tolerance. Symptoms can develop acutely or evolve over time.

Dyspnea is the most common presenting symptom. Initially, most patients only experience dyspnea with marked exertion, but as the disease progresses, dyspnea occurs with even normal ambulation, such as climbing stairs in the home. Other common symptoms include:

- Difficulty breathing unless upright (orthopnea), because of increased venous return to the heart with recumbency
- Paroxysmal nocturnal dyspnea
- Fatigue
- Dependent edema
- Cough, often an early symptom related to increased left ventricular filling pressures

Right-sided symptoms can be subtle, with right upper quadrant fullness or pain, anorexia, and abdominal bloating occasionally described.

SIGNS AND SYMPTOMS

A variety of physical signs of CHF can be noted on examination (Table 13.3).

- Rapid heart beat (tachycardia) and a narrow pulse pressure (occasionally with a low systolic pressure) are present when the stroke volume is low.
- Quick, shallow breathing (tachypnea) may result when there is pulmonary edema or high left ventricular filling pressures.
- Elevated central venous pressure, common in CHF, can be estimated by careful inspection of the neck veins.
- Prominent V-waves are noted when significant tricuspid valve regurgitation is present.

Physical Signs of Congestive Heart Failure	**TABLE 13.3**

Tachycardia
Narrow pulse pressure
Tachypnea
Pulsus alternans
Hypotension
Increased jugular venous pressure (+/− prominent V-waves)
Enlarged, tender liver (pulsatile when significant TR exists)
Ascites
Pedal edema
Basilar rales
Dullness to percussion at the bases
Bronchial breath sounds
Egophony
Laterally displaced apical impulse
Apical heave
Parasternal lift
Increased P_2 component of second heart sound
Cardiac gallops (S_3 and S_4)
Holosystolic murmur at the apex

TR, tricuspid regurgitation.

Other right-sided findings include:

- Enlarged, tender liver (which may be pulsatile when significant tricuspid regurgitation exists)
- Ascites
- Pedal edema

Basilar rales (caused by fluid passing into the alveoli) and signs of pleural effusions (dullness to percussion at the bases, bronchial breath sounds, and egophony) can be discovered on lung examination.

Cardiac gallops are often detected by careful auscultation. These low-pitched sounds are best detected by listening over the apex with the bell of the stethoscope. Jugular venous distension and a third heart sound (S_3) are nearly diagnostic when associated with the symptoms described previously. An S_3 gallop occurs during the rapid filling phase of the ventricle, shortly after S_2. Although an S_3 can be a normal finding in children, young adults, and pregnant women, in older patients it is usually indicative of CHF. An S_4 may also be noted just prior to S_1, coinciding with atrial contraction in late diastole. This sound may be caused by an increase in the force or volume of atrial contraction, as seen in thyrotoxicosis, but more commonly is related to a reduction in ventricular compliance that occurs in long-standing hypertension or ischemia. Mitral regurgitation is commonly present when the left ventricle is dilated. A loud, holosystolic murmur at the apex, usually radiating to the axilla or occasionally the lower left sternal border, is suggestive of mitral regurgitation.

Functional Classification

Physicians commonly classify patients' symptoms of CHF according to the New York Heart Association system of functional classification. This system divides patients with CHF into four classes according to symptom severity:

- **Class I** patients are asymptomatic. They have evidence of cardiac disease but suffer no limitations and have no symptoms of heart failure.
- **Class II** patients have mild symptoms of heart failure. Their symptoms are notable only on significant exertion, and thus they are only slightly limited by their disease.
- **Class III** patients have heart failure of moderate severity. Their heart failure results in significant limi-tations, with symptoms that are noted on mild exertion, such as walking.
- Class IV patients have severe heart failure that renders them unable to perform any physical activity and produces symptoms at rest.

Testing

Echocardiography and Radionuclide Ventriculography

Because the physical signs of heart failure are not specific, patients with symptoms suggestive of CHF should have an assessment of left ventricular function by echocardiography or radionuclide ventriculography, even in the absence of physical signs. Physical findings support but do not independently confirm the presence of CHF.

Chest Radiograph and Electrocardiogram

The goal of testing in the patient with CHF is to not only provide supportive evidence of CHF but also define the substrate and characterize the hemodynamic derangements that result from abnormal ventricular performance. The chest radiograph and electrocardiogram are invaluable tools for evaluating patients with known or suspected CHF. They are readily available to physicians and relatively inexpensive.

The chest radiograph assists in discerning the presence and/or cause of CHF and aids in differentiating CHF from other conditions. In mild heart failure, the chest radiograph may show evidence of cardiomegaly

and dilatation of the pulmonary veins in the upper lobes. The cardiac silhouette is typically enlarged in patients with systolic dysfunction. A ratio of the diameter of the cardiac silhouette to the thoracic diameter greater than 0.5 on a postero-anterior (PA) chest film suggests cardiomegaly. Evidence of pulmonary congestion with a normal cardiac silhouette suggests noncardiogenic pulmonary edema or diastolic dysfunction. As CHF worsens in severity, interstitial edema, Kerley B lines, perivascular edema, and subpulmonic effusions can be seen.

The electrocardiogram may provide important clues to the etiology of CHF. Evidence of acute or previous myocardial infarction may suggest the mechanism for reduction in left ventricular performance. Acute ST-T wave changes can be indicative of myocardial ischemia. Tachyarrhythmias or bradyarrhythmias might represent a trigger for the development of decompensated heart failure. Tachyarrhythmias, such as atrial fibrillation, may raise suspicion for the presence of thyroid dysfunction and/or inadequate cardiac output caused by the rapid ventricular rate. Conversely, bradyarrhythmias can result in inadequate cardiac output because of slow ventricular rate. Low electrocardiographic voltage may suggest pericardial effusion. Left ventricular hypertrophy or enlargement is a common feature seen in patients with renal disease, given their chronic state of pressure and volume overload.

Assessment of Left Ventricular Function

Assessment of left ventricular function is necessary for all patients who present with signs of CHF; this is especially important in patients with renal disease because their incidence of diastolic dysfunction is high. The most common parameter used to describe systolic function is the ejection fraction. The ejection fraction reflects the volume of blood ejected during systole divided by the volume of blood present in the ventricle at end diastole, and is expressed as a ratio or percentage. A normal ejection fraction is approximately 60%. The ejection fraction reflects left ventricular contractility, preload, and afterload. The ejection fraction is highly dependent on the loading conditions placed on the ventricle; it may change significantly without any intrinsic changes in cardiac status should the loading conditions vary.

Left ventricular function may be evaluated by one of three techniques.

1. Multigated radionuclide ventriculography
2. Echocardiography
3. Left ventricular angiography

Each test has advantages and disadvantages; which study to do depends on the clinical situation and on the expertise at one's institution.

Multigated radionuclide ventriculography (MUGA) MUGA scans provide a precise and reliable measurement of left ventricular ejection fraction. Regional wall motion can be assessed. As the entire ventricle is imaged, it is probably the best technique available to assess ejection fraction. Its limitations include an inability to evaluate valvular function, ventricular hypertrophy, and diastolic properties. A time delay is required to develop the images, limiting its utility in urgent situations. MUGA is also more expensive than echocardiography.

Echocardiography   The echocardiogram uses ultrasound to image the ventricular walls in two dimensions. End-diastolic and end-systolic volumes are calculated, and the ejection fraction is determined. In addition to measuring systolic function, echocardiography provides concomitant evaluation of regional wall motion, left ventricular hypertrophy, left atrial size, severity of valvular disease, detection of pericardial effusions, and ventricular thrombus formation. Echocardiography is noninvasive, less expensive than MUGA, and provides instantaneous information. A particular advantage of this test in patients with renal disease is the ability to assess diastolic properties by measuring mitral in-flow velocities. Its drawbacks are few: the study is technically inadequate in a subset of patients, especially those with obstructive pulmonary disease, and it provides only a semiquantitative estimate of ejection fraction. In patients with renal disease, echocardiography is probably superior to nuclear imaging as an initial diagnostic modality.

Left ventricular angiography   Cardiac catheterization provides the clinician with a tremendous amount of information; however, the decision to proceed with catheterization must be balanced against its risks. It carries a 1 in 1000 chance of a serious complication such as stroke, myocardial infarction, or death. Angiography carries a risk of dye toxicity, causing renal failure, especially in patients with preexisting renal insufficiency. Its advantages include a precise determination of the hemodynamic derangements that result from the decompensated cardiac status, assessment of the severity of valvular stenosis and insufficiency, measurement of cardiac output by planimetry or the Fick method, assessment of regional and global left ventricular function, and, more importantly, definition of the coronary artery anatomy. Cardiac catheterization should be strongly considered in patients with a high likelihood of coronary artery disease as the cause of their CHF.

Because dye toxicity is a significant concern in patients with preexisting renal insufficiency and CHF, the clinician can assess the regional and global function noninvasively with echocardiography or MUGA scan, defining the hemodynamics and coronary anatomy, when necessary, with catheterization. This approach reduces the volume of dye that patients receive, thus diminishing their likelihood of contrast-induced nephrotoxicity. Patients already on hemodialysis or peritoneal dialysis may need adjustment in their regimen pre- and post-dye infusion to remove the additional intravascular volume.

The decision to evaluate coronary anatomy depends on the clinician's determination of the probability of finding significant coronary artery disease. If the patient has anginal symptoms or multiple risk factors for atherosclerosis, coronary angiography is indicated. If the pretest probability of coronary artery disease is moderate, a stress test (using exercise or pharmacologic means such as dipyridamole) with an imaging modality is likely the best initial study. Patients with a high-risk positive stress study result are then referred for catheterization. In a patient with low likelihood of coronary disease, no further evaluation is indicated.

Other Tests

Severe anemia (hemoglobin less than 8 gm/dL) can worsen heart failure symptoms by decreasing the body's oxygen-carrying capacity. The clinician may consider increasing hemoglobin, thereby improving oxygen-carrying capacity by packed red blood cell transfusion. Erythropoietin may be administered in cases of anemia caused by renal failure.

Electrolytes and renal function must be measured. Inappropriate elevation of blood urea nitrogen to serum creatinine ratio suggests renal failure caused by increased renal vascular resistance, resulting in inadequate renal perfusion.

Thyroid dysfunction can produce or aggravate heart failure. Hence, thyroid function studies should be obtained, especially if CHF is accompanied by atrial fibrillation or clinical evidence of thyroid disease or if it occurs in patients older than 65 years of age.

Arterial blood gas examination will determine the severity of hypoxemia and the presence of respiratory acidosis or alkalosis. It is especially useful in patients in respiratory distress.

Serial cardiac enzyme measurement may be indicated to exclude or confirm a diagnosis of suspected myocardial infarction. The clinician must remember that renal insufficiency can cause false elevation of creatine phosphokinase and MB fraction, mimicking myocardial injury.

Urinalysis should be done to evaluate for heavy proteinuria suggesting renal disease, and for infection that may exacerbate CHF.

Differential Diagnosis

A variety of pulmonary disorders can produce dyspnea similar to that seen in CHF. Thus, even in patients with a known history of CHF, alternative and concomitant pulmonary causes of dyspnea (such as asthma, pneumonia, pneumothorax, and chronic obstructive pulmonary disease) should be considered.

Exertional dyspnea may represent cardiac ischemia or be caused by peripheral deconditioning in sedentary individuals. Lower extremity edema is often the result of chronic venous insufficiency, especially in obese individuals. Finally, because both hypothyroidism and hyperthyroidism can produce or exacerbate CHF, thyroid function tests should be obtained in patients with CHF.

Summary of Diagnosis

- CHF is common in patients with chronic renal failure, with or without dialysis treatment.
- CHF is most commonly the result of impaired left ventricular function caused by hypertension and fluid overload.
- As cardiac output declines, the kidneys attempt to maintain adequate volume by increased proximal tubular sodium reabsorption.
- Distal renal tubular reabsorption is marked in CHF because of excessive aldosterone activity.
- Dyspnea is the most common presenting symptom of CHF.
- Tachycardia with narrow pulse pressure as a result of low stroke volume is an accompaniment.
- New York Heart Association's functional classification system yields prognostic information.
- A chest radiograph is helpful in showing cardiomegaly, pulmonary congestion, and pleural effusion. Pulmonary congestion without cardiomegaly suggests noncardiogenic pulmonary edema.
- The electrocardiogram may provide important clues to the cause of CHF.
- Anemia should be treated with erythropoietin. Thyroid function test can be helpful.

TREATMENT

General Principles

The management of CHF is akin to that for acute renal failure in that evaluation and treatment must take place concurrently. Treatment of CHF depends on the cause and acuity of illness at the time of presentation.

Cardiogenic shock and acute cardiogenic pulmonary edema reflect acute catastrophic cardiac conditions that require urgent cardiology consultation. Patients with cardiogenic shock should be placed on a cardiac monitor, administered oxygen, and intubated, if necessary. If volume overload is not present, a fluid challenge should be given.

If pulmonary congestion is present in the setting of hypotension, intravenous inotropic agents such as dopamine and dobutamine should be instituted, and an intra-aortic balloon pump should be considered in patients unresponsive to other treatment.

In the setting of acute myocardial ischemia or injury, urgent revascularization with thrombolytic therapy or percutaneous transluminal coronary angioplasty should be done.

Acute Cardiogenic Pulmonary Edema

As initial therapy, patients with acute cardiogenic pulmonary edema with normal or elevated systemic blood pressure should be given oxygen and placed on a cardiac monitor. Initial pharmacologic therapy is directed at preload reduction.

Nitrates, given sublingually, topically, or parenterally, result in venodilation, and consequently alleviate congestive symptoms in patients with ischemic or nonischemic causes of CHF.

Loop diuretics should be administered in generous doses, especially in patients with preexisting renal insufficiency. In addition to their diuretic effect, these agents exert some venodilating effect, thereby acutely reducing preload.

Morphine, given intravenously in doses of 2 to 5 mg, can be effective in causing venodilation and reducing pulmonary congestion. The doses may be repeated as needed, provided the patient is not developing respiratory failure and is maintaining an adequate blood pressure.

If symptoms of pulmonary edema persist and the blood pressure is normal or elevated, intravenous nitroprusside can be initiated to reduce afterload.

Rotating tourniquets, phlebotomy, or urgent dialysis may be necessary for patients unresponsive to other therapies.

An urgently administered echocardiogram may be useful in patients who are in extremis or who don't respond to initial therapy.

Patients with Mild Symptoms

Patients with mild symptoms can be treated less aggressively initially. Loop diuretics may be sufficient to improve symptoms. Once the patient has been stabilized, further diagnostic evaluation can be done.

Most patients should be admitted to the hospital on their initial presentation of CHF, especially if there is a suspicion of cardiac ischemia or injury, a need for repeated doses of intravenous therapy, or if hypoxia is present. Patients who have mild symptoms and a low suspicion for myocardial ischemia may be evaluated and treated as outpatients. Patients with an established diagnosis of CHF may be treated in the office or emergency department and discharged if symptoms resolve and no concern of an acute coronary syndrome exists.

Hypertensive Crisis

In the situation of hypertensive crisis, aggressive treatment of the hypertension will improve cardiac performance and pulmonary edema. Hypertensive patients tend to have lowered fluid volume at the time of presentation, and excessive use of diuretics should be avoided.

Medical Therapy for Left Ventricular Systolic Dysfunction

The treatment of CHF concurrent with systolic dysfunction in a patient with renal disease is similar to that for the patient without renal disease. Pharmacologic intervention consists of a three-pronged attack (Table 13.4):

1. Volume reduction to decrease preload
2. Afterload reduction to reduce the work of the heart
3. Improve pump function

Volume Reduction

Diuretics   The goal of diuretic therapy is to prevent symptoms caused by volume overload. No data exists regarding its impact on mortality.

Control of fluid status is important in the patient with renal disease, especially in those with CHF. Diuretics are instrumental in maintaining an euvolemic status in patients who are not anuric.

Thiazide diuretics, with the exception of metolazone, are not very effective as monotherapy in patients whose creatinine clearance is less than 30 mL/min.

A loop diuretic is likely more effective in patients with impaired renal function, but higher doses must be employed.

Adding a thiazide diuretic, such as hydrochlorothiazide or metolazone, 30 minutes before the loop diuretic may improve urine output in unresponsive patients. Serum potassium must be carefully monitored in these patients, however.

If renal function is poor and diuretic therapy ineffective, peritoneal or hemodialysis must be considered. Patients already on dialysis can be managed by alterations in their dialysis regimen.

Afterload Reduction

Angiotensin-converting enzyme (ACE) inhibitors ACE inhibitors are the mainstay of therapy for heart failure caused by systolic dysfunction. Patients started on ACE inhibitors may experience a progressive rise in serum creatinine. The patients at the highest risk are those who are intravascularly volume-depleted. This risk can be minimized in these patients by gently increasing fluid and salt intake (or decreasing their diuretic dosage) before initiating therapy with ACE inhibitors. In the patient with renal disease, low doses of ACE inhibitors may be tried. The incidence of acute renal failure is very high in CHF patients treated with a combination of ACE inhibitors and diuretics. Serum potassium and creatinine concentrations should be periodically checked in those patients treated with ACE inhibitors.

ACE inhibitors are beneficial for patients with CHF. These agents have been shown to reduce mortality and morbidity in patients with class III and IV heart failure, as well as patients with class I and II heart failure whose left ventricular ejection fractions are less than 35%. For the patient requiring ongoing dialysis, ACE inhibitors lead to decreased daily fluid intake, resulting in less weight gain between dialysis sessions.

Medical Therapy for Systolic Dysfunction		TABLE 13.4
Preload Reduction	**Afterload Reduction**	**Inotropic Agents**
Diuretics	ACE inhibitors	Digoxin
Nitrates	Hydralazine	Dobutamine
Morphine		
Dialysis		

ACE inhibitor contraindications   In patients who cannot tolerate or have contraindications to ACE inhibitors, a combination of isosorbide (a long-acting nitroglycerin preparation that reduces preload) and hydralazine (an afterload reducer) may be used. This combination has been shown to improve exercise capacity and mortality in patients compared with placebo, although it was less effective than enalapril in reducing mortality.

Pump Function Improvement

Inotropic agents   Inotropic agents comprise the third arm of therapy for systolic dysfunction. Digoxin is most effective in patients with significant ventricular dysfunction who have a third heart sound or who are in atrial fibrillation. Care must taken in the patient with kidney disease because digoxin is renally excreted. Alternate-day dosing is typically recommended. Dobutamine is an intravenous inotrope, which may be used in the hospital for patients with severe or refractory symptoms. Patients may benefit symptomatically for months after a three-day infusion of dobutamine (usually 5 to 10 μg/kg/min). The cardiac rhythm must be monitored during the infusion because dobutamine can induce ventricular arrhythmias, made all the more likely by the electrolyte disturbances that can occur in CHF.

Beta blockers have been suggested to be effective in systolic heart failure by interrupting the "vicious circle" of sympathetic overload. Favorable data regarding metoprolol and carvedilol have been published. At this time, these therapies should only be used by a cardiologist experienced in treating CHF patients.

Patients with CHF and refractory volume overload may benefit from intravenous dopamine or dobutamine to improve renal perfusion. Hemodialysis or continuous ambulatory peritoneal dialysis (CAPD) is considered for those patients unresponsive to medical therapy. Those individuals with especially poor left ventricular function may benefit from intra-aortic balloon pumps in the acute setting or from left ventricular assist devices in the chronic setting. These devices are used only as a bridge to angioplasty, surgery, or transplant. Suitable candidates with refractory symptoms may be considered for transplantation. Combined kidney-heart transplants have been done successfully in rare cases.

Medical Therapy for Left Ventricular Diastolic Dysfunction

Diastolic dysfunction is caused by abnormal ventricular compliance, typically secondary to hypertensive heart disease or ischemia. Aggressive treatment of hypertension is important to promote regression of ventricular hypertrophy. Therapy for pulmonary congestion in diastolic dysfunction is accomplished with diuretics and/or nitrates. Care must be taken not to reduce preload too much because cardiac output depends heavily on preload in these patients. Beta blockers and calcium channel blockers of the nondihydropyridine type (diltiazem or verapamil) have also been shown to be beneficial in diastolic dysfunction, perhaps by increasing diastolic relaxation.

Associated Conditions

Once the cause has been determined, subsequent therapeutic intervention can be addressed. Surgically correctable causes of CHF such as valvular disease, pericardial disease, or coronary disease that are amenable to revascularization should be considered. Restoration of sinus rhythm should be contemplated in patients with underlying atrial dysrhythmias. Blood pressure must be well controlled and fluid and sodium restriction implemented. Many patients with renal disease will already have been instructed to restrict fluids and sodium. The appropriate maintenance medical therapy of CHF initiated depends on whether the patient has systolic or diastolic dysfunction of the left ventricle.

Electrolyte and Acid-Base Abnormalities

Patients with CHF experience a wide variety of acid-base and electrolyte disturbances. Metabolic acidosis, caused by lactate, can occur from hypoxemia or circulatory failure and is exacerbated by the kidney's reduced ability to excrete acid in renal dysfunction. Although bicarbonate therapy may be beneficial in patients who are hyperkalemic and whose serum bicarbonate levels are less than 12 mEq/L, bicarbonate therapy is not generally recommended because of the sodium load that accompanies the bicarbonate.

Hyponatremia

Hyponatremia often develops in patients with CHF. Although patients with CHF have low urinary sodium excretion and tend to retain sodium, they retain even more free water, partly because of the effect of ADH. Consequently, their hyponatremia is dilutional. Thiazide diuretics can aggravate this problem. Usually hyponatremia will respond to free water restriction.

Hypokalemia and Hyperkalemia

Depending on the circumstances, hypokalemia or hyperkalemia may develop. Hypokalemia is caused by several factors. Activation of the renin-angiotensin-aldosterone axis leads to increased potassium excretion and sodium retention, caused by the effects of aldosterone. Diuretics also cause urinary excretion of potassium. The excess fluid retention in CHF may also contribute slightly to hypokalemia. Because hypokalemia can precipitate arrhythmias, it is essential to keep the serum potassium above 4 mEq/dL. Patients with significantly reduced renal function or impaired renal perfusion caused by low cardiac output can develop hyperkalemia as a result of the kidney's inability to excrete enough potassium. ACE inhibitors, by decreasing the release of aldosterone by angiotensin II and decreasing renal perfusion, can also contribute to hyperkalemia.

Hypomagnesemia

Hypomagnesemia also complicates CHF if patients have adequate renal function. Both loop and thiazide diuretics cause magnesium wasting. Some clinicians argue that hypomagnesemia may precipitate arrhythmias in the setting of abnormal cardiac substrate. Patients with significant renal dysfunction tend to have diminished magnesium excretion, thus hypomagnesemia is typically not seen in the patient with significant renal insufficiency.

Asymptomatic Individuals

Asymptomatic individuals with a left ventricular ejection fraction less than 40% may benefit from ACE inhibitor therapy.

REFERRAL

Patients who develop CHF should be seen by a cardiologist. The urgency to obtain a consultative opinion depends on the severity of the illness. The cardiologist can not only assist with the initial evaluation but also provide the patient and primary care physician with therapeutic and prognostic information.

PREVENTION

Because CHF represents a physiologic state of decompensation that often requires hospitalization, prevention is preferred to treatment of the established condition. The known risk factors for development of coronary artery disease should be identified and modified whenever possible. Risk factors that can be modified include:

- Hypertension
- Diabetes mellitus
- Cigarette smoking
- Hyperlipidemia

KEY POINTS

- Assessment of left ventricular function is important. Diastolic dysfunction is high in patients with chronic renal failure.

- Systolic function is determined by ejection fraction. Normal ejection fraction is 60%.

- Left ventricular function can be evaluated by MUGA, echocardiography, or left ventricular angiography.

- Therapeutic options are essentially limited to maintenance of fluid and electrolyte balance and to improvement in left ventricular pump function.

- Fluid and electrolyte balance is difficult with compromised renal function. Dialysis, CAPD, or hemodialysis is the mainstay of therapy.

- A variety of inotropic agents are used to improve cardiac output. Their roles are less clear in achieving patient well-being or improving survival in the presence of renal dysfunction.

- Obesity
- Sedentary lifestyle

Hypertension should be aggressively treated in all patients, but especially in African-Americans, who have a higher incidence of complications related to their blood pressure.

Patients with Systolic or Diastolic Dysfunction

Patients with systolic or diastolic dysfunction must be educated on the appropriate use of their medications. Dietary counseling regarding sodium intake is vitally important, and patients should be instructed to follow a 2-gram sodium (4 gm sodium chloride) diet. If coronary artery disease is part of their clinical profile, a low fat, low cholesterol diet such as the American Heart Association Step One Diet should be implemented. Patients need to weigh themselves every morning. Should their weight increase by more than 3 pounds, they should contact their physician. Patients on dialysis must be instructed on the importance of complying with their regimen. Finally, patients must pay close attention to any symptoms that develop. Treatment of mild decompensation can be done on an outpatient basis with minor medical adjustments, saving the expense of hospitalization.

SUMMARY

CHF is commonly seen in patients with renal disease. The precise determination of the presence and extent of underlying cardiac disease requires a careful history, physical examination, electrocardiographic and radiographic interpretation, and appropriate use of further imaging studies. Appropriate treatment depends on the etiology and severity of cardiac disease. With appropriate education, judicious use of medications, and longitudinal follow-up, the patient will not only live longer but also enjoy a better quality of life.

COMMONLY ASKED QUESTIONS

Why does a patient with congestive heart failure require measurement of left ventricular function?

We believe every patient should have one assessment of left ventricular function because treatment varies depending on the cause of congestive heart failure and on the systolic and diastolic function of the left ventricle. When the underlying substrate has been characterized, clinical judgment should determine the necessity of a repeat evaluation. Patients with documented poor systolic dysfunction caused by cardiomyopathy with an ejection fraction of 20% would likely not require repeat assessment of left ventricular function, should they be readmitted in congestive heart failure. Conversely, patients with left ventricular hypertrophy and diastolic dysfunction who present with recurrent congestive heart failure and electrocardiogram evidence of a recent myocardial infarction may benefit from repeat echocardiography. The echocardiogram may now exhibit significant systolic dysfunction, which would result in a change in medical therapy and potentially signify the need for further diagnostic studies.

What if the patient with systolic dysfunction cannot tolerate ACE inhibitors?

Currently, the combination of isosorbide and hydralazine is recommended as second-line therapy. This combination was shown to improve symptoms and survival, although the V-Heft II trial found it to be less effective in promoting survival as compared with ACE inhibitors. Much research is ongoing in the new class of agents, which are direct angiotensin II receptor antagonists. Currently, there is little clinical data regarding the long-term outcome of patients with congestive heart failure. Further research may alter this recommendation by the time of publication.

How should digoxin be dosed in patients with renal failure?

Digitalis is excreted via the kidneys, therefore the dose must be adjusted in most patients with underlying renal insufficiency.

Typically, a dosage of digoxin of 0.125 mg every other day does not lead to toxicity. However, this patient population is one of the few that truly benefits from measurement of a serum digoxin level when the agent is presumed to be at steady state.

SUGGESTED READINGS

Bonow R, Udelson J. Left ventricular diastolic dysfunction as a cause of CHF: mechanisms and management. Ann Intern Med 1992;117:502.

Cohn JN, Johnson G, Ziesche S, et al. A comparison of enalapril with hydralazine-isosorbide dinitrate in the treatment of chronic CHF. New Engl J Med 1991; 35:303–310.

CONSENSUS Trial Study Group. Effects of Enalapril on mortality in severe CHF. New Engl J Med 1987; 316:1425–1435.

Guidelines for the evaluation and management of heart failure: report of the American College of Cardiology/American Heart Association Task Force on Practice Guidelines. Circulation 1995;92:2764–2784.

Heart Failure Guideline Panel. Heart failure: management of patients with left ventricular systolic dysfunction. Am Family Phys 1994,50(3):603–616.

Kanel WB. Epidemiological aspects of heart failure. Cardiol Clin 1989;7(1):19.

Leier CV, Boudoulas H. Cardiorenal Diseases and Disorders. 2nd ed. Mt. Kisco, NY: Futura Publishing Company, 1992.

Mair FS. Management of heart failure. Am Family Phys 1996;54(1):245–254.

Mandal AK, Markert RJ, Saklayen MG, et al. Diuretics potential angiotensin-converting enzyme inhibitor-induced acute renal failure. Clin Nephrol 1994;42: 170–174.

McElroy PA, Shroff SG, Weber KT. Pathophysiology of the failing heart. Cardiol Clin 1989;7(1):25–38.

Pfeffer MA, Braunwald E, Moy LA, et al. Effect of captopril on mortality and morbidity in patients with left ventricular dysfunction after myocardial infarction: results of the survival and ventricular enlargement trial. N Engl J Med 1992;327:669–677.

Riley DJ, Weir ML, Bakris GL. Renal adaptation to the failing heart: understanding the cascade of responses. Postgrad Med 1994;95(8):141–146, 149–150.

Seamens CM, Wrenn K. Breathlessness: strategies aimed at identifying and treating the cause of dyspnea. Postgrad Med 1995;98(4):215–216, 219–222, 225–227.

Unverferth D, Magorien R, Leier CV, et al. The hemodynamic and metabolic advantages gained by a three-day infusion of dobutamine in patients with congestive cardiomyopathy. Am Heart J 1983;106:29–34.

Weber KTI, Janicki JS. Pathogenesis of heart failure. Cardiol Clin 1989;7(1):1–24.

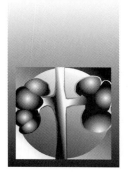

Generalized Edema

Anil K. Mandal

BACKGROUND

Anatomy and Physiology

Edema is defined as the presence of excessive fluid in the tissues of the body. Fluid accumulates mainly in the extracellular fluid compartment (ECFC), but it can also accumulate in the intracellular fluid compartment (ICFC).

The ECFC consists of intravascular fluid space and interstitial fluid space. The total amount of body fluid is 60% of total body weight; two-thirds (40%) reside in the ICFC and one-third (20%) reside in the ECFC. In the ECFC, 40% of the fluid is in the intravascular space as blood or plasma and 60% is in the interstitial space. Fluid is filtered from the intravascular space into the interstitial space at the arteriolar end of a capillary. The fluid then returns into the intravascular space at the venous end of the capillary; this action is due primarily to the difference in the gradient between the hydrostatic pressure at the venous end of the capillary and the oncotic pressure exerted by plasma albumin. Under normal circumstances, fluid does not accumulate in the interstitial space because interstitial fluid pressure remains negative. Hence, no edema is discernible.

The total "edema safety factor" against edema formation is 17 mm Hg negative pressure and includes:

Interstitial fluid pressure	−7 mm Hg
Lymphatic flow	−6 mm Hg
Lymphatic washout of proteins	−4 mm Hg

As fluid continues to accumulate in the interstitial space and the interstitial fluid volume increases, interstitial fluid pressure increases in parallel with the volume. The negative interstitial fluid pressure is dissipated and the pressure rises into the positive range when edema becomes evident. Lymph flow can increase as much as 10- to 50-fold. The lymph vessels can carry away large amounts of fluid and help prevent the interstitial fluid pressure from rising into the positive pressure range. As the lymph flow increases, it carries protein away from the interstitium, thus reducing the interstitial fluid colloid osmotic pressure. This is called "washdown" of the interstitial fluid protein. As washdown occurs, the differential gradient between plasma colloid osmotic pressure and the colloid osmotic pressure in the interstitium increases, thus increasing the osmotic absorption of fluid from the interstitium into the capillaries. Therefore, excessive fluid accumulation in the interstitial space initially may occur in one of the following two ways: (*a*) abnormal leakage of fluid from the blood capillaries or (*b*) reduced plasma oncotic pressure caused by low plasma albumin.

Conditions Causing Edema

Abnormal leakage of fluid from the capillaries can occur in the following conditions:

- CHF
- Acute glomerulonephritis
- Angioedema
- Venous obstructions (inferior vena cava obstruction caused by thrombosis or extrinsic compression by a tumor, and subclavian vein stenosis caused by a catheter placement for temporary access to hemodialysis)

Low serum albumin as in cirrhotics or nephrotics reduces the oncotic pressure gradient and hinders return of filtered plasma water at the venous end. When fluid begins to accumulate, further fluid accumulation occurs through renal retention of sodium and water. The main stimulus for renal retention of sodium and water is decreased effective arterial blood volume (EABV), which causes activation of two major hormones, aldosterone and vasopressin. Aldosterone and vasopressin act on the kidney to cause sodium and water retention, respectively, and result in sustained edema. The renal mechanism of edema is presented in Figure 14.1.

EABV is made up of three components:

- Absolute volume of the intravascular space
- Cardiac output
- Systemic vascular resistance

A change in one of the components without a compensatory change in the others will affect the volume of the circulation. Thus, in generalized edema, a major disturbance occurs in the regulation of extracellular volume. The disturbance is characterized by renal retention of sodium and water, with expansion of interstitial space and, frequently, plasma volume.

The pathogenesis of severe renal retention of sodium and water is unclear, although many factors have been proposed. These factors include aldosterone, vasopressin, and atrial natriuretic factor (ANF).

To investigate the pathogenesis of sodium retention in chronic liver disease, 19 patients with chronic liver disease were studied: 13 without (group 1) and 6 with (group 2) histories of clinical sodium retention (ascites or edema) by varying dietary sodium intake.

The patients were placed on a 20 mmol/day sodium-constant diet for 1 week, followed by a 100 mmol/day sodium-constant diet for 1 week. After 5 days of equilibration on each diet, blood and urine samples were collected for plasma ANF and urinary sodium excretion. Group 1 patients achieved near-sodium balance in 5 days on both low-sodium (urinary sodium 17 ± 3 mmol/day) and normal sodium diet (urinary sodium 80 ± 5 mmol/day). ANF levels tended to be elevated, but the increase was not significantly greater than that in the control subjects (10 ± 4 pg/mL to 19 ± 4 pg/mL) on the same diets. Group 2 patients showed significantly positive sodium balance on both the 20 mmol/day (urinary sodium 9.5 ± 3.3 mmol/day) and 100 mmol/day sodium diet (urinary sodium 37 ± 13 mmol/day). This occurred despite significantly elevated baseline ANF and plasma ANF levels after sodium challenge (62 ± 9 pg/mL on a 100 mmol/day sodium diet).

Effective Circulating Blood Volume

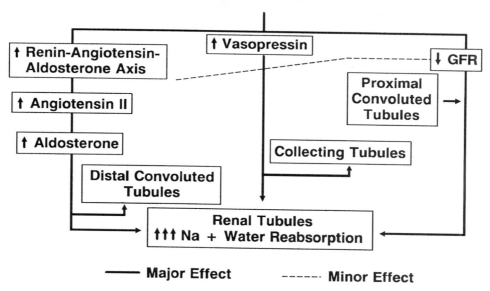

——— **Major Effect**   ------ **Minor Effect**

FIGURE 14.1.

Effective circulating blood volume (ECBV). If ECBV is diminished, there is increased production of renin-angiotensin and aldosterone, which promotes excessive sodium reabsorption. As a result, serum sodium should increase, but, in reality, in most edematous states serum sodium is below normal, which is caused by increased AVP causing water retention. The latter is the cause of dilutional hyponatremia. *GFR,* glomerular filtration rate.

CAUSES

Edema may be associated with significant proteinuria (>0.5 g/24 hr), present in such conditions as renal disease and unilateral or bilateral renal vein thrombosis. Edema may also be associated with slight or no proteinuria (<0.5 g/24 hr). Associated conditions are:

- CHF
- Cirrhosis of the liver
- Malnutrition
- Inferior vena cava thrombosis below the renal veins
- Hypothyroidism

Causes of generalized, massive edema (anasarca) include the following:

- Nephrotic syndrome
- CHF
- Cirrhosis of the liver
- Microcystic disease in newborns

Generalized edema with orthopnea, paroxysmal nocturnal dyspnea is caused by CHF. Generalized edema with massive ascites can be caused by one of the following:

- Cirrhosis of the liver
- Pelvic malignancy with spread into peritoneum, inferior vena cava, superior vena cava (e.g., lymphoma, metastasis).
- Lymphedema caused by lymphatic obstruction by tumor or parasite (filaria). In this case, ascites is chylous.

In one study, the common causes of leg edema in the elderly population were venous stasis (63.2%), drug-induced edema (13.8%), and CHF (15.1%). Less frequent causes of leg edema include:

- Thrombophlebitis
- Cirrhosis of the liver
- Lymphedema
- Prostatic carcinoma
- Ovarian mass

On comparison of the circumference of leg edema on initial visit and four weeks after treatment, both the exercise and nonexercise groups showed significant decreases in the measurement of the leg edema, except in those caused by lymphedema.

Idiopathic Edema

Idiopathic edema is commonly seen in menstruating females. In some females, prolonged upright posture may be a cause; in others, diuretic abuse may be a primary factor in initiating edema. Females abuse diuretics to lose weight. Chronic diuretic use leads to secondary hyperaldosteronism, with sustained sodium retention and worsening of ankle swelling for as long as 2 weeks after cessation of diuretics. In some females, because edema develops with the onset of menstruation, a relationship with estrogen may be postulated.

DIAGNOSIS

Renal Disease Edema

Percutaneous renal biopsy and histopathologic studies of the renal tissue are the surest means to establish a diagnosis of renal disease. However, history, associated findings, and renal function testing can help to indirectly assess the type of renal disease in a given patient. Degree of proteinuria helps to differentiate between glomerular and tubulointerstitial diseases.

Glomerular Diseases

Severity of 24-hour proteinuria does not distinguish between primary and secondary glomerular diseases.

Primary glomerular diseases include:

- Minimal lesion disease
- Membranous glomerular nephritis
- Membranoproliferative glomerular nephritis
- Focal glomerular sclerosis

Secondary glomerular diseases include:

- Diabetic nephropathy
- Lupus nephritis
- Vasculitis (e.g., Wegener's granulomatosis, polyarteritis nodosa)

Tubulointerstitial Diseases

Twenty-four hour proteinuria less than 1 gram is common in association with acute and chronic tubulointerstitial renal disease and uncontrolled hypertensive renal disease (essential hypertension). Thus, in a given patient with heavy proteinuria (≥ 3 g/24 hr), the presence of generalized edema (anasarca) and normal or near-normal renal function (serum creatinine <1.4 mg/dL) and the absence of associated conditions such

as hypertension and retinopathy suggests minimal lesion disease. Another patient who has heavy proteinuria and, in addition, shows moderate to severe hypertension and mild to moderate impairment of renal function (serum creat-inine ≥ 2 mg/dL) may show membranous glomerulonephritis, membranoproliferative glomerulonephritis, or focal glomerular sclerosis. These conditions and the presence of exudative retinopathy suggest diabetic ne-phropathy, while the presence of cardiomegaly or glossomegaly suggest amyloidosis.

The common causes of nephrotic syndrome (by definition, proteinuria ≥ 3.5 g/24 hr) are:

- Minimal lesion disease
- Membranous glomerulonephritis
- Membranoproliferative glomerulonephritis
- Focal glomerular sclerosis
- Diabetic nephropathy
- Amyloidosis

Congestive Heart Failure

In the case of edema caused by CHF, persistent and moderate to severe shortness of breath is a consistent accompaniment. Other consistent findings include:

- Inability to lie flat in bed (orthopnea)
- Distended neck veins
- Gallop rhythm
- Diminished air entry with rales at the lung bases

Recommended investigations include a chest radiograph, an echocardiogram, and a multigated angiogram (MUGA) scan.

Chest Radiograph

Chest radiograph reveals the extent of cardiomegaly, severity of pulmonary congestion, and presence or absence of pleural effusion. If pleural effusion is present, a chest radiograph can determine the massiveness of the effusion and the necessity for therapeutic thoracentesis.

Echocardiogram and MUGA Scan

Echocardiogram and MUGA scan will provide estimates for ventricular function and left ventricular ejection fraction. The MUGA scan provides more accurate assessment of left ventricular ejection fraction than does the echocardiogram. The lower the ejection fraction, the lesser the renal function and the more marked the sodium retention. As a result of sustained sodium retention, edema and pulmonary congestion are likely to worsen and become progressively resistant to treatment.

MUGA scan or equilibrium radionuclide angiocardiography has become the widely used technique for radionuclide monitoring of left ventricular function (ejection fraction). This study is of clinical value in the management of patients with myocardial infarction, valvular heart disease, and cardiomyopathy. In normal individuals, left ventricular ejection fraction is 50% or higher. With automated or semiautomated methods, variability between ejection fraction determination is less than 2%, with a variability of 5% in separate studies repeated in the same patient.

Cirrhosis of the Liver

Hypoalbuminemia causing decreased effective circulating volume is perhaps the most important stimulus for excessive renal sodium retention in cirrhosis of the liver. Enhanced distal sodium reabsorption caused by elevated circulating aldosterone level further aggravates edema and ascites.

Summary of Complete Workup for Edema

- Comprehensive history
- Physical examination including rectal examination for prostate in males and pelvic examination in females
- Complete blood count
- Chemistry profile
- Thyroid function tests with thyroid stimulating hormone (TSH)
- Electrocardiogram
- Chest radiograph
- When indicated, pelvic or leg ultrasound and pelvic CT scan, circumference of the leg with the maximum amount of edema initially and after 4 weeks of treatment
- Echocardiogram and MUGA scan as indicated

TREATMENT

Therapeutic options for edema include the following:

- Bed rest
- Variable restriction of salt and fluid intake
- Diuretic therapy
- Treatment of the cause
- Adjuvant therapy

Bed Rest

Bed rest alone helps to mobilize fluid from the dependent portions of the body and results in mild diuresis. Supportive stockings add further to the mobilization of fluid. The mechanism of diuresis induced by bed rest and/or supportive stockings is not clearly under-

Summary of Diagnosis

- In generalized edema, a major disturbance occurs in the normal regulation of extracellular volume, characterized by renal retention of sodium and water.
- The pathogenesis of excessive renal retention of sodium and water is not clear, although many factors are involved, including aldosterone, vasopressin, and ANF.
- Most common causes of generalized edema include nephrotic syndrome, CHF, and cirrhosis of the liver.
- The renin-angiotensin-aldosterone axis appears to exert an important role in chronic edematous conditions.
- Idiopathic edema is commonly seen in menstruating females. In some females, prolonged upright posture may be a cause; in others, diuretic abuse may be a primary factor in initiating edema.
- Degree of proteinuria does not distinguish between primary and secondary renal diseases, whereas associated findings do. For instance, nephrotic range proteinuria (≥ 3 g/24 hr) with no associated findings suggests primary renal disease. However, nephrotic range proteinuria in association with diabetic retinopathy in a patient with a long history of diabetes mellitus is generally attributed to diabetic nephropathy.
- Moderate to severe shortness of breath is a consistent accompaniment in cases of edema caused by CHF.
- A thiazide diuretic alone may be adequate in cirrhotics but is ineffective in CHF or nephrotic syndrome.
- The adverse effects of thiazide and loop diuretics are similar and relate to fluid, electrolyte, and metabolic disturbances.

stood but appears to be caused by an increase in EABV and renal perfusion.

Variable Restriction of Salt and Fluid Intake

Unless salt and fluid intake are restricted, sodium and water balance will remain positive. Salt intake should be determined by sodium excretion rate. Thus, at least one 24-hour urinary sample should be obtained for sodium excretion after 2- and 4-gram sodium intake, respectively, for 3 days each. These urinary collections should be obtained in the absence of diuretic use. (Urinary electrolytes are not interpretable if urinary samples are collected during diuretic therapy.) If 24-hour urinary sodium excretion is less than 20 mEq on 2- or 4-gram daily sodium intake, daily sodium intake should be reduced to 1 (23 mEq) or 0.5 gram, which is essentially a salt-free diet. Such stringent reductions in salt intake are not generally necessary with the availability of a variety of potent diuretics. However, some patients develop resistance to diuretic therapy, and restriction of salt and fluid intake remains the mainstay of therapy.

Patients with massive edema are unable to excrete free water and develop concomitant hyponatremia. Therefore, free water intake should be limited to an amount equal to daily urine output plus insensible loss (500 to 1500 mL/day, depending on living conditions) plus additional loss.

Diuretic Therapy

Three classes of diuretics are commonly used: thiazide (sulfonamide) diuretics, loop-acting diuretics, and potassium-sparing diuretics. Acetazolamide is an inhibitor of proximal bicarbonate reabsorption and therefore is not classified as a diuretic.

Thiazide Diuretics

Thiazide diuretics actions are attributable solely to inhibition of sodium and chloride reabsorption in the distal convoluted tubule. Thiazide diuretics act independently of carbonic anhydrase inhibition. They partially decrease free water clearance or the ability to maximally dilute urine. They do not interfere with the ability to concentrate urine. Thiazide diuretics induce natriuresis to the extent of 5 to 7% of filtered sodium and therefore are considered relatively mild diuretics. A thiazide diuretic alone may be adequate in cirrhotics but is ineffective in CHF or nephrotic patients.

Thiazide diuretics include hydrochlorothiazide (available as 25, 50, or 100 mg tablets alone, or in combination with potassium-sparing agents), indapamide (available as 2.5 mg tablets), and metolazone (available as 0.5, 2.5, 5, or 10 mg tablets). The recommended dosages are hydrochlorothiazide 12.5 to 25 mg twice daily, indapamide 2.5 to 5 mg once daily in the morning, and metolazone 2.5 to 10 mg once daily in the morning.

Loop-acting Diuretics

The sulfonamide derivative loop-acting diuretics include:

- Furosemide, available as 20, 40, and 80 mg tablets
- Bumetanide, available as 0.5, 1, and 2 mg tablets

The phenoxyacetic acid derivative is ethacrynic acid, available as 25 and 50 mg tablets.

The mode of action of loop-acting diuretics is both hemodynamic and tubular. Hemodynamically, loop-acting diuretics have been shown to increase renal blood flow and, in some instances, glomerular filtration rate (GFR). These effects appear to be mediated by prostaglandins (PGs), since the natriuretic and diuretic effects are blunted by prostaglandin synthesis inhibitors (such as indomethacin). In the renal tubules, loop-acting diuretics act on the ascending thick limb of loop of Henle and inhibit chloride and sodium transport, amounting to excretion of 15 to 20% of filtered sodium. Therefore, the natriuresis and diuresis can be marked. One bolus of intravenous injection of furosemide 40 mg could result in diuresis of 5 to 6 liters in a few hours. Furosemide has a slight inhibitory effect on sodium transport in the proximal tubule; ethacrynic acid has a slight inhibitory effect on sodium transport in the collecting tubule.

Thus, loop diuretics are potent diuretics and, by inhibiting sodium chloride transport in the ascending thick limb, impair formation of hypertonic medullary interstitium. Hypertonicity in the medullary interstitium generates the gradient for final concentration of urine. Final concentration of urine is determined by arginine vasopressin (AVP) concentrations. Therefore, a patient treated with a loop diuretic will be unable to maximally concentrate the urine during hydropenia. Loop diuretics also markedly reduce renal diluting capacity during water diuresis.

Dosage and administration The most commonly used loop diuretic is furosemide, and oral administration is the most common method of treatment. Recommended dosage is 40 mg, orally, twice daily for nephrotic syndrome or CHF, and 40 mg once daily for cirrhosis of the liver.

The equivalent dosage of bumetanide is 0.5 mg twice daily or ethacrynic acid 25 mg twice daily.

In acute CHF with pulmonary edema, an intravenous bolus of furosemide 40 mg twice daily produces prompt relief of shortness of breath. An intravenous bolus of a loop diuretic reduces left ventricular filling pressure and pulmonary vascular congestion, minimizing pulmonary edema. A bolus of a loop diuretic given intravenously is not as effective in chronic CHF as it is in acute CHF.

Relief of pulmonary edema as an outcome of intravenous furosemide therapy is not observed with oral furosemide therapy. In the event an intravenous loop diuretic is a recommended therapy, furosemide is preferable to ethacrynic acid because of the high risk of ototoxicity with ethacrynic acid.

Adverse Effects of Thiazide and Loop-acting Diuretics

The adverse effects of thiazide and loop-acting diuretics are similar and relate to fluid, electrolyte, and metabolic disturbances. The electrolyte disturbances include:

- Hyponatremia
- Hypochloremia
- Hypokalemia
- Hypomagnesemia

Renal insufficiency with elevated blood urea nitrogen (BUN) to serum creatinine ratio suggestive of volume depletion is a concomitant feature of diuretic therapy.

Two common metabolic disturbances are hyperglycemia and hyperlipidemia. Hyperglycemia is associated with hypokalemia or dehydration, either of which blunts insulin release and gives rise to hyperglycemia. The relationship of hyperglycemia with dehydration may be more important than with hypokalemia because fluid therapy generally corrects hyperglycemia, whereas increasing serum potassium levels does not always do so. Hyperlipidemia, mostly elevated serum cholesterol, is common with diuretic therapy. However, cholesterol elevation levels off after years of diuretic use. Although cardiovascular risk of hyperlipidemia with diuretic therapy has been stressed, it has not been documented.

In almost all cases, the adverse effects (including hyperglycemia and hyperlipidemia) caused by diuretic therapy reverse on discontinuation of diuretics. These will be exemplified in the following case studies.

CASE STUDY

H.S., a 69-year-old white male, visited the hypertension clinic on July 7, 1993 for treatment of hypertension. He was receiving maxzide 25 (hydrochlorothiazide 25 mg + triamterene 37.5 mg), one tablet daily, and nifedipine, 10 mg orally, three times daily. A laboratory study was done on the day of the visit. Based on the results, maxzide was discontinued and a laboratory study was repeated two weeks later. The laboratory results are presented in Case Study Table 1. From the table, note that the patient had hyperglycemia and mild renal insufficiency. Two weeks after discontinuation of diuretic therapy, blood glucose returned to normal levels and renal function improved. The latter changes are likely the result of volume repletion, which is evident by the increase in urinary sodium concentration and the slight decrease in urinary creatinine concentration.

Adverse Effects of Diuretic Therapy on Serum Values CASE STUDY TABLE 1

	July 07	July 21
Glucose (mg/dL)	200	105
BUN (mg/dL)	30	19
Creatinine (mg/dL)	2.1	1.7
Sodium (mEq/L)	140	143
Potassium (mEq/L)	3.7	3.9
Chloride (mEq/L)	104	107
CO_2 (mEq/L)	26	28
Urinary values (spot urine)		
Sodium (mEq/L)	37.4	86.5
Creatinine (mEq/L)	165	149.4

CASE STUDY

R.H., a 72-year-old white male, is a follow-up patient in the hypertension clinic. He gave a history of CHF. He was receiving furosemide 40 mg, orally, twice daily. In a visit on August 13, the furosemide dose was increased to 60 mg twice daily, and metolazone 2.5 mg was added to the regimen. Blood samples were drawn on May 12, August 13, August 23. The results are presented in Case Study Table 2. From this table, note that the patient had progressive loss of weight, increase of hemoglobin and hematocrit, hypokalemia, hypochloremia, metabolic alkalosis, and renal insufficiency. The increases in hemoglobin and hematocrit are caused by hemoconcentration, which is the result of volume depletion. However, despite hypokalemia and dehydration, his blood glucose did not increase. Uric acid and cholesterol levels were elevated.

Diuretic (furosemide) therapy is probably the most common cause of hypochloremic hypokalemic metabolic alkalosis today. In most cases, patients are asymptomatic or mildly symptomatic and generally require no aggressive treatment except adjustment of the dosage or discontinuation of diuretic therapy.

CASE STUDY TABLE 2   Adverse Effects of Diuretic Therapy

Parameters	Dates		
	May 12	August 13	August 23
Furosemide	40 mg PO BID	40 mg PO BID	60 mg PO BID
Metolazone	No	No	2.5 mg PO daily
Weight (LB)	191	187	180
Sitting BP (mm Hg)	122/63	125/68	129/76
Hemoglobin (g/dL)	11.9	13.2	14.5
Hematocrit (%)	36.3	40.5	43.5
BUN (mg/dL)	37	35	67
Serum creatinine (mg/dL)	1.6	1.5	1.8
Serum Na^+ (mEq/L)	139	139	141
Serum K^+ (mEq/L)	4	3.8	3
Serum CL^- (mEq/L)	104	99	88
Serum CO_{2^-} (mEq/L)	29	32	39
Serum glucose (mg/dL)	92	ND	89
Furosemide to 60 mg BID			
Metolazone 2.5 mg P.O.			
Serum uric acid (mg/dL)	8.4	ND	13.2
Serum cholesterol (mg/dL)	151	ND	200

PO, per oral; BID, twice daily.

Postassium-sparing Diuretics

Potassium-sparing diuretics include:

- Spironolactone
- Triamterene
- Amiloride

These diuretics inhibit sodium reabsorption by acting on the cortical collecting tubules, but they may have an effect on the outer medullary collecting tubules. These potassium-sparing agents induce a mild natriuresis to the extent of 2 to 3% of filtered sodium. Spironolactone acts by competing with aldosterone for binding receptor sites. Although amiloride has a pronounced effect in the presence of aldosterone, triamterene inhibits sodium reabsorption independent of aldosterone.

Dosage and administration of potassium-sparing diuretics   The usual dosage of spironolactone is 50 to 200 mg/day, with a maximal dose of 400 mg/day.

CASE STUDY

J.M., a 60-year-old white male, is a hypertension clinic follow-up patient. His diagnoses include alcoholic cirrhosis, acute and chronic CHF, and chronic atrial fibrillation. Physical examination revealed slight shortness of breath, bilateral lower extremity edema, and ascites. He was treated with captopril, digoxin, and furosemide, which was substituted by bumetanide. The results of his arterial blood gas studies and other laboratory studies are presented in Case Study Table 3.

This table demonstrates that the patient had severe hypochloremia and hypokalemia and associated metabolic alkalosis. The markedly elevated BUN to serum creatinine ratio strongly suggests severe volume depletion that, along

with hypochloremia, has resulted in metabolic alkalosis.

Diuretic therapy, especially loop diuretics, can reduce renal function to a great extent in patients with chronic renal insufficiency mainly caused by volume depletion. Reducing the dose of the diuretic often promptly improves renal function to baseline levels. For example, a patient with chronic renal failure was treated with 40 mg oral furosemide daily. His serum creatinine as of October 6, 1993 was 5.9 mg/dL, when furosemide was reduced to 20 mg daily. Three weeks later, his serum creat-inine decreased from 5.9 to 5.4 mg/dL. During the same period, his serum glucose decreased from 150 to 127 mg/dL.

Serum Values	Adverse Effects of Diuretic Therapy Blood Gas Analysis	CASE STUDY TABLE 3 Normal Range
Glucose	114 mg/dL	
BUN	44 mg/dL	pH 7.51	7.35-7.45
Creatinine	1.0 mg/dL	PCO_2 46.7	34-45
Sodium	132 mg/dL	PO_2 71	75-108
Potassium	2.9 mEq/L	bicarbonate 38	18-23
Chloride	83 mEq/L		
CO_2	36.8 mEq/L		

The drug may be given in single or divided doses, and the effect does not start for 48 hours.

Triamterene dosage is 50 mg twice daily. The dosage may be increased to 100 mg twice daily.

Amiloride dosage is 5 mg twice daily. The dosage may be increased to 10 mg twice daily.

Adverse effects of potassium-sparing diuretics Potassium-sparing diuretics should be avoided under the following conditions:

- Impaired renal function
- Concomitantly with angiotensin-converting enzyme (ACE) inhibitors
- Concomitantly with nonsteroidal anti-inflammatory drugs (NSAIDs)
- Underlying diabetic nephropathy
- Concomitantly with potassium supplement, especially in the presence of impaired renal function

The adverse effects of spironolactone include:

- Hyperkalemia
- Gynecomastia
- Impotence
- Painful breasts and decreased libido in females

The adverse effects of triamterene include:

- Hyperkalemia
- Folic acid deficiency leading to megaloblastic anemia
- Triamterene renal calculi

The adverse effects of amiloride include:

- Hyperkalemia
- Hyperchloremic metabolic acidosis

Carbonic anhydrase inhibitors   Acetazolamide is a carbonic anhydrase inhibitor. Acetazolamide acts mainly in the proximal tubule to cause bicarbonate diuresis. Bicarbonate excretion secondarily leads to sodium excretion and water diuresis. Because of chiefly bicarbonate diuresis, acetazolamide is recommended in CHF with metabolic alkalosis and refractory to diuretic therapy. It is also indicated in chronic respiratory acidosis with metabolic alkalosis. Other indications include hyperuricemia and cystine stone formers. The goal is to keep the urine alkaline, which will increase urinary uric acid and cystine excretion, respectively. Acetazolamide is a common drug used for glaucoma.

Adverse effects of acetazolamide include:

- Hypokalemia
- Hyperchloremic non-anion gap metabolic acidosis
- Nephrocalcinosis
- Nephrolithiasis

Refractory Edema

The recommended therapy for refractory edema with normal or slightly impaired renal function includes promoting diuresis. One of the following combinations may be chosen:

For normal renal function (serum creatinine < 1.5 mg/dL): A loop diuretic orally and a potassium-sparing diuretic orally.

For mild to moderate impairment of renal function (serum creatinine > 1.5 mg/dL, < 3 mg/dL), choose one of the following combinations: A loop diuretic orally plus a thiazide diuretic orally; acetazolamide intravenously or orally plus a loop diuretic orally or intravenously; acetazolamide intravenously or orally plus a loop diuretic orally plus a thiazide diuretic orally.

Treatment of the Cause

Treatment of the cause will depend on treatability of the primary cause. In general, specific treatments for CHF and cirrhosis of the liver are limited. When renal disease is present, some glomerular diseases (e.g., minimal lesion disease) are treatable and generally respond well to corticosteroid therapy. Other glomerular diseases, such as membranous glomerulonephritis or membranoproliferative glomerulonephritis, which typically give rise to nephrotic syndrome, do not respond to corticosteroid therapy in most cases.

Adjuvant Therapy

For nephrotic or cirrhotic edema (serum albumin < 2.5 g/dL), administer 25% albumin 100 to 200 mL infusion, or furosemide 40 to 80 mg intravenous bolus during or immediately following albumin infusion.

For refractory CHF, treatment includes:

- Nitroprusside infusion (preload and afterload effect)
- Digoxin
- Furosemide and dopamine infusion to promote natriuresis and diuresis

KEY POINTS

- Although a reduced GFR is frequently observed in edematous patients, many edematous patients with normal GFR retain sodium markedly.

- Aldosterone appears to play a permissive role in excessive sodium retention. Aldosterone antagonist spironolactone consistently induces natriuresis and diuresis and thus, potentiates the effect of loop diuretics.

- Therapeutic options consist of bed rest, variable restriction of fluid and salt, diuretic therapy, treatment of the cause, and adjuvant therapy.

- Hyponatremia is a common finding in edematous conditions such as cirrhosis of the liver or nephrotic syndrome as a result of free water retention from elevated plasma vasopressin levels. Rigid fluid restriction should be avoided to increase free water excretion.

- Bed rest alone helps to mobilize fluid from the dependent portions and results in mild diuresis.

- Thiazide diuretics alone may be adequate in cirrhotic patients but are ineffective in patients with CHF or nephrotic syndrome.

- An intravenous bolus of 40 mg furosemide could result in diuresis of 5 to 6 liters in a few hours.

- Intravenous bolus of a loop diuretic reduces left ventricular filling pressure and pulmonary vascular congestion, minimizing pulmonary edema and relieving shortness of breath.

- The two common metabolic disturbances associated with diuretic therapy are hyperglycemia and hyperlipidemia; both almost always reverse on discontinuation of diuretic therapy.

- Although cardiovascular risk of hyperlipidemia with diuretic therapy has been stressed, it has not been documented.

- Dobutamine infusion to improve ejection fraction

Furosemide 480 mg is added in a liter bag of 5% dextrose in water and infused at a rate of 42 mL/hr, which will deliver 20 mg furosemide per hour. Dopamine is infused separately at a rate of 1 to 3 μg/kg/min. The net result is decreased pulmonary venous congestion, leading to relief of shortness of breath.

Dobutamine is considered a selective β_1-adrenergic agonist. In therapeutic doses, dobutamine also had mild β_2- and α_1-adrenergic receptor agonist effects. Unlike dopamine, dobutamine does not cause release of norepinephrine. The main effect of therapeutic doses of dobutamine is cardiac stimulation. Dobutamine is used to increase cardiac output in the short-term treatment of patients with cardiac decompensation caused by depressed contractility from organic heart disease. Adverse effects include an increase in heart rate and systolic blood pressure. The recommended dosage is 2.5 to 15 μg/kg/min.

The therapy for refractory edema with markedly impaired renal function (GFR $\leq$20 mL/min) includes:

- Intermittent hemodialysis
- Continuous ambulatory peritoneal dialysis (CAPD)
- Continuous venovenous hemofiltration (CVVH)
- Continuous venovenous hemodiafiltration (CVVHD)

Of the aforementioned modalities, CAPD appears to be the most effective method for treating generalized edema with impaired renal function. It is a simple technique done by the patients themselves; however, a support system is helpful. Loss of albumin through CAPD exchanges, especially during peritonitis, is a serious drawback of this technique. In patients with severe proteinuria and hypoalbuminemia, hemodialysis is preferable. Proteinuria can be arrested with an ACE inhibitor such as enalapril.

REFERRAL

Referral of patients with generalized edema will depend on the associated findings. Thus, a patient with generalized edema and proteinuria should be referred to a nephrologist. A patient with generalized edema with massive ascites but no evidence of CHF may be referred to a nephrologist or a gastroenterologist; a patient with edema and distended neck veins who cannot lie flat in bed should be referred to a cardiologist. Edema limited to lower extremities, no proteinuria, and no other associated findings should raise a question of malignancy, and consultation with a hematologist or oncologist is appropriate.

PREVENTION

Prevention of chronic edematous states consists of restricting salt and fluid intake, resting frequently in bed, wearing supportive stockings, keeping legs clean and dry, and seeking medical attention if soreness, ulceration, or blisters are noted. In male patients with normal renal function, using scrotal support for minimizing scrotal swelling, low-dose thiazide diuretics such as hydrochlorothiazide 12.5 mg or metolazone 2.5 mg, and spironolactone 25 mg twice daily are helpful to keep them free of edema.

COMMONLY ASKED QUESTIONS

What is causing my body to swell?
Although the initial cause of swelling may differ from one disease process to another, persistent swelling is the result of sodium and water retention by the kidney.

Will persistent swelling cause any harm to my body?
Swelling (edema) does not typically do any long-term harm to the body. However, massive swelling may cause breakdown of the skin and local infection (cellulitis).

Can the swelling be kept under control even though the cause of the swelling may not be completely eradicated?
Yes, by lying down more frequently than assuming an upright posture, and by reducing salt and fluid intake.

Is there any medicine that I can take to keep my swelling down?
Yes, you can take a diuretic (water pill) alone or in combination with other drugs that your doctor will prescribe. The diuretic increases sodium and water excretion by the kidney and helps to reduce the swelling.

Is there any treatment that can make my swelling go away permanently?
It depends on the initial cause of the swelling. If congestive heart failure or renal disease that has given rise to the swelling is cured, the swelling will disappear permanently.

SUGGESTED READINGS

Bichet DG, Anderson RJ, Schrier RW. Renal sodium excretion, edematous disorders, and diuretic use. In: Schrier RW, ed. Renal and Electrolyte Disorders. Boston: Little, Brown and Company, 1992:89-159.

Ciocon JO, Galindo-Ciocon D, Galindo DJ. Raised leg exercises for leg edema in the elderly. Angiology 1995;46:19-25.

de Jonge JW, Knottnerus JA, van Zutphen WM, et al. Short-term effect of withdrawal of diuretic drugs prescribed for ankle edema. Br Med J 1994;308(6927):511-513.

Guyton AC. The body fluid compartments: extracellular and intracellular fluids; interstitial fluid and edema. In: Textbook of Medical Physiology. Philadelphia: WB Saunders, 1991:274-285.

Karnad DR, Temtulkar P, Abraham P, et al. Head-down as a physiologic diuretic in normal controls and in patients with fluid-retaining states. Lancet 1987;2(8558): 525-528.

Pockros PJ, Reynolds TB. Rapid diuresis in patients with ascites from chronic liver disease: the importance of peripheral edema. Gastroenterology 1986;90:1827-1833.

Ritz E, Fliser D, Wiecek A, et al. Pathophysiology and treatment of hypertension and edema due to renal failure. Cardiology 1994;84(suppl 2):143-154.

Warner LC, Campbell JC, Morali GA, et al. The response of atrial natriuretic factor and sodium excretion to dietary sodium challenges in patients with chronic liver disease. Hepatology 1990;12:460-466.

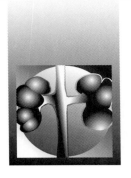

CHAPTER 15

Diabetes and the Kidney

Nabil Farhan
N. Stanley Nahman, Jr

BACKGROUND

Diabetic nephropathy leads to dialysis or transplantation in 30 to 40% of patients with type I diabetes and is the most common cause of end-stage renal disease (ESRD) in the United States. In patients with diabetic nephropathy, understanding the clinical syndromes, appropriate diagnostic evaluation, and approach to therapy is thus critical for minimizing patient morbidity and mortality, and may have a significant impact on the utilization of health care dollars.

Effects of Diabetes on the Kidney: Chronic and Acute

See Table 15.1.

Chronic Effects

Chronic diabetes may result in progressive renal insufficiency and lead to ESRD. Diabetic nephropathy leading to progressive renal failure generally refers to diabetic glomerulosclerosis; that is, a progressive glomerulopathy beginning first as proteinuria followed later by progressive azotemia and the need for renal replacement therapy.

Chronic effects of diabetes on the kidney may manifest in other ways, including:

- Chronic interstitial nephritis
- Nephrosclerosis with hyporeninemic hypoaldo-steronism
- Papillary necrosis
- Large-vessel renovascular disease
- Autonomic dysfunction with neurogenic bladder, resulting in functional obstructive nephropathy

Acute Effects

Acute effects of diabetes on the kidney may be caused by diabetic ketoacidosis and hypertonic, nonketotic coma. Both syndromes can result in pre-renal failure as a consequence of volume depletion, but with appropriate therapy, most cases are reversible.

RENAL SYNDROMES OF CHRONIC (TYPE I) DIABETES

Diabetic Glomerulosclerosis

Diabetic glomerulosclerosis occurs in patients with type I or type II diabetes, but the natural history of the disease has been established primarily through study of patients with type I diabetes (Fig. 15.1). The glomerulopathy of diabetic glomerulosclerosis does not generally manifest before diabetes has been present for at least 7 to 10 years.

TABLE 15.1	Effect of Diabetes on the Kidney	
Condition	Pathophysiology	Potential Clinical Sequelae
Chronic Conditions		
Diabetic nephropathy from diabetic glomerulosclerosis	Glomerulopathy; nephrotic syndrome accompanied by azotemia	Most common cause of ESRD requiring dialysis or kidney transplantation
Chronic interstitial nephritis or nephrosclerosis	Interstitial disease resulting from ischemia; commonly with hypertension and minimal proteinuria	Unusual cause of progressive kidney failure in diabetes
Large-vessel renovascular disease	Atherosclerotic RAS	Hypertension, progressive renal failure in a single kidney, bilateral RAS or with a damaged contralateral kidney
Neurogenic bladder with incomplete bladder evacuation	Bilateral ureteral dilatation with reflux nephropathy from inability to empty bladder	ARF, less common cause of progressive renal failure
Acute Conditions		
Diabetic ketoacidosis	Volume depletion, factitious elevation of serum creatinine	Reversible with appropriate therapy
Nonketotic, hyperosmolar coma	Severe volume depletion resulting from osmotic diuresis	ARF

ESRD, end-stage renal disease; RAS, renal artery stenosis; ARF, acute renal failure.

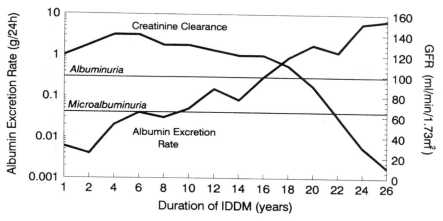

FIGURE 15.1.

Natural history of diabetic glomerulosclerosis in patients with type I diabetes. In patients developing diabetic glomerulosclerosis, microalbuminuria typically develops between 5 and 15 years after onset of diabetes. Over the next decade, there is a greater than 80% chance of developing macroscopic albuminuria ("dipstick-positive" proteinuria). At the onset of macroscopic albuminuria there is a steady, linear decline in GFR (approximately 1 mL/min/month), leading to a need for renal replacement therapy in 3 to 5 years. (Modified with permission from Molich ME. ACE inhibitors and diabetic nephropathy. Diabetes Care 1994;17:756-760.)

The alteration in renal function and glomerular permeability that results from diabetic nephropathy can be summarized as follows: early in the course of the disease, patients tend to have hyperfiltrating glomeruli with a supernormal glomerular filtration rate (GFR). This is presumably caused by the osmotic effects of hyperglycemia and/or alterations in periglomerular vascular tone. During this early phase, urinary protein excretion is typically normal. The emergence of glomerulosclerosis manifests with progressive increases in urinary protein excretion. The demonstration of macroscopic proteinuria (detectable via the dipstick test) indicates advanced disease and is associated with a progressive loss of GFR, leading to ESRD in approximately 7 to 8 years. In those patients developing ESRD, the loss of GFR is nearly linear and occurs at a rate of approximately 1 mL/min/month. Thus, with an initial GFR of 100 mL/min, the progressive loss of renal function will lead to the need for dialysis in approximately 90 months, or 7 to 8 years (at which time GFR is approximately 10 mL/min). The linear loss of GFR can be slowed significantly with effective glycemic control (hemoglobin A_{1C} levels $\leq$7%), tight control of blood pressure (systolic blood pressure <130 mm Hg), and dietary protein restriction (0.6-0.8 gm/kg/day). Angiotensin-converting enzyme (ACE) inhibitors may be used cautiously in this endeavor.

Chronic Interstitial Nephritis or Nephrosclerosis

Chronic interstitial nephritis or nephrosclerosis may accompany diabetic glomerulosclerosis; they are caused by long-standing interstitial ischemia. Fixed small vessel disease results from hyaline deposition in the walls of renal arterioles, or the periglomerular capillaries, resulting in glomerular ischemia and tubular atrophy. Hyporeninemic hypoaldosteronism or papillary necrosis may result from chronic ischemia of the juxtaglomerular apparatus or renal medulla, respectively. The decrease in plasma aldosterone levels may manifest as hyperkalemia and non-anion gap metabolic acidosis. Papillary necrosis may lead to sloughing of medullary tissue and present as flank pain, gross hematuria, and acute urinary tract obstruction.

Chronic interstitial nephritis or nephrosclerosis may occasionally result in progressive renal insufficiency and the need for dialysis. Clinically, patients exhibit a steady rise in serum creatinine concentration, with only minimal proteinuria.

Large-Vessel Renovascular Disease

Accelerated development of atherosclerosis in diabetes may promote development of large-vessel renal artery stenosis. Renal artery stenosis (RAS) may cause hypertension and azotemia or may worsen preexisting conditions. RAS results from accumulation of atheromatous plaque, leading to lumenal compromise and decreased renal perfusion pressure. Glomerular perfusion pressure (and thus GFR) may be directly dependent on systemic blood pressure in patients with fixed vascular lesions from RAS. Clinically, this may manifest as an increase in serum creatinine concentrations following pharmacologic control of hypertension.

CHRONIC EFFECTS OF TYPE I AND II DIABETES

Neurogenic Bladder and Obstructive Uropathy

Autonomic neuropathy is a common complication of diabetes and may lead to the development of a neurogenic bladder. Neurogenic bladder dysfunction results in a decreased sensation to void and bladder overfilling. Bilateral ureteral dilatation with reflux nephropathy may result, with an associated loss of GFR. Thus, neurogenic bladder with obstructive uropathy should be considered when evaluating diabetic patients with unexplained increases in serum creatinine concentrations.

RENAL SYNDROMES OF ACUTE (TYPE II) DIABETES

Hyperosmolar Nonketotic Coma

Hyperosmolar nonketotic coma is an acute metabolic complication seen in patients with type II diabetes. The disease is characterized by extreme hyperglycemia, profound dehydration, and increased plasma osmolality in the absence of overt ketoacidosis. It can occur in a patient without prior history of diabetes mellitus.

Hyperosmolar nonketotic coma may be precipitated by acute medical illnesses, such as:

- Infection
- Cerebrovascular accident
- GI bleeding
- Myocardial infarction
- Pancreatitis

It has also been associated with hyperalimentation and high concentrations of intravenous glucose, and is associated with patients receiving hemodialysis or peritoneal dialysis. Extreme intracellular and extracellular hyperosmolarity leads to the development of central nervous system dysfunction, ranging from mild confusion to generalized seizure activity or coma.

Plasma glucose levels are usually at least 1000 mg/dL and may exceed 2000 mg/dL. Serum hypertonicity accompanies the increase in serum glucose. Many patients with hyperosmolar nonketotic coma have a slight increase in their anion gap with a plasma bicarbonate level in the range of 20 mEq/L.

The mortality rate from hyperosmolar nonketotic coma may exceed 50%. It is crucial to identify all precipitating factors and correct the reversible disorders. Large volumes of intravenous normal saline are indicated initially in patients with hemodynamic instability. As the hemodynamic status of the patient improves,

TABLE 15.2	Diagnostic Approach to Diabetic Conditions Affecting the Kidney

Condition	Signs and Symptoms	Diagnosis
Diabetic nephropathy from diabetic glomerulosclerosis	Early: none Later: volume overload, edema, hypertension, CHF, uremia	Early: microalbuminuria Later: macroalbuminuria, diabetic retinopathy; renal biopsy in unusual cases
Chronic interstitial nephritis or nephrosclerosis	Hypertension, azotemia with minimal (< 1 gm) proteinuria, hyperkalemia, hyperchloremic metabolic acidosis, papillary necrosis	Azotemia with minimal proteinuria, leukocyte casts on urinalysis, appropriate serologic or radiographic studies
Large-vessel renovascular disease	Hypertension and/or unexplained azotemia	IVDSA
Neurogenic bladder with nonobstructive uropathy	Symptoms of bladder neck obstruction, recurrent UTI, bladder distension on examination	Foley catheter placement, renal ultrasound to assess obstruction, bladder cystometrics, diuresis renography

CHF, congestive heart failure; IVDSA, intravenous digital subtraction angiography; UTI, urinary tract infection.

attention to the water deficit can be given. In general, half of the water deficit is replaced in the first 24 hours. Correction attempted more quickly than 24 hours may lead to cerebral edema and worsening of neurologic deficits. For more information on water deficit correction, refer to Chapter 5, "Hyponatremia and Hypernatremia."

Insulin replacement, in smaller doses than used in diabetic ketoacidosis, is frequently indicated. Potassium replacement therapy is frequently more urgent in hypertonic, nonketotic coma than in diabetic ketoacidosis because a more rapid intracellular shift of potassium occurs with therapy.

DIAGNOSIS

See Tables 15.2 and 15.3.

Diabetic Glomerulosclerosis

Early diagnosis of diabetic glomerulosclerosis is essential for effective therapeutic intervention. Type I diabetics should have blood pressure and urinary albumin levels checked on an annual basis if the diabetes has been present for at least 5 years. Urinary protein excretion should be assessed by urinalysis and routine dipstick test for albuminuria. Assessment of microalbuminuria is indicated in patients lacking macroscopic proteinuria.

The presence of microalbuminuria is an established risk factor for the development of macroscopic proteinuria. Microalbuminuria is measured in a 6- to 8-hour urine collection specimen. Normal rates of

microalbuminuria excretion are equal to or less than 25 μg/min (>30 mg/24 hr).

Despite reports demonstrating that persistent microalbuminuria may be associated with biopsy-proven diabetic glomerulosclerosis (i.e., a late finding), treatment of microalbuminuria is strongly justified for the following reasons:

- Microalbuminuria may be reversible with aggressive therapy.
- If left untreated, microalbuminuria almost invariably leads to macroscopic proteinuria and the eventual development of renal insufficiency.

Thus, aggressive treatment of microalbuminuria is an important first step in attempting to slow the development of diabetic glomerulosclerosis.

An empiric diagnosis of diabetic glomerulosclerosis can be made on the following clinical grounds:

- Presence of macroscopic proteinuria
- History of diabetes of at least 5 to 7 years
- Documented diabetic retinopathy

The lack of retinopathy in a proteinuric diabetic raises the possibility of the presence of other glomerular diseases. In the authors' hands, these patients frequently undergo renal biopsy to establish the diagnosis. Patients with diabetic nephropathy and macroscopic proteinuria may have normal or near-normal serum creatinine levels (<2.0 mg/dL) for up to 5 years. Patients with heavy proteinuria and elevated serum creatinine levels represent a more complex medical problem. This

Clinical Characteristics and Diagnostic Considerations in Patients with Diabetic Nephropathy — TABLE 15.3

Duration of Diabetes	Retinopathy	Nephrotic Syndrome	Azotemia	Diagnostic or Therapeutic Options
Appropriate	Present or absent	Absent	Absent	Assess microalbuminuria, if positive: early diabetic glomerulosclerosis
Appropriate	Present	Present	Absent	Advanced diabetic glomerulosclerosis
Appropriate	Present	Present	Present	Very advanced diabetic glomerulosclerosis
Too short	Present	Present	Absent	Likely diabetic glomerulosclerosis, but consider renal biopsy
Appropriate	Absent	Absent	Present	Likely diabetic glomerulosclerosis, but consider renal biopsy
Appropriate	Present or absent	Absent	Present	Not typical of diabetic glomerulosclerosis; must exclude acute renal failure (Table 15.4)

presentation represents an advanced form of diabetic glomerulosclerosis or, alternatively, underlying diabetic glomerulosclerosis with a superimposed, secondary cause of acute renal failure (ARF). If the patient's serum creatinine levels exceed the expected linear loss of GFR, an evaluation for ARF is required (Table 15.4). ARF may result from potentially reversible diseases such as nonsteroidal anti-inflammatory drug (NSAID) ingestion, large-vessel RAS, or urinary tract obstruction, and thus should be pursued aggresively.

Chronic Interstitial Nephritis or Nephrosclerosis

The diagnosis of chronic interstitial nephritis or nephrosclerosis is suggested in patients with elevated serum creatinine concentrations and minimal proteinuria (<1 gm). Acute interstitial nephritis should be excluded. Urinalysis may show slight proteinuria and the presence of leukocyte casts and eosinophiluria.

Hyporeninemic hypoaldosteronism is suggested by the presence of low plasma renin activity, low plasma aldosterone levels, and hyperkalemia and hyperchloremic metabolic acidosis. Twenty-four hour urinary potassium excretion will be inappropriately low, reflecting the decrease in plasma aldosterone.

Chronic interstitial nephritis may cause medullary ischemia and papillary necrosis. Papillary necrosis can manifest clinically as flank pain, hematuria, and/or acute urinary tract obstruction. The diagnosis is made by demonstrating papillary tissue (may appear in conjunction with a blood clot) in the urine or by characteristic radiographic findings seen following intravenous or retrograde urography. The latter study is preferred, given the nephrotoxic potential of intravenous contrast agents. Other risk factors for papillary necrosis should be considered, including:

- Excessive analgesic ingestion
- Recurrent ureteral obstruction
- Chronic pyelonephritis
- History of sickle cell disease

Large-Vessel Renovascular Disease

The diagnosis and therapy of RAS is described in detail in Chapter 12. In brief, RAS should be suspected in any patient with hypertension refractory to therapy (having failed the co-administration of at least three drugs) or in any hypertensive patient with an unexplained elevation in serum creatinine concentrations. The authors perform arteriography in any patient fitting either of these diagnoses. Intravenous digital subtraction angiography (IVDSA) provides acceptable visualization of the

renal arteries and requires less than 10 mL of intravenous contrast material. Patients in whom there is only a moderate level of clinical suspicion for RAS may not require angiography and thus can be screened using noninvasive testing (the captopril stimulation test or captopril renography). Clinical suspicion is increased in patients with a history of large-vessel renovascular disease, vascular bruits on clinical examination, or renal asymmetry by ultrasound. In general, the authors would subject these patients to diagnostic arteriography (IVDSA).

Neurogenic Bladder and Obstructive Uropathy

Patients with autonomic dysfunction and a neurogenic bladder may complain of overflow incontinence or recurrent urinary tract infection. Bladder cystometric studies are used to make the diagnosis. Renal ultrasound may demonstrate hydroureter and hydronephrosis. Diuresis renography can further distinguish between the obstructive versus nonobstructive cause of hydronephrosis.

Summary of Diagnosis

- Diabetic glomerulosclerosis occurs in patients with type I or type II diabetes.
- Diabetic nephropathy does not generally manifest before diabetes has been documented for 8 to 15 years.
- Macroscopic proteinuria (detectable via dipstick test) indicates advanced disease and is associated with a progressive loss of renal function.
- Linear loss of renal function may be slowed with good glycemic control, tight blood pressure control, and dietary protein restriction. The cautious use of ACE inhibitors may be additive.
- Hyperosmolar nonketotic coma is an acute metabolic complication seen in patients with type II diabetes. Hyperosmolar nonketotic coma may be precipitated by an acute medical illness.

TREATMENT

Diabetic Glomerulosclerosis

The therapy for diabetic glomerulosclerosis (Table 15.5) includes:

- Control of hyperglycemia
- Control of hypertension

Common Causes of Acute Renal Failure in Diabetic Patients   TABLE 15.4

Prerenal causes
   Volume depletion
   Congestive heart failure
   Nonsteroidal anti-inflammatory drug ingestion
Renal parenchymal disease
   Vascular disorders
      Large-vessel renal artery occlusion
      Small vessel vasculitis
      Hemolytic uremic syndrome/thrombotic thrombocytopenic purpura (HUS/TTP)
      Atheroembolic disease
   Acute glomerulonephritis
   Tubular interstitial diseases
      Allergic interstitial nephritis
         Antibiotics
      Acute tubular necrosis
         Intravenous contrast administration
         Aminoglycoside antibiotics
         Sepsis
         Pigment toxicity: hemoglobinuria, myoglobinuria
Post-renal obstruction
   Neurogenic bladder
   Nephrolithiasis
   Papillary necrosis

Therapeutic Approach to Diabetic Renal Diseases   TABLE 15.5

Condition	Therapeutic Options
Diabetic nephropathy from diabetic glomerulosclerosis	Glycemic control: Hb $A_{1c} \leq 7\%$ Hypertension control: systolic BP of 130 mm Hg ACE inhibitor therapy (cautious use) Dietary protein restriction: 0.6–0.7 gm/kg/day
Chronic interstitial nephritis or nephrosclerosis	Hypertension control Correct hyperkalemia: loop diuretic, mineralocorticoid Correct acidosis: bicarbonate, 1 mEq/kg/day Correct obstruction from papillary necrosis
Large-vessel renovascular disease	Balloon angioplasty or surgical bypass of critical lesions Anticipate progression of medically treated lesions
Neurogenic bladder with obstructive uropathy	Frequent voiding Cholinergics Self-catheterization Incision of internal sphincter
Diabetic ketoacidosis	Fluid resuscitation, insulin, correct electrolyte disorders, identify cause for event
Nonketotic, hyperosmolar coma	Fluid resuscitation, insulin, correct electrolyte disorders, identify cause for event

- Dietary protein restriction, when appropriate
- Cautious use of ACE inhibitors

Each of the aforementioned modalities is presented in the sections that follow.

Glycemic Control

The Diabetes Control and Complications Trial demonstrated that blood sugar control, with a target hemoglobin A_{1C} less than or equal to 7%, reduced the occurrence of both microscopic and macroscopic proteinuria. Improved glycemic control can be attained from:

- Frequent blood sugar testing and appropriate adjustments in insulin dosing
- Use of subcutaneous insulin pump delivery systems
- Pancreas transplantation

It is the authors' practice to reserve transplantation for patients who have concurrent ESRD from diabetic nephropathy. In this setting, the patient receives a combined pancreas/kidney transplant.

Control of Hypertension

Blood pressure is a critical determinant of the progression of diabetic nephropathy. Decreasing the systolic blood pressure from 144 to 128 mm Hg resulted in a decrease in the rate of GFR loss from 0.9 to .4 mL/min/month.

Note that a systolic blood pressure of 128 mm Hg is well below the 135 mm Hg quoted as "normal" by the Joint National Commission on High Blood Pressure. On this basis, "hyper" control of blood pressure is indicated. The authors target all proteinuric diabetics to a systolic blood pressure of 120 to 125 mm Hg. Aggressive antihypertensive therapy should be used to attain this goal. In addition, the antihypertensive regimen should include ACE inhibitors whenever possible (see next section).

Dietary Protein Restriction

In selected patients, limiting the dietary protein intake to 0.6-0.7 gm/kg/day may further help to slow the progression of diabetic glomerulosclerosis.

Angiotensin-converting Enzyme (ACE) Inhibitors

The ACE inhibitor trial in type I diabetics shows a significant effect of ACE inhibitors in slowing the progression of diabetic glomerulosclerosis. When compared with placebo, ACE inhibitor therapy decreased mortality and comorbid events, such as the need for dialysis. Therefore, in all patients with diabetic glo-

merulosclerosis and normal renal function, cautious use of ACE inhibitors is worthy of trial.

ACE inhibitors are indicated in any hypertensive, proteinuric diabetic patient. This includes hypertensive patients with microalbuminuria or macroscopic proteinuria. ACE inhibitors may also decrease proteinuria in normotensive (systolic blood pressure <120 mm Hg) patients. Low doses of the drugs are used and the patient is monitored for signs or symptoms of hypotension. The response to therapy is assessed by measuring urinary protein excretion. Urinary protein excretion may decrease as soon as 1 month following therapy, but a therapeutic response can take up to 1 year to manifest. The authors do not empirically treat normotensive patients with normal urinary protein excretion.

Complications of ACE Inhibitors

ACE inhibitor therapy should be used with caution in patients with preexisting azotemia and/or a tendency toward hyperkalemia. By inhibiting the production of angiotensin II, the drugs subsequently decrease aldosterone and urinary excretion of potassium. Thus, patients with azotemia and/or hyperkalemia may have a tendency to develop life-threatening hyperkalemia. The drugs should be used with extreme caution or not at all in these patient subgroups. If ACE inhibitors are used, serum potassium levels should be monitored frequently. Pregnant females should not take ACE inhibitors because of potential teratogenic effects.

Chronic Interstitial Nephritis or Nephrosclerosis

The therapy of patients with chronic interstitial nephritis or nephrosclerosis is directed at blood pressure control and correction of electrolyte and acid-base abnormalities. Hyperkalemia associated with hyporeninemic hypoaldosteronism may be treated with dietary potassium restriction. If hypertension accompanies the hyperkalemia, a loop diuretic (such as furosemide) may help control the hypertension as well as the hyperkalemia.

When hyperchloremic metabolic acidosis is present, instituting sodium bicarbonate therapy (1 mEq/kg/day) will help maintain normal acid-base status. In extreme cases, mineralocorticoids (9-L-fluorohydrocortisone) may be necessary in patients with autonomic neuropathy and hypotension complicated by hyporeninemic hypoaldosteronism. 9-L-fluorohydrocortisone may be given in a dose of 0.1 to 0.3 mg orally once daily. The maximum dose is 1 mg daily. All patients should be followed closely for evidence of congestive heart failure (CHF) because of their increased sodium retention.

Patients with papillary necrosis and unilateral ureteral obstruction need urologic intervention. Cystoscopic removal of obstructing tissue may be necessary. In patients not amenable to cystoscopy, percutaneous nephrostomy tube placement may be indicated to relieve the obstruction. The obstructing tissue can then be removed using an anterograde approach.

Large-Vessel Renovascular Disease

Angiographically proven RAS should be treated with balloon angioplasty or vascular bypass surgery. High-grade lesions (>90%, as assessed by visual inspection of the angiogram) and lesions in which the renal artery systolic blood pressure gradient exceeds 50 mm Hg should be treated. Judgment on whether to treat lower grade lesions is typically based on the clinician's experience, but progression of atherosclerotic RAS should be anticipated, regardless. Restenosis of surgically or medically treated RAS must be considered if hypertension worsens or if there is an unexpected rise in serum creatinine concentrations. (See also Chapter 12.)

Neurogenic Bladder and Obstructive Uropathy

In the event of acute urine retention, an indwelling Foley catheter should be placed in the bladder. After decompressing the bladder and establishing the diagnosis, subsequent episodes can be prevented by asking the patient to void frequently, by using cholinergic therapy, or by intermittent bladder catheterization. Surgical options include incision of the internal sphincter.

ASSOCIATED CONDITIONS

Diabetic Ketoacidosis

Diabetic ketoacidosis is an acute metabolic complication characteristic of insulin-dependent diabetes, but it may also occur in type II diabetes. Insulin deficiency and hyperglycemia, accompanied by an increase in counter-regulatory hormones (primarily epinephrine and glucagon), are the essential factors in the pathogenesis of diabetic ketoacidosis (Table 15.6).

Precipitating causes of diabetic ketoacidosis include:

- Interruption of insulin administration
- Physical stress (infection, myocardial infarction, trauma, surgery, inflammation)
- Emotional stress with an associated increase in counter-regulatory hormones

The main characteristics of diabetic ketoacidosis are hyperglycemia, ketosis, and acidosis. Hyperglycemia is the result of increased liver production of glucose by stimulation of gluconeogenesis and inhibition of glycolysis, and impaired peripheral glucose utilization. Ketosis results from increased fatty acid production in adipose tissue and subsequent beta oxidation in the

Hormonal Mediators in Diabetic Ketoacidosis		TABLE 15.6
Hormone	**Target Organ(s)**	**Physiologic Effects**
Insulin	Liver	Stimulates glycogenesis
		Inhibits glycogenolysis
	Muscle	Increases glucose uptake
		Stimulates glycogenesis
		Inhibits glycogenolysis
	Adipose tissue	Increases free fatty acid synthesis and storage
		Inhibits intracellular lipolysis
Epinephrine	Pancreas	Suppresses insulin release
		Increases glucagon secretion
	Muscle	Stimulates glycogenolysis
		Inhibits glycogenesis
Glucagon	Liver	Stimulates gluconeogenesis
		Inhibits glycolysis
		Stimulates ketone body production

liver. Anion gap metabolic acidosis is mainly caused by accumulation of ketoacids (β-hydroxybutyrate and acetoacetate) resulting from increased production and decreased peripheral utilization.

Underestimation of the ketoacid burden may result from serum samples tested with reagent strips or tablets. These methods detect mainly acetoacetate and do not give an accurate indication of β-hydroxybutyrate levels. Acetoacetate is the oxidized form of β-hydroxybutyrate. During periods of hypoxemia or tissue hypoperfusion, acetoacetate is reduced to β-hydroxybutyrate, and serum acetoacetate levels may underestimate the true ketone burden. Conversely, the ketone load may appear to increase during therapy because the β-hydroxybutyrate pool is converted to acetoacetate.

Approximately 15% of patients with diabetic ketoacidosis have elevated lactic acid levels (>5 mEq/L). Increased lactate production results from hypoperfusion (with increased peripheral pyruvate production) and insulin deficiency (resulting in an inhibition of pyruvate degradation leading to increased lactate production).

A hyperchloremic, non-anion gap metabolic acidosis may develop in up to 50% of patients following therapy of ketoacidosis. This is primarily the result of volume expansion during treatment that leads to increased renal excretion of ketones, which are a substrate for bicarbonate regeneration. Urinary loss of ketones in this setting is equivalent to bicarbonate wasting and generates the hyperchloremic acidosis.

Effect of Diabetic Ketoacidosis on Serum Creatinine Concentration

Determination of serum creatinine levels frequently depends on the formation of a chromogenic complex between picrate and creatinine. Thus, the level of creatinine is proportional to the degree of color change in the reaction. The accuracy of this method is limited because both creatinine and noncreatinine chromogens are detected with this reaction and thus may cause a false elevation in the serum creatinine. Automated, enzymatic, one-slide-based assays avoid this problem and give an accurate indication of the true serum creatinine. One-slide assays do not yield the false increase in creatinine at serum glucose levels above 600 mg/dL that is common with two-slide assays.

Electrolyte Abnormalities

Osmotic diuresis that results from glycosuria leads to volume contraction and depletion of body potassium and phosphate stores. Despite a total body potassium deficit (up to 400 mEq), serum potassium levels may be high or normal as a result of acidosis, insulin deficiency, and hyperosmolarity, all which cause a shift of intracellular potassium to the extracellular space. Potassium deficits should be anticipated and aggressively replaced because, with treatment of ketoacidosis, extracellular potassium will move back into the intracellular compartment, potentially causing hypokalemia.

Phosphate depletion may also exist despite elevation of serum phosphate levels because of phosphate shifting from the intracellular to the extracellular compartment. Low phosphate levels cause shifting of the oxygen dissociation curve to the left (indicating no unloading of oxygen), as a result of depleted 2,3-diphosphoglycerate levels. This effect is countered by the presence of acidosis, which causes a shift of the curve to the right (indicating unloading of oxygen). Phosphate depletion should be anticipated and treated accordingly because, during reversal of acidosis, phosphate deficiency may manifest with an unopposed leftward shift of the oxygen dissociation curve, indicating that no unloading of oxygen is occurring.

Hyponatremia in diabetic ketoacidosis may result from osmotic diuresis with an associated decrease in total body sodium, or from dilutional hyponatremia in conjunction with hyperglycemia (pseudohyponatremia). Dilutional hyponatremia results from the movement of free water from the intracellular space, in response to the hypertonic environment induced by hyperglycemia.

TREATMENT

Fluid deficits from diabetic ketoacidosis may be substantial, depending on the duration of the illness and on other confounding factors (fever, vomiting, diarrhea, etc.). Fluid replacement with normal saline, insulin infusion, and potassium and phosphorus administration is the mainstay of therapy. Bicarbonate replacement is indicated for a serum pH less than 7.0 mEq/L or a serum bicarbonate less than 5 mEq/L, particularly in patients with hemodynamic instability and/or cardiac arrhythmias. When indicated, small amounts of intravenous bicarbonate replacement (50 mEq/amp) are recommended but should be discontinued when the pH reaches 7.2. Patients with advanced renal insufficiency or ESRD who develop diabetic ketoacidosis may not develop diuresis to the same extent as patients with normal renal function, thus limiting the extent of volume contraction.

These patients may become more severely acidotic. Replacement fluid should be administered judiciously to avoid volume overload and pulmonary edema. Significant renal impairment in patients with advanced ESRD minimizes potassium and phosphorus losses so that replacement of these electrolytes should be closely monitored. In this setting, insulin replacement therapy is the chief modality of treatment. Hypoglycemia may complicate therapy in these patients because renal insufficiency leads to decreased insulin catabolism and impaired renal gluconeogenesis.

KEY POINTS

- Diagnosis of diabetic nephropathy can be reasonably made on the basis of a history of diabetes mellitus for 5 to 7 years, diabetic retinopathy, and the presence of gross proteinuria.

- Aggressive treatment of microalbuminuria is an important first step in attempting to slow the development of diabetic glomerulosclerosis.

- Decline in renal function usually parallels an increase in proteinuria.

- Acute deterioration of renal function can occur from reversible conditions, such as ingestion of NSAIDs, large-vessel RAS, or urinary tract obstruction and/or infection.

- ACE inhibitors may be used cautiously, in particular in patients with impaired renal function. Regular monitoring of serum creatinine and potassium levels is essential if ACE inhibitors are used. The editor does not recommend ACE inhibitor therapy in patients with impaired renal function.

- No therapy is known to halt the progressive deterioration of renal function or proteinuria; patients should be referred to a nephrologist without any delay for dialysis intervention.

REFERRAL

Nephrology consultation can be useful in evaluating patients with ARF or in those exhibiting an unusual presentation of diabetic nephropathy. Patients with un-

controllable hypertension requiring frequent monitoring or additional diagnostic evaluation may benefit from nephrology consultation.

Renal replacement options for diabetics with ESRD include hemodialysis, continuous ambulatory peritoneal dialysis (CAPD), or kidney transplantation. The authors pursue transplantation in all diabetics, assuming there is no contraindication to the procedure. Transplantation options available to patients in most institutions include cadaveric renal transplantation, live donor (related and unrelated) renal transplantation, and combined cadaveric (single donor) pancreas/kidney transplantation. Many patients can directly undergo transplantation without requiring dialysis. Early referral (creatinine approximately 2-3 mg/dL) to the nephrologist or transplant program is important to facilitate this approach.

Azotemic diabetics should be referred to the nephrologist in preparation for transplantation. Activities and procedures that need to be coordinated include preparing the patient psychologically for dealing with renal failure, referral to the transplant program in anticipation of transplantation, and, if transplant is not anticipated before the need for dialysis, establishment of vascular or peritoneal access. It is generally accepted that, in diabetics, renal replacement therapy should be instituted before the onset of severe uremic or congestive symptoms; diabetics with uremia or CHF tend to be sicker than nondiabetic patients with kidney failure.

COMMONLY ASKED QUESTIONS

What is a typical time frame between developing diabetes and needing dialysis or transplantation?
Renal failure develops in only 30 to 40% of type I diabetics; thus, not all patients will develop this complication. Microalbuminuria usually does not ensue before the disease has been present at least 5 years, and macroscopic proteinuria generally appears after 7 to 10 years. GFR is lost at a linear rate after the appearance of macroscopic proteinuria, with renal replacement therapy required in approximately 90 months (7 to 8 years). Uncontrolled hypertension can greatly accelerate the loss of GFR and bring patients to dialysis in half that time.

How successful is dialysis or transplantation in treating diabetic renal failure?
The 1-year survival rate for dialysis patients with end-stage renal disease secondary to diabetes mellitus is approximately 70%. The 1-year patient survival rate following living-related donor kidney transplant approaches 96%, and 91% with cadaveric renal transplantation. The 5-year patient survival in diabetic patients after living-related kidney transplant is approximately 85%, and 80% following cadaveric kidney transplantation.

What can be done to cure or slow the progression of diabetic glomerulosclerosis?

Diabetic glomerulosclerosis cannot be cured, but the loss of GFR may be slowed by therapies such as tight hypertension and glycemic control, correction of hyperkalemia and acidosis, ACE inhibitors, cholinergics, fluid replacement, and insulin. A list of therapies is outlined in Table 15.5.

SUGGESTED READINGS

Diabetes Control and Complications Trial. The effect of intensive treatment of diabetes on the development and progression of long-term complications in insulin-dependent diabetes mellitus. N Engl J Med 1993;329: 977-986.

Lewis E, Hunsicker L, Bain R, et al. The effect of angiotensin-converting enzyme inhibition in diabetic nephropathy. N Engl J Med 1993;329:1456-1462.

Mauer S, Steffes M, Ellis E, et al. Structural-functional relationships in diabetic nephropathy. J Clin Invest 1984; 74:1143.

Mogensen C. Microalbuminuria as a predictor of clinical diabetic nephropathy. Kidney Int 1987;31:673-689.

Mogensen C, Christensen C. Predicting diabetic nephropathy in insulin-dependent patients. N Engl J Med 1984;311: 89-93.

Parving H, Smidt U, Anderson A, et al. Early aggressive antihypertensive treatment reduces rate of decline in kidney function in diabetic nephropathy. Lancet 1983;1:1175-1179.

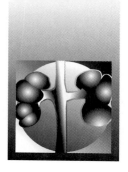

Hypercalcemia

Anil K. Mandal

BACKGROUND

Physiology

Normal ranges of total serum calcium vary from 8.5 to 10.5 mg/dL. Approximately 50% of total serum calcium is protein-bound, mostly bound with albumin (40%), but a small amount is bound with globulins (10%). Only the free or ionized calcium (50%) is essential for neuromuscular function and glandular secretion. Ionized calcium ranges from approximately 1.16 to 1.32 mmol/L.

Calcium is poorly absorbed from the intestinal tract. Approximately 80 to 90% of daily dietary calcium intake (1 gm = 1000 mg) is excreted in the feces, the remaining 10 to 20% in the urine. Calcium excretion (CaE) in the urine conforms to the same principles as sodium excretion. Approximately two-thirds of the filtered calcium is reabsorbed in the proximal tubules. In the ascending limb of loop of Henle and in the distal convoluted and collecting tubules, reabsorption of the remaining calcium varies, depending on the calcium concentration in the blood. When calcium concentration is low, reabsorption in these nephron segments is very high, so that little to no calcium appears in the urine. Conversely, an increase in calcium concentration above normal increases urinary CaE markedly.

Parathyroid hormone (PTH), together with vitamin D, is the principal regulator of serum calcium concentration. In the normal physiologic regulation of serum calcium, a decrease in serum calcium leads to an increase in PTH, which increases release of calcium from the skeleton and its delivery to the extracellular fluid (ECF). PTH also acts on the kidney to increase distal tubular reabsorption of calcium and stimulate the renal 1-α hydroxylase enzyme that increases the production of 1α,25-dihydroxyvitamin D_3. 1α,25-dihydroxyvitamin D_3 acts on gut epithelium to increase the fractional absorption of calcium from the gut. Tubular reabsorption of calcium has a less vital role than osteoclastic bone reabsorption in the pathogenesis of hypercalcemia. In states of fluid dehydration, however, the capacity for excretion of a large bone-derived filtered load of calcium is impaired because of enhanced proximal reabsorption of calcium along with sodium. PTH-related protein (PTHrP), the recently identified peptide factor, further aggravates hypercalcemia by increasing distal tubular calcium reabsorption.

CAUSES

Two major causes of hypercalcemia are primary hyperparathyroidism and hypercalcemia of malignancy.

Hypercalcemia may be a manifestation of a variety of disorders, including the following:

- Primary hyperparathyroidism
- Primary malignancy
- Metastatic malignancy, including multiple myeloma
- Sarcoidosis
- Familial benign hypercalcemia
- Hyperthyroidism
- Hypervitaminosis D
- Acute osteoporosis
- Milk-alkali syndrome
- Adrenal insufficiency

Hypercalcemia may be seen in as many as 1.5% of all patients with malignant disease, with or without bony metastases. The malignant neoplasms most commonly associated with hypercalcemia include carcinoma of the lung (all cell types), breast cancer, squamous cell carcinomas, hematologic malignancies, and renal cell carcinoma.

Lung and breast cancers account for 60% of all cancers associated with hypercalcemia.

Pathophysiology

Hypercalcemia is the most common metabolic complication of cancer. Malignancy-associated hypercalcemia can be divided into the following three syndromes:

1. Humoral hypercalcemia of malignancy (HHM)
2. Local osteolytic hypercalcemia (LOH), based on whether a circulating hormone or local paracrine factors mediate accelerated bone resorption
3. Calcitriol-mediated hypercalcemia

PTHrP plays a dominant role in the pathogenesis of HHM. The stimulation of increased osteoclastic bone reabsorption by PTHrP is a principal feature of HHM. Neoplasms that metastasize widely to bone and induce local osteoclastic bone reabsorption-such as multiple myeloma-also are capable of inducing hypercalcemia. Besides osteoclastic bone reabsorption, enhanced calcium absorption by kidney and intestine under the influence of PTHrP may be an important factor in the pathogenesis of hypercalcemia in certain neoplasms.

Based on existing data, it is unclear what percentage of neoplasms metastasizing to bone and stimulating local bone resorption are also capable of stimulating hypercalcemia by systemic factors.

Hypercalcemia is a rare complication of prostate cancer, and no definite association with any histologic subtype of prostatic malignancy has been documented. All cases of hypercalcemia resulting from prostate cancer reported in the literature are well-documented cases of neuroendocrine carcinoma of the prostate. Gastric and colorectal cancer are virtually never associated with hypercalcemia.

Another mechanism for induction of hypercalcemia in malignancy is 1α,25-dihydroxyvitamin D_3 or calcitriol. Calcitriol seems to contribute significantly to hypercalcemia in hematologic malignancies and in chronic granulomatous diseases, including sarcoidosis and tuberculosis.

A distinct syndrome of calcitriol-mediated hypercalcemia is seen in patients with Hodgkin's or non-Hodgkin's lymphoma. This syndrome is characterized by the following:

- Hypercalcemia
- Intestinal hyperabsorption of calcium
- Normal or slightly elevated serum PO_4 level
- Absence of renal PO_4 wasting
- Elevated serum calcitriol level
- Increased renal excretion of calcium
- Suppressed PTH and PTHrP levels
- Normal nephrogenous cAMP

Extrarenal production of calcitriol appears to be the underlying defect in Hodgkin's or non-Hodgkin's lymphoma, although it is unclear whether the lymphoma cells or the infiltrating host monocytes and macrophages are the primary source. There is some evidence that other osteolytic factors such as interleukin-1 and tumor necrosis factor may, with calcitriol, exacerbate the hypercalcemia in these malignancies.

Associated Conditions

Renal Transplant Recipients

Hypercalcemia occurs in 10 to 30% of renal transplant recipients, most often caused by persistent hyperparathyroidism in these patients. However, a low to normal PTH level and virtually undetectable levels of PTHrP were reported in a patient who had recurrent hypercalcemia for 7 years. An elevated level of $1\alpha,25$-dihydroxyvitamin D_3 (calcitriol) leads to the diagnosis of an underlying lymphoma in this patient.

The possibility of an underlying lymphoproliferative disorder should therefore be considered in the differential diagnosis of hypercalcemia in renal transplant patients. Also, elevated levels of $1\alpha,25$-dihydroxyvitamin D_3 should be a key indication for considering underlying non-Hodgkin's lymphoma, which is common in transplant patients.

A combination of elevated serum $1\alpha,25$-dihydroxyvitamin D_3 value, a normal 25-hydroxyvitamin D value, plus low values for PTH and PTHrP has been found in a variety of neoplastic and granulomatous diseases and in infective conditions with hypercalcemia. The infective conditions include AIDS, with cryptococcosis, *Pneumocystis carinii*, *Candida albicans*, and disseminated fungal infections.

Hyperparathyroidism

Hyperparathyroidism is associated with an increased occurrence of malignancy. On occasion, hypercalcemia has been attributable to cancer when underlying hyperparathyroidism is responsible.

Milk-Alkali Syndrome

Milk-alkali syndrome had almost vanished but has surged again with the growing popularity of the use of calcium carbonate as an antacid or as calcium supplementation to prevent osteoporosis.

CASE STUDY: MILK-ALKALI SYNDROME

A 69-year-old white male was brought by friends into the emergency room of VA Medical Center, Dayton, Ohio, because he was confused and disoriented. He gave a vague history of nausea and vomiting for several days before his arrival at the emergency room. Physical examination revealed no abnormalities except for confusion and disorientation.

Laboratory examination revealed hemoglobin 12.2 g/dL, hematocrit 36.3%, total WBC count 11,600 m^3 with normal differential, and platelet count 391,000 m^3. Serum chemistry showed sodium 133 mEq/L, potassium 3.4 mEq/L, chloride 84 mEq/L, bicarbonate 38 mEq/L, urea nitrogen 81 mg/dL, and creatinine 8.3 mg/dL. Other laboratory tests include serum calcium 15.6 mg/dL, serum phosphate 5.4 mg/dL, serum albumin 3.7 g/dL, and total protein 6.7 g/dL. Serum osmolality was 308 mOsm/kg. Twenty-four hour urinary calcium was 432 mg, and uric acid 565 mg. A spot urinary electrolytes showed sodium 113 mEq/L, chloride 84 mEq/L, potassium 13 mEq/L, and creatinine 23.9 mg/dL. Chest radiograph showed no mass or infiltrate. Electrocardiogram showed no abnormalities.

This patient had a triad of hypercalcemia, hyperbicarbonatemia (metabolic alkalosis), and renal

failure, which is consistent with milk-alkali syndrome. He was initially infused with isotonic saline at a rate of 150 mL/hr. After several hours of hydration, furosemide 40 mg was given intravenously every 6 hours for 24 hours, then every 12 hours for another 24 hours. Furosemide was discontinued after 48 hours. He was also given calcitonin 4 IU/kg by intravenous infusion, one dose on day one; and prednisone orally 20 mg on day one, 10 mg on day two, 5 mg on day three, and 2.5 mg on day four. Serum calcium returned to normal on day five of hospital admission, and serum urea nitrogen and serum creatinine decreased to almost normal levels on day eight (Fig. 16.1).

The patient's mental status improved in parallel with the decrease of serum calcium on day two of hospital admission. He became fully oriented to time and space and was able to give relevant history. He stated that he felt bloated in the abdomen. He was consuming one gallon of milk daily along with ice cream and up to 50 tablets of Tums. (Tums are rich in calcium carbonate.) Thus, a history of excessive intake of calcium-containing products and heavy consumption of dairy products, along with complete reversal of hypercalcemia, metabolic alkalosis, and renal failure substantiated a diagnosis of milk-alkali syndrome.

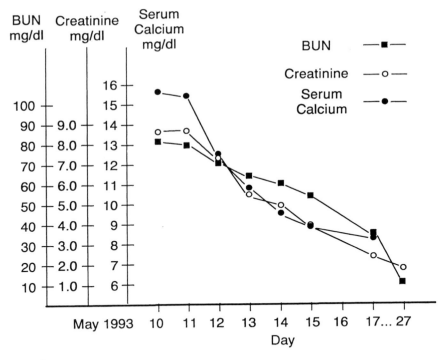

FIGURE 16.1.

A 69-year-old white male was brought to the emergency room by a friend who noted him to be confused and disoriented. No previous history or laboratory studies were available. Serum calcium was 15.6 mg/dL, BUN was 81 mg/dL, and serum creatinine was 8.3 mg/dL at the time of admission. With hydration and furosemide, when serum calcium decreased to 13 mg/dL in 24 hours, the patient became alert and oriented and was able to give a relevant history. All the values returned to normal in the course of several days (see text for details of management). (Adapted with permission from Mandal AK. Management of Acute Renal Failure in the Elderly: Treatment Options: Drugs and Aging, Vol. 4. New Zealand: Adis International, Ltd, 1996: 226-250.)

SYMPTOMS

Symptoms of hypercalcemia are often related to the underlying cause for hypercalcemia, the time course for the development of hypercalcemia, the severity of hypercalcemia, and intercurrent medical conditions. Hypercalcemia generally gives rise to neuromuscular, renal, and gastrointestinal manifestations.

When serum calcium concentration rises above normal, the nervous system is depressed, and the reflex activities of the central nervous system become sluggish. The depressive effects begin to appear when total calcium level rises above 12 mg/dL, and they become more marked when the level rises above 15 mg/dL. When the total calcium level rises above 17 mg/dL, the patient is symptomatic, and calcium phosphate product is likely to precipitate throughout the body. Elevated calcium decreases the Q-T interval of the heart and causes constipation and loss of appetite because of decreased contractility of smooth muscles of the gastrointestinal tract.

In elderly or critically ill patients, significant cognitive impairment may be seen with mild degrees of hypercalcemia.

Marked dehydration and profound mental status changes accompany greater degrees of hypercalcemia. Nephrolithiasis, peptic ulcer disease, and joint manifestations suggest primary hyperparathyroidism as the cause of hypercalcemia. An increasingly recognized presentation of hyperparathyroidism, particularly in the elderly population, is severe hypercalcemia. In a study of 111 hypercalcemic hyperparathyroid patients found in an urban population of one million people in the United Kingdom, 14 subjects presented with acute hypercalcemic syndrome. The majority of patients with primary hyperparathyroidism have long-standing hypercalcemia, very large parathyroid adenomas, radiographic evidence of osteitis fibrosa cystica (50%), and a history of nephrolithiasis (60%). Osteitis fibrosa cystica is virtually never seen in hypercalcemia associated with malignancy.

Acute hypercalcemic syndrome develops in association with severe hypercalcemia and occurs in malignancy and primary hyperparathyroidism. Patients with malignancy-associated hypercalcemia are usually symptomatic, and hypercalcemia adds significantly to their morbidity and mortality. More often, individuals with known malignancy are diagnosed with hypercalcemia during the course of the disease. The symptoms of hypercalcemia may masquerade as symptoms of the underlying malignancy or its therapy. For example, weight loss, anorexia, muscle weakness, constipation, and altered mental status are attributed to progressive cancer. Impaired mental function, lethargy, and disorientation may be thought to be caused by narcotic analgesics or anxiolytic therapy, but, in fact, may be caused by hypercalcemia.

Hypercalcemic crisis is characterized by the following symptoms, which may be the first clinical manifestations of hypercalcemia associated with malignancy:

- Dehydration
- Renal insufficiency
- Mental obtundation

In general, the higher the level of serum calcium, the more likely that malignancy is the underlying cause for hypercalcemia.

Familial benign hypercalcemia (FBH) resembles primary hyperparathyroidism but shows slight parathyroid hyperplasia or overactivity. Hypercalcemia is associated with hypocalciuria and persists even after parathyroidectomy. Familial transmission is of autosomal dominant type. A high incidence of neonatal primary hyperparathyroidism occurs among the offspring of the affected families. This is a benign condition and does not cause nephrolithiasis or bone disease. Pancreatitis is an infrequent occurrence.

DIAGNOSIS

The differential features of primary hyperparathyroidism versus hypercalcemia of malignancy, the two major causes of hypercalcemia, are summarized in Table 16.1.

The following laboratory tests are essential in patients with hypercalcemia:

Differential Diagnosis of Major Causes of Hypercalcemia   **TABLE 16.1**

Features	Primary Hyperparathyroidism	Malignancy
Duration	Long history	Short history
History of underlying malignancy	Absent	Present
Symptoms	Bone pain, renal stones common Rarely, symptoms of hypercalcemia	Symptoms related to hypercalcemia: cognitive dysfunction, vomiting, constipation, renal failure
Intact PTH level	Elevated	Normal or low
PTHrP (n = 2.7 pmol/L)	Normal (95%)	Elevated (82%) without detectable bone metastases; elevated (38%) with metastatic bone disease
Serum calcitriol level	Normal	Elevated in Hodgkin's or non-Hodgkin's lymphoma
Correlation between serum urate and serum calcium	Significant	Nonsignificant
Correlation between serum creatinine and serum calcium	Significant	Nonsignificant
Elevation of serum urea nitrogen	Uncommon	Common (mostly caused by dehydration)
Urinary cAMP	Elevated	Suppressed
Glucocorticoid suppression test (prednisone 40 mg TID) for 2 days	No effect	Effective in decreasing serum calcium (breast cancer, lymphoma, myeloma)

PTH, parathyroid hormone; PTHrP, PTH-related protein.

- Serum-intact PTH level
- PTHrP
- Serum level of calcitriol or $1\alpha,25$-dihydroxyvitamin D_3
- Urinary cAMP

   Additional tests include:

- Correlation curve between serum urate and serum calcium
- Correlation curve between serum creatinine and serum calcium
- Glucocorticoid suppression test: prednisone is given orally 40 mg three times daily for 5 days. Serum calcium is obtained before and after completion of therapy.

- Bone survey
- Bone marrow
- Bone biopsy

   Bone survey and bone marrow studies are considered in cases of myeloma. Bone biopsy is considered in cases with suspected primary hyperparathyroidism.

Familial Benign Hypercalcemia

This condition is best defined by doing an oral calcium-loading test. A result of a serum PTH concentration greater than 2.6 pmol/L in a hypercalcemic patient is suggestive of hyperparathyroidism. Fasting serum PTH concentrations in 58 patients with surgically and histologically proven primary hyperparathyroidism were well above 2.7 pmol/L, with a range of 3.2 to 84.5 pmol/L. In contrast, 13 of 20 patients with FBH had fasting serum PTH concentrations greater than 2.6 pmol/L, but the range was much smaller: only 1.6 to 6.1 pmol/L. There was a significant correlation between serum PTH and age in the FBH patients only. Fasting urine CaE ranged from 280 to 4440 μg/L of glomerular filtrate in primary hyperparathyroidism and 60 to 680 μg/L of glomerular filtrate in FBH. The best biochemical differentiation between patients with primary hyperparathyroidism and those with FBH is to plot fasting serum PTH against CaE.

TREATMENT

General measures include:

- Hydration
- Avoidance of prolonged immobilization
- Identification of the underlying cause of hypercalcemia

   Specific measures include:

- Inhibiting bone resorption
- Increasing renal sodium and CaE

Summary of Diagnosis

- PTH, in combination with vitamin D, is the principal regulator of serum calcium concentration.
- Dehydration is an important factor in the pathogenesis of hypercalcemia by means of its enhancing proximal tubular reabsorption of calcium.
- Hypercalcemia is the most common metabolic complication of cancer.
- The malignant neoplasms most commonly associated with hypercalcemia include carcinoma of the lung and breast, squamous cell carcinomas, hematologic malignancies, and renal cell carcinoma.
- PTHrP plays a dominant role in the pathogenesis of HHM. The stimulation of increased osteoclastic bone reabsorption by PTHrP is a principal feature of HHM.
- A distinct syndrome of calcitriol-mediated hypercalcemia is seen in patients with Hodgkin's or non-Hodgkin's lymphoma.
- Marked dehydration and profound mental status changes are common presenting features of severe hypercalcemia (serum $Ca^{2+} \geq 17$ mg/dL).
- Rehydration is the essential first step of treatment.
- Calcium is cotransported with sodium; hence, inhibition of sodium reabsorption with a diuretic will result in inhibition of calcium reabsorption and CaE. Loop diuretics are the preferred diuretics.
- The cornerstone of therapy in severe hypercalcemia is inhibition of osteoclastic bone reabsorption by calcitonin, biphosphonates, or mithramycin.

- Decreasing intestinal absorption of calcium (suppressing vitamin D metabolism)
- Treating the underlying cause

Hydration

Because depletion of ECF volume aggravates hypercalcemia by stimulating excessive reabsorption of calcium through renal tubules, rehydration is the essential first step to offset this process. The benefit of rehydration is shown in a schematic diagram in Figure 16.2.

Rehydration
|
↑ ECF volume
|
↑ GFR
↑ Proximal tubule delivery
↓ Reabsorption of sodium and calcium (co-transport)
↑ Urinary excretion of calcium and sodium

FIGURE 16.2.
The benefit of rehydration. *ECF,* extracellular fluid; *GFR,* glomerular filtration rate.

The recommended fluid for rehydration is isotonic (normal) saline, which should be given at a rate of 1 liter every 4 to 6 hours for the first 24 hours, then at a slower rate. The rate of fluid administration should be determined by serial recording of supine and upright blood pressures, pulse rate, urine output, and serum calcium level.

Calcium Diuresis

Calcium is cotransported with sodium; hence, inhibition of sodium reabsorption with a diuretic will result in inhibition of calcium reabsorption. Loop diuretics that include furosemide, ethacrynic acid, or bumetanide can inhibit reabsorption of up to 15% of filtered sodium in the ascending thick limb of loop of Henle. In so doing, a loop diuretic can promote urinary CaE up to 800 or even 1000 mg/day.

Calcium diuresis with a loop diuretic is recommended after ECF volume is considered repleted, based on clinical assessment such as improvements in supine systolic blood pressure and urine output and in decreases in serum urea nitrogen.

There is no set dosage regimen of a loop diuretic; however, 40-mg intravenous bolus every 6 hours may be considered. Severe volume depletion accompanied by hyponatremia, hypokalemia, and hypomagnesemia may develop promptly after administration of the loop diuretic. These electrolyte disorders may be severe and could prove dangerous, particularly in elderly patients. Therefore, serum electrolytes should be monitored frequently during the course of treatment with a loop diuretic. Urinary volume should be measured hourly. Fluid and electrolytes should be replaced in quantities appropriate to avoid volume depletion and electrolyte disorders. Sudden hyponatremia could lead to cerebral edema and convulsions; hypokalemia could lead to dangerous cardiac arrhythmias, especially in those with underlying heart disease.

Inhibit Osteoclastic Bone Reabsorption

The principal pathophysiologic alteration in severe hypercalcemia is enhanced osteoclastic bone reabsorption. Therefore, the cornerstone of therapy to control severe hypercalcemia is to inhibit osteoclastic bone reabsorption. The following agents have been known to do so:

- Calcitonin
- Biphosphonates
- Plicamycin (mithramycin)
- Gallium

Calcitonin

Calcitonin is the most rapidly acting agent; it acts within minutes of its administration, decreasing the release of skeletal calcium, phosphorus, and hydroxyproline. In addition, calcitonin's action of decreasing renal tubular calcium reabsorption may, in part, explain its rapid onset of action. In doses of 2 to 8 IU/kg of body weight intravenously, subcutaneously, or intramuscularly every 6 to 12 hours, calcitonin rapidly lowers serum calcium. Administration of glucocorticoids in combination with calcitonin may prolong the action of calcitonin. Tachyphylaxis often develops on calcitonin administration and is a distinct disadvantage for repeated use of calcitonin. However, calcitonin's lack of toxic properties has a distinct advantage over other agents. Nevertheless, it does cause minor, though usually transient, side effects, including nausea, abdominal cramps, and flushing.

Biphosphonates (Diphosphonates)

The biphosphonates are analogs of pyrophosphate. The first-generation biphosphonate is etidronate (EHDP). A new generation of aminobiphosphonates includes pamidronate (ADP). These drugs have high affinity for hydroxyapatite of bone, especially in areas of bone turnover, such as those that occur at metastatic lesions. These bone-seeking biphosphonates are stable in the body because phosphatase enzymes cannot hydrolyze their central carbon-phosphorus-carbon bond. Concentrated in areas of high bone turnover, the biphosphonates are taken up by osteoclasts and inhibit osteoclast action. Biphosphonates are poorly absorbed and must be given intravenously to be effective in hypercalcemia. Both EHDP and ADP are approved for use.

Etidronate   EHDP given in doses of 7.5 mg/kg/day intravenously for 3 days normalized serum calcium in 30 to 40% of patients. In some cases, continuation of oral EHDP after intravenous therapy may control hypercalcemia. At sustained oral doses of 25 mg/kg/day for more than 6 months, EHDP causes a mineralization defect.

Pamidronate   ADP is extremely potent in inhibiting osteoclast-mediated skeletal reabsorption yet does not cause mineralization defect. The efficacy, dose-response relationship, and safety of 30 mg, 60 mg, and 90 mg of a single, intravenous 24-hour infusion of ADP for the treatment of moderate to severe hypercalcemia of malignancy were studied. Serum calcium corrected for albumin, urine hydroxyproline, and CaE, and serum PTH levels were determined before and after ADP therapy. Corrected serum calcium normalized in 40% of patients who received 30 mg, in 61% of patients who received 60 mg, and in 100% of patients who received 90 mg.

The decline in the serum calcium level was associated with decreased osteoclastic skeletal resorption evidenced by a decrease in urinary calcium and hydroxyproline excretion. Clinical improvement, including mental well-being and appetite, paralleled the fall in serum calcium, whether patients received 30 mg, 60 mg, or 90 mg of ADP.

Side effects included:

- Low-grade fever
- Asymptomatic hypocalcemia
- Hypophosphatemia
- Hypomagnesemia

Thus, ADP has a pharmacologic profile similar to that of EHDP, but ADP is more potent and remains effective over a longer time. In hypercalcemia of malignancy, ADP appears to be as effective as established agents with the advantage that a single dose of ADP 90 mg intravenously provides a durable response.

Plicamycin (Mithramycin)
Plicamycin, derived from an actinomycete of the genus *Streptomyces,* is a tumoricidal antibiotic. Marked hypocalcemia was observed when plicamycin was administered at 50 μg/kg for 5 consecutive days. Plicamycin localizes in areas of active bone resorption and has been shown to directly inhibit bone resorption in vitro. Urinary calcium and hydroxyproline excretion decrease in patients treated with plicamycin. Plicamycin may also inhibit renal tubular reabsorption of calcium.

Plicamycin administered by infusion in doses of 15 to 25 μg/kg over 4 to 24 hours lowers serum calcium within 24 to 48 hours. Total serum calcium is restored to normal within 48 hours in approximately 75% of patients. If serum calcium does not normalize within 48 hours, a second dose should be administered. An alternative treatment schedule consists of infusion of 15 to 25 μg/kg plicamycin for 3 to 4 consecutive days.

Plicamycin has cumulative toxic effects and is less potent than the aminobiphosphorates. Hemorrhage caused by thrombocytopenia and renal insufficiency accompanied by proteinuria may occur in patients.

Renal insufficiency often accompanies severe hypercalcemia. Therefore, potential nephrotoxicity of plicamycin should preclude its use when there is moderate impairment of renal function.

Gallium Nitrate
Gallium nitrate is effective in hypercalcemia of malignancy. Normocalcemia, sustained for a mean period of 11 days, can be achieved in approximately 75% of patients treated with 200 mg/m² of gallium nitrate infused over 5 days. Comparative trials with calcitonin and EHDP demonstrate the greater efficacy of gallium over these agents. The major concern, however, is renal function impairment. Caution must be exercised with concomitant use of aminoglycoside antibiotics and other nephrotoxic drugs.

Glucocorticoids
Glucocorticoids are the most effective agents in hypercalcemia associated with elevated $1\alpha,25$-dihydroxyvitamin D_3 (calcitriol) and normal to low PTH and PTHrP levels. Glucocorticoids are the most effective inhibitors of calcitriol production. Glucocorticoids are given in the form of prednisone 60 mg orally daily for 5 to 7 days. Thereafter, the dose should be tapered to a maintenance dose of 10 to 20 mg daily or on alternate days. Lower dosages and alternate-day schedules are effective in the hypercalcemia of granulomatous diseases. Side effects are uncommon with lower dosages or alternate-day schedules.

Phosphate
Phosphate given intravenously has a dramatic effect on severe hypercalcemia. Phosphate therapy leads to a decline in urinary and fecal excretion of calcium. Calcium kinetic studies show a rapid disappearance of calcium from the circulation within minutes of beginning

a phosphate infusion. Calcium-PO$_4$ product precipitates in the skeleton; however, it also precipitates in the kidneys, soft tissues, and heart.

Intravenous phosphate is an effective treatment of severe hypercalcemia in hypophosphatemic individuals, but should be used with caution in normophosphatemic patients because it may cause hyperphosphatemia. The dose is 3.1 gm of phosphate by intravenous infusion for 24 hours.

Hypercalcemia accompanied by hypophosphatemia, which occurs in hyperparathyroidism and HHM, may be treated with oral phosphate. Phosphate therapy should not be used if renal insufficiency exists with hyperphosphatemia or even with normal PO$_4$ level.

Hypercalcemia and Renal Stones   Renal effects of hypercalcemia are:

- Increased CaE (hypercalciuria)
- Tubular defect
- Stone formation

Hypercalciuria causes an impairment in urinary concentration. The exact mechanism of urinary concentrating defect is not known; however, osmotic diuresis and resistance to vasopressin (nephrogenic diabetes insipidus) are considered plausible mechanisms. Hypercalciuria can cause nephrocalcinosis. This metastatic calcification of the renal parenchyma, most severe in the medulla and corticomedullary areas, may be asymptomatic but can lead to progressive tubulointerstitial disease and renal insufficiency.

Hypercalciuria also predisposes to stone formation within the collecting system, especially if recurrent urinary infection develops with Proteus organism, and causes persistent alkaline urine. Intermittent treatment with the Bactrim, nitrofurantoin, or quinolone group of drugs should minimize the risk of recurrent urinary tract infection, alkalinization of urine, nephrocalcinosis, and stone formation.

Dialysis

Hemodialysis with no or low calcium dialysate is recommended in severe symptomatic hypercalcemia (hypercalcemic crisis) associated with moderate to severe renal failure, such as that seen in multiple myeloma. Calcium may be removed by hemodialysis to the extent of 250 mg per hour.

Hemodialysis is not recommended for hypercalcemia of malignancy that has given rise to chronic urinary tract obstruction and chronic renal failure. In such cases, only palliative treatment with fluid and plicamycin (mithramycin) can be recommended. Unilateral or bilateral nephrostomy can be done to relieve azotemia and provide symptomatic relief.

Treatment of the Cause

Despite advances in therapy for hypercalcemia, acute hyperparathyroidism is most often a surgical emergency. Medical management, beyond stabilization in preparation for surgery, has virtually no role in the management of acute hyperparathyroidism.

Hypercalcemia of malignancy warrants tumor-specific chemotherapy and/or radiation therapy that should be supplemented by adjuvant treatment of hypercalcemia.

Pregnancy   Since the treatment of asymptomatic hyperparathyroidism itself is controversial, it is even more difficult to define the treatment plan for an asymptomatic pregnant woman who has primary hyperparathyroidism. However, a recent consensus panel has recommended that young patients with asymptomatic hyperparathyroidism be treated surgically. The preferable period for surgical treatment is in the second trimester. Whether a patient is treated medically or surgically in these situations, the pregnancy should be considered high risk. The neonate should be monitored carefully for signs of hypocalcemia or impending tetany. If the mother is treated medically to term (or if spontaneous or elective abortion occurs), she should be monitored for hyperparathyroid crisis postpartum. Sudden worsening of hypercalcemia can result from the loss of the placenta and dehydration.

The diagnosis of hyperparathyroidism should be suspected during pregnancy if the following conditions exist:

- Appropriate clinical symptoms or signs (especially nephrolithiasis or pancreatitis)
- Hyperemesis beyond the first trimester
- History of recurrent spontaneous abortions or stillbirths or neonatal deaths
- Neonatal hypocalcemia or tetany or a total serum calcium concentration greater than 10.1 or 8.8 mg/dL during the second or third trimester, respectively

REFERRAL

Hypercalcemic patients may be referred for consultation to a nephrologist, an endocrinologist, a hematologist, an oncologist, and a neck surgeon for advice on

KEY POINTS

- Lung and breast cancers account for 60% of all cancers associated with hypercalcemia.

- Hypercalcemia is a rare complication of prostate cancer.

- Gastric and colorectal cancer are virtually never associated with hypercalcemia.

- Hypercalcemia associated with normal or elevated serum PO_4 level and with or without abnormal renal function is mostly caused by malignancy.

- Hypercalcemia associated with low serum PO_4 despite abnormal renal function strongly suggests primary hyperparathyroidism.

- The triad of hypercalcemia, acute renal failure, and metabolic alkalosis suggests milk-alkali syndrome.

- In elderly or critically ill patients, significant cognitive impairment may be seen even with mild hypercalcemia ($\leq$ 12 mg/dL).

- In general, the higher the level of serum calcium, the more likely malignancy is the underlying cause of hypercalcemia.

- Good hydration is a vital preventive measure because dehydration aggravates hypercalcemia.

- Osteoclastic bone reabsorption is the principal pathophysiologic alteration in severe hypercalcemia associated with hyperparathyroidism and malignancy.

- Hypercalcemia impairs renal excretion of sodium, which is a cotransport for calcium, thereby further aggravating hypercalcemia. This is further worsened by volume depletion.

- PTH and PTHrP enhance further renal tubular reabsorption of calcium.

- Rehydration with intravenous infusion of isotonic saline is the essential first step of treatment of hypercalcemia, regardless the etiology.

- The cornerstone of therapy is inhibition of osteoclastic bone reabsorption by one of the following agents: calcitonin, a biphosphonate, plicamycin (mithramycin), and/or corticosteroids. A biphosphonate preparation, ADP 90-mg intravenous single infusion is considered most effective. The action lasts longer than other agents and side effects are mild.

- Corticosteroids are effective in hypercalcemia caused by myeloma and lymphoproliferative disorders. Corticosteroids can be combined with calcitonin or a biphosphonate.

- The most important part of treatment of hypercalcemia is to identify and treat the cause so that recurrent hypercalcemia is prevented or minimized.

the diagnosis and further management of hypercalcemia. Consultation with all the different medical subspecialists is not essential. A consultation with a nephrologist may be sufficient for the immediate treatment of hypercalcemia. However, consultation with an endocrinologist and a neck surgeon should be considered *if* primary hyperparathyroidism is highly suspected. If the patient has an identifiable malignancy that could account for hypercalcemia, consultation with a hematologist is essential.

PREVENTION

Good hydration is a vital preventive measure because dehydration aggravates hypercalcemia. Biphosphonates or corticosteroids given orally on a long-term basis may mitigate the severity of hypercalcemia. Intake of calcium-rich foods, such as dairy products, should be limited. Multivitamins should be avoided. However, eradication of the cause, if possible, should be the best prevention for hypercalcemia.

PROGNOSIS

Prognosis in hypercalcemia resulting from causes other than malignancy is good, if treated on time and adequately with appropriate therapy.

For hypercalcemia of malignancy, the decision to treat aggressively or not all will depend on the type of malignancy. In malignancy with one or more years of survival, hypercalcemia should be treated aggressively to reduce morbidity and improve survival. In malignancy with widespread metastasis and limited survival, a compassionate decision may be to withhold therapy for hypercalcemia.

COMMONLY ASKED QUESTIONS

In case of hypercalcemia resulting from primary hyperparathyroidism, patients are likely in severe distress. Naturally, they will ask questions about relief. Interestingly, patients do not experience pain in hypercalcemia of malignancy, which is more common than hypercalcemia caused by primary hyperparathyroidism among hospitalized patients. Hypercalcemia tends to hasten the patient's demise. Many such patients as described before are mentally obtunded or poorly responsive and are almost incapable of asking the doctor any direct question(s).

SUGGESTED READINGS

Carella MJ, Gossain VV. Hyperparathyroidism and pregnancy: case report and review. J Genet Intern Med 1992;7:448-453.

Glenn JF. Hypercalcemia and urologic malignancies. Urology 1995;45:139-141.

Nussbaum SR. Pathophysiology and management of severe hypercalcemia. Endocrinol Metab Clin North Am 1993;22:343-362.

Nussbaum SR, Younger J, Vandepol CJ, et al. Single-dose intravenous therapy with pamidronate for the treatment of hypercalcemia of malignancy: comparison of 30-, 60-, 90-mg dosages. Am J Med 1993;95:297-304.

Rosol TJ, Capen CC. Mechanisms of cancer-induced hypercalcemia. Lab Invest 1992;67:680-702.

Seymour JF, Gagel RF. Calcitriol: the major humor mediator of hypercalcemia in Hodgkin's disease and non-Hodgkin's lymphoma. Blood 1993;82:1383-1394.

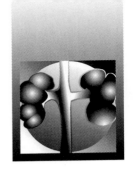

17
CHAPTER

Glomerulonephritis

Gerhard H. Wirnsberger

BACKGROUND

Glomerulonephritis (GN) is the consequence of a variety of immune pathologic processes that result in inflammation of the glomerulus as well as other components of the renal parenchyma.

Considerable recent advances in the field of immunopathology have improved our understanding of the dysregulation in the immune system and diverse interactions with renal parenchyma.

Analysis of immunologic dysfunction has focused on three different concepts:

- Formation of an immune complex deposited into the glomerular mesangium
- Cross-reactivity of antibody with endogenous determinants within the glomerulus
- Binding of circulating antibodies in situ by an extrinsic antigen that is trapped within the glomerulus

Each of these concepts is supported by results of experimental work in animals and by studying the disease in humans. The immunopathogenetic factors and possible antigens responsible for the immune-induced injuries and the diversity of histopathologic changes are briefly reviewed in Table 17.1.

When clinical manifestations arise from alterations in the glomerular structure and function, primary GN exists. Primary GN includes minimal lesion disease, membranous GN, IgA nephropathy, etc. The secondary forms of GN are most commonly associated with various systemic immune complex, infectious, and neoplastic disorders (Table 17.2). The principal clinical features are characterized by varying degrees of hematuria, proteinuria, flank pain, active urinary sediment, and reduction of the glomerular filtration rate. However, many types of GN also give rise to edema, hypertension, or signs of uremia.

Before 1950, the diagnosis of GN was based on different clinical presentations, including blood in the urine, hypertension, and buildup of fluid in the tissue. With the introduction of percutaneous needle biopsy in the early 1950s, the histologic classification became an integral part of the management and prognosis of renal diseases. The importance of the role of renal biopsy in clinical nephrology is underscored by the fact that a large number of histopathologic entities lead to different clinical features.

In general, the inflammatory process in the glomeruli can be separated into several distinct histopathologic types of GN (Fig. 17.1). Besides patient history and careful physical examination, the major noninvasive diagnostic tools available to the clinician to establish a correct diagnosis and to assess severity and course of the underlying disease are urinary examination and serologic studies (Table 17.3). Renal function is estimated mainly by measurement of the serum creatinine concentrations and, in some cases, by the creatinine clearance. The presence of cellular and granular casts and dysmorphic erythrocytes (i.e., acanthocytes, which typically appear as fragmented cells with blebs and budding) generally represent more severe disease than does isolated hematuria or proteinuria alone.

CLINICAL PATTERNS

Based on the course of the disease and the combination of different signs and symptoms, four major clinical patterns of GN can be identified:

Possible Immunopathogenetic Factors and Antigens Involved in Glomerulonephritis   **TABLE 17.1**

Exogenous	Endogenous
Foreign proteins (e.g., serum sickness, vaccines)	Structural components (e.g., basement membrane antigens)
Drugs (e.g., penicillamine, gold, captopril, methicillin)	DNA
Infections (e.g., streptococcus and staphylococcus, hepatitis virus, HIV)	Tumor antigens
	Rheumatoid factors

Most Common Causes of Secondary Glomerulonephritis   **TABLE 17.2**

Morphologic Types	Causative Factors
Endocapillary proliferative GN	*Streptococci, Staphylococci, Pneumococci*
IgA nephropathy	Hepatitis B infection (in Asia)
Minimal change nephropathy	Hodgkin's disease, NSAIDs
Focal segmental glomerulosclerosis	Heroin abuse, HIV infection
Membranous GN	Carcinomas, gold, penicillamine, lupus, hepatitis B or C
Membranoproliferative GN	Hepatitis B or C infection, non-Hodgkin's lymphomas, shunt nephritis

GN, glomerulonephritis; NSAIDS, nonsteroidal anti-inflammatory drugs.

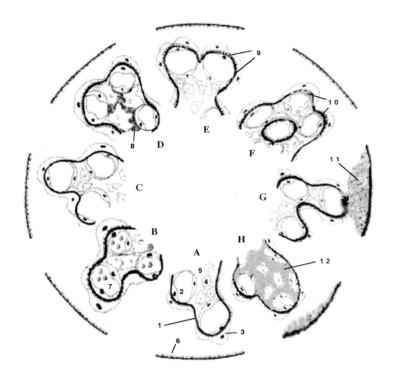

FIGURE 17.1.
Schematic representation of possible histomorphologic changes in glomerulonephritis. **A.** Capillary tuft from a normal glomerulus: *1.* Glomerular basement membrane; *2.* Endothelial cells; *3.* Visceral epithelial cells ("podocytes"); *4.* Mesangial cells; *5.* Mesangial matrix; *6.* Parietal epithelial cells. **B.** Exudative leukocytic: Predominance of numerous neutrophilic granulocytes (*7*) and occasionally some eosinophils, and swelling of mesangial and endothelial cells. **C.** Minimal proliferative (minimal change): Minimal proliferation of mesangial cells with loss of podocyte foot processes (revealed by electron microscopy). **D.** Proliferative endocapillary and/or mesangioproliferative: Marked cellular proliferation with an increase in the mesangial matrix (*8*). **E.** Membranous: Subepithelial deposition of immune complexes with interposed spikelike basement membrane protuberances on the outer surface of the capillary tuft (*9*). **F.** Membranoproliferative: Proliferation of predominantly mesangial cells and largely diffuse thickening of the glomerular capillary wall (*10*). **G.** Mesangioproliferative with crescents: Crescent formation of proliferative parietal epithelial cells (*11*). **H.** Segmental or global scarring: Fibrous scarring with obliteration of the capillary tuft (*12*).

- Nephritic syndrome
- Rapidly progressive syndrome
- Nephrotic syndrome
- Asymptomatic urinary abnormalities (proteinuria and/or hematuria)

These patterns of GN will be briefly described in the following sections for the purpose of primary care.

Nephritic Syndrome

Nephritic syndrome is characterized by sudden onset of diffuse GN affecting most or all the glomeruli. Diffuse GN includes postinfectious GN, lupus GN, membranoproliferative GN, and vasculitis, which includes Wegener's granulomatosis. The cardinal clinical features include:

- Nephritic urinary sediment
- Moderate to heavy proteinuria (which may be in the nephrotic range)
- Edema
- Hypertension
- Moderate to severe renal function impairment

In serologic studies, hypocomplementemia is commonly associated with postinfectious GN, lupus nephritis, or membranoproliferative GN. Some serologic findings are highly suggestive of the underlying disorders, such as:

- Antistreptococcal antibodies in postinfectious GN
- Antibodies to glomerular basement membrane in Goodpasture's disease
- Antinuclear antibodies in lupus nephritis

Noninvasive Diagnostic Tests	TABLE 17.3

Ultrasonography
Assessment of renal function
  Serum creatinine (creatinine clearance)
Urinalysis
  Dipstick
  24-hour urine collection
Urine microscopy
  Red cell morphology
  Leukocytes
  Fat-laden macrophages ("foam cells")
  Granular casts
  Cell casts
Serologic parameters
  ASO and AHase titers
  Antibasement membrane antibody
  ANCA
  ANA dsDNA antibodies
  Hepatitis B/C battery
  Plasma complement levels (CH50, C3, C4)
  Cryoglobulins

ASO, antistreptolysin-O; AHase, antihyaluronidase; ANCA, anti-neutrophilic cytoplasmic antibody; ANA, antinuclear antibody.

- Antineutrophilic cytoplasmic antibodies (ANCA) in Wegener's granulomatosis

Rapidly Progressive Syndrome

Initially, the clinical manifestations of rapidly progressive syndrome are similar to those of nephritic syndrome. Without therapeutic intervention, rapid loss of renal function occurs within weeks or months. Biopsy reveals extensive cellular crescents with or without immune complex formation on immunofluorescence microscopy. When glomerulosclerosis, crescents, or interstitial fibrosis is extensive, the lesions are usually irreversible.

Based on serologic and immunohistochemical findings, three different histologic subtypes could be distinguished:

- Antiglomerular basement membrane disease (Goodpasture's disease; 20% of all cases), characterized by linear pattern of IgG deposits along the glomerular basement membrane
- ANCA-associated microscopic vasculitis (40% of all cases), showing sparse positive or negative results in immunohistology (pauci immune deposits)
- A heterogenous group distinct from the aforementioned two groups (40% of all cases), revealing a granular pattern of immune-complex deposits (IgG, IgA, or IgM)

Nephrotic Syndrome

By definition, the nephrotic syndrome is characterized by the presence of heavy proteinuria (usually ≥ 3.5 g/24 hr/ 1.73 m^2 body surface area). Associated findings include lipiduria, hypoalbuminemia (serum albumin < 3.5 g/dL), hypercholesterolemia, and peripheral edema.

Many different histologic appearances can be identified. Table 17.4 details the most frequent causes of nephrotic syndrome, primary and secondary. Analysis of urinary protein should quantify and qualify urine protein loss as selective (loss of albumin and other low

Major Causes of Nephrotic Syndrome	TABLE 17.4

Primary (idiopathic)

Minimal change disease
Membranous GN
Proliferative GN
Focal segmental glomerulosclerosis
Membranoproliferative GN

Secondary (systemic)

Autoimmune
  SLE
Neoplastic
  Hodgkin's and non-Hodgkin's lymphomas, multiple myeloma, lymphocytic leukemia, gastrointestinal carcinomas
Endocrine
  Diabetic glomerulosclerosis
Cardiovascular
  Renal vein thrombosis, inferior vena cava obstruction, constrictive pericarditis
Drugs
  Probenecid, lithium, tolbutamide, fenoprofen, naproxen, penicillamine
Nephrotoxins
  Mercury, bismuth, gold
Allergens
  Bee stings, wool, poison oak, poison ivy, variety of pollens
Infection
  Syphilis, schistosomiasis, malaria, tuberculosis
Miscellaneous
  Amyloidosis, hereditofamilial nephritis, obesity, pregnancy, sickle cell anemia, spherocytosis

GN, glomerulonephritis; SLE, systemic lupus erythematosus.

molecular weight [MW] proteins) or nonselective (loss of high MW proteins). Selective proteinuria is associated with minimal change glomerular disease; unselective proteinuria is associated with other histologic types (Table 17.4). As a result of persistent hypoalbuminemia caused by markedly increased protein excretion, and even with a compensatory enhanced hepatic synthesis of proteins, a variety of pathophysiologic derangements and complications are seen, such as malnutrition, increased risk of infections (peritonitis, urinary tract infection), and deep venous thrombosis in patients with nephrotic syndrome.

Another complication of the nephrotic syndrome is caused by a variety of disturbances in the pharmacokinetics of protein-bound drugs including anticoagulants and lipid lowering agents. Abnormalities of vitamin D metabolism may result in secondary hyperparathyroidism and osteomalacia. The type of glomerular lesion in a given patient with nephrotic syndrome can be established only by renal biopsy and by studying the renal tissue with light, transmission electron, and immunofluorescent microscopy techniques.

Asymptomatic Proteinuria and Hematuria

Asymptomatic proteinuria and hematuria are often discovered by chance on routine physical examination. Urinalysis often reveals red cells that have a dysmorphic appearance, occasionally red cell casts, and mild proteinuria (usually < 1 g/day). The majority of these patients can be reassured of a good prognosis, and they do not need further examination or treatment. They should be followed closely if they develop evidence of progression, characterized by increased proteinuria, hypertension, or renal insufficiency.

The prognosis of a particular GN depends on the histologic subtype and the severity of the interstitial fibrosis (and not merely on the number of glomeruli affected). The presence of a chronic form of GN is suspected from a patient's history of acute nephritis or the nephrotic syndrome, along with an increase in systemic blood pressure, elevated serum creatinine concentrations, and impairment of the kidneys' concentrating ability. Proteinuria and hematuria are rarely severe. The degree of proteinuria tends to decrease because of the decline in the glomerular filtration rate caused by declining renal function. In some cases, however, the persistence of a heavy proteinuria despite declining renal function caused by interstitial fibrosis can be explained by atrophy of tubular epithelium, which is unable to absorb the filtrated protein sufficiently. Urine microscopy and ultrasonography yield valuable information about a patient's clinical course. Thus, the finding of waxy casts in urine sediment are typical for a chronic process, whereas granular casts and renal tubular cells suggest an "active" disease.

Summary of Diagnosis

- Salient clinical features of GN include hematuria, proteinuria, active urinary sediment, and reduction of the glomerular filtration rate.
- Abnormal urinalysis concomitant with upper respiratory tract infection or without systemic manifestations suggests IgA nephropathy.
- Renal function in terms of serum creatinine may be normal.
- Abnormal urinalysis preceded by upper respiratory tract infection or sore throat of 1 to 2 weeks suggests poststreptococcal GN. Acute poststreptococcal GN is more commonly associated with scabies and impetigo in tropical climates. Renal function in terms of serum creatinine is usually diminished.
- Diffuse GN is characterized by nephritic urinary sediment, edema, hypertension, and moderately to severely impaired renal function.
- Presentation of poststreptococcal GN in adults may be asymptomatic or mildly symptomatic.
- Presentation of poststreptococcal GN is usually severe in young children, with edema, hypertension, and even hypertensive complications such as encephalopathy or congestive heart failure.
- Abnormal urinalysis accompanied by abnormal renal function in patients with the complaint of cough productive of sputum and/or hemoptysis suggests Wegener's granulomatosis. One or more densities in the chest radiograph are supportive.

POSTINFECTIOUS GLOMERULONEPHRITIS

Postinfectious GN typically presents as an acute inflammatory disease with recovery occurring in most or all patients. The typical form is acute poststreptococcal GN, which can occur in populations sporadically or in an epidemic manner. Lancefield group A streptococci are responsible for the majority of all cases. Other causes of infection-associated GN are *Staphylococcus*, hepatitis B and C virus, and HIV (Table 17.1). In most adults the signs and symptoms are often mild, but rapidly progressive renal failure can occur in less than 1% of adults.

Pathophysiology

Immunohistologic and electron microscopic investigations and corresponding experimental data from animal models support the theory that most of the infectious agents serve as planted antigen for immune complex formation with specific antibodies in addition to the circulating immune complexes. Immune complex formation in situ can also play a role in the pathogenesis of the inflammatory process. Nevertheless, these events lead to further complement fixation and recruitment of additional inflammatory mediators and cells. Infectious antigens have been detected within the affected glomeruli independent of immunoglobulin deposits. In cases of virus-associated glomerulopathies, recent evidence suggests a direct cytopathogenic effect on endothelial and mesangial cells. The capillary tufts are enlarged with predominant swelling of the endothelial and mesangial cells. The existence of numerous granulocytes may be a reaction to subepithelial deposits ("humps") of immune complex. Renal tubules usually appear unremarkable. Conversely, severe tubular damage typically results in changes of the renal excretory function.

Symptoms

Acute poststreptococcal GN can occur at any age, with a male to female ratio of 2:1. The latent interval from acute infection to clinical onset may be as short as 2 days or as long as 8 weeks, depending on the site of infection. The latent period following pharyngitis is 1 to 2 weeks, whereas the latent period after skin infection is usually 3 weeks or longer. The presentation is commonly acute in children, with the appearance of "nephritic signs" in the form of gross hematuria, edema, and hypertension. Oliguria or anuria frequently dominates the early phase. Nephrotic syndrome may be the presenting feature in 25% of adults with acute poststreptococcal GN. In some patients, no clinical signs or symptoms except a nephritic urine sediment are seen, or the infectious disorder will be dominated by nonrenal symptoms but related to gastrointestinal, pulmonary, or central nervous system signs and symptoms. The presence of dysmorphic erythrocyturia should alert the physician to pursue the diagnosis of acute (postinfectious) GN. Elevations in blood pressure are characteristically mild; fewer than 1% of patients will have a hypertensive encephalopathy with headache, nausea, and

vomiting. Hypertension can be severe and give rise to acute left ventricular failure, particularly in children.

The course and prognosis of acute poststreptococcal GN is usually better for children than for adults, depending on the severity of the acute disease and on epidemiologic considerations. The presence of numerous glomerular crescents, tubular atrophy, and interstitial fibrosis found on renal biopsy indicates a less favorable prognosis. Gross hematuria can persist for months. After the infection has been controlled with antibiotics, proteinuria decreases during recovery. Infrequently, a mild proteinuria may persist but does not adversely affect the outcome. The delayed remission of proteinuria probably reflects the slow rate of resolution of subepithelial deposits.

Diagnosis

During the early phase of the disease, the C1q, C3, C4, C5, and properdin levels are depressed in most patients. The complement profile returns to normal within a few weeks. However, reduced C3 for months either correlates with rapid progression or suggests another diagnosis. The glomerular filtration rate may decrease, but the serum creatinine levels return toward normal with disease resolution. Hematuria and unselective proteinuria (ranging from 1 to 4 g/day) are invariably present. In fresh urine sediment, granular, pigmented, and red blood cell casts, as well as dysmorphic erythrocytes indicative of glomerular injury, may be seen. White cell casts, although more typical of pyelonephritis, are occasionally observed in severe exudative process. Oval fat bodies and foam cells may be detected in patients with nephrotic syndrome.

Bacterial cultures of the throat or of skin lesions should be obtained. The incidence of elevated titers of streptococcal antibodies ranges up to 80% in patients with skin diseases and to more than 95% in patients with pharyngitis. The most common nephritogenic streptococcal strains involved are types 12, 9, 25, and 49. For differential diagnostic reasons, the serum concentrations of antistreptolysin-O (ASO), antistreptokinase (ASK), and antihyaluronidase (AHase) should be measured also. Streptozyme is a combination of all three titers and is readily available. These antibodies indicate streptococcal infection but not necessarily GN. In a typical case, a renal biopsy is not required to assess the pathologic process but may be indicated in patients with rapidly progressive renal failure.

Treatment

Therapy depends on the symptoms and the clinical course of acute poststreptococcal GN. Patients with positive throat cultures or those with scabies and impetigo should be treated with appropriate antibiotics. For streptococcal infection, benzathine penicillin 1.2 million units by intramuscular injection is adequate therapy. Prophylactic treatment is controversial because recurrences of acute poststreptococcal GN are rare. The major aims of therapy are control of blood pressure and treatment of fluid volume overload. Furosemide usually provides prompt diuresis with reduction of blood pressure. For hypertension not controlled by diuretics, vasodilators are usually effective. Furthermore, daily sodium intake should be restricted to 2 to 4 grams. In patients with progressive renal function deterioration, the serum potassium concentration should be carefully monitored and treated appropriately. To minimize rapid increase of blood urea nitrogen, dietary protein restriction to 0.5 g/kg/day and intake of proteins of high biologic value might be necessary until renal function improves.

OTHER BACTERIAL INFECTION-RELATED GLOMERULONEPHRITIS

Although a variety of organisms may be involved in infectious GN, the following are most commonly implicated:

- *Staphylococcus aureus* in acute bacterial endocarditis
- *Streptococcus viridans* in subacute bacterial endocarditis
- *Staphylococcus epidermidis* in shunt nephritis

With earlier recognition and more effective antibiotic therapy, the overall incidence of GN and death from renal failure has decreased.

Pathology

The pathogenesis and the histologic findings resemble those in poststreptococcal GN. In all forms, glomerular hypercellularity with endogenous cell proliferation and subendothelial immune deposits in the glomerular tufts are typical.

Symptoms

Patients most commonly present with microscopic hematuria and mild proteinuria. An initial finding of nephrotic syndrome is unusual in endocarditis but occurs in up to 30% of patients with shunt nephritis. Systemic signs and symptoms include:

- Fever
- Petechial hemorrhage
- Arthralgias
- Hepatosplenomegaly

Treatment

In comparison with poststreptococcal disease, the duration of antigenemia is often prolonged in patients with endocarditis or an infected shunt because of delays in diagnosis and treatment. Control of the infection usually leads to rapid improvement in renal function to nearly the former baseline. However, progressive renal failure can occur in patients who have not received appropriate antibiotic therapy. In laboratory investigation, the plasma C3, C4, and C2 levels are usually depressed. Therapy is directed at eradication of the underlying cause, with adequate antimicrobial therapy and removal of an infected shunt.

VIRAL INFECTION-RELATED GLOMERULONEPHRITIS

Chronic hepatitis B and C virus infection is associated with several types of glomerular diseases, particularly the following:

- Essential mixed cryoglobulinemia
- Membranoproliferative GN
- Membranous nephropathy
- IgA nephropathy

At present, it remains unclear why only some patients develop these complications. Clinicians postulate that the glomerular lesions are caused by formation of pre-formed antigen-containing immune complex deposits from the circulation within the capillaries. Patients often have proteinuria in the nephrotic range accompanied by elevated serum transaminase levels. However, infection may be asymptomatic in some cases, and a history of chronic persistent hepatitis is often absent. Thus, a relatively normal liver histology does not exclude the presence of a chronic hepatitis.

Patients may improve in cryoglobulin titers and in the renal function from therapeutic regimens that include steroids, cytotoxic agents, or plasma exchange. Hepatitis C virus-associated GN may benefit from treatment with interferon alpha (IFN-α), which suppresses viremia and reduces the urinary protein loss. The optimal dose and duration of IFN-α therapy, however, is not yet established.

HIV virus-associated nephropathy occurs in symptomatic and asymptomatic HIV-seropositive patients and has become one of the most common causes for renal complications. At onset, nephropathy can be identified by varying degrees of proteinuria (often in the nephrotic range) or by clinical signs of acute or chronic renal insufficiency. However, slight information is available regarding the treatment of this population. Although in some cases nephrotic syndrome has been partially treated with steroids, it is wise not to administer prolonged courses of such immunosuppressive medications because of possible side effects. The effect of antiviral agents, specifically Zidovudine (AZT), on the natural history of HIV-associated renal diseases is also mostly unknown.

ASSOCIATED SYSTEMIC CONDITIONS

Lupus Nephritis

Systemic lupus erythematosus (SLE) is a chronic multisystem disorder of unknown cause with a marked predominance in females, especially during the reproductive years (ratio of females to males is 5:1). SLE is an autoimmune process with concurrent formation of antibodies against DNA and other nuclear structures, leading to the deposit of immune complexes in different organs. The reported prevalence of renal manifestations ranges between 40 and 90%, in which glomerular lesions are most commonly observed, reflecting different forms of GN.

Pathophysiology

Different types of GN observed in SLE do not differ morphologically from idiopathic GN, and they are not pathognomonic for the underlying disease. These histopathologic changes may be characterized by a mesangial, focal, or diffuse proliferative GN. The latter type correlates clinically with an active urine sediment, proteinuria, and, often, with acute decline in renal function. The severity of the tubulointerstitial involvement is an important prognostic sign, correlating positively with the presence of hypertension, an elevated plasma creatinine concentration, and a progressive clinical course.

Symptoms

The clinical features of generalized lupus erythematosus is polymorphic. In 80% of patients, the disease begins gradually with extrarenal symptoms. Most patients present with symptoms such as fever and fatigue, skin manifestations including malar (butterfly) rash, alopecia, discoid (scarring) lesions, or Raynaud's phenomenon.

Although characteristic immunoserologic findings already indicate the presence of multiple clinical and laboratory criteria of lupus as defined by the American Rheumatism Association, it is important to know that SLE can mimic many other multisystem disorders, including:

- Drug interactions
- Systemic vasculitis
- Infectious mononucleosis
- Rheumatoid arthritis

Lupus tends to be milder in the elderly, who often have a presentation more similar to that of drug-induced lupus. The elderly have a lower incidence of malar rash, antilupus (LE) antibody, and fewer signs and symptoms of renal and central nervous system involvement; however, they have more sicca symptoms, serositis, and musculoskeletal manifestations. In the majority of patients with renal involvement, blood pressure is within the normal range. In general, the severity of clinical signs correlates with the severity of morphologic changes.

Diagnosis

Although the clinical picture, with its extrarenal and renal signs and symptoms, is not specific to SLE, immunoserologic tests and urinalysis possess diagnostic relevance and help to determine the severity of tissue damage. Thus, diagnosis of SLE is based on the evidence of antinuclear antibodies (ANA) and antibodies against cytoplasmic antigens. In virtually all patients, antibodies to native DNA are present. Hypocomplementemia is another laboratory hallmark for the severity of renal alterations. The rheumatoid factor is often positive in SLE patients and may lead to diagnostic confusion in patients with arthritis. Cryoglobulins can also appear in the serum, especially in the case of severe renal changes.

In patients with active nephritis, the urine sediment may show hematuria, various degrees of proteinuria, and red blood cell casts. Proteinuria will be observed in more than 70% of patients, with an average of 3 to 5 grams per day. An abnormal urinalysis with or without an elevated serum creatinine concentration is present in approximately 50% of patients at the time of diagnosis; however, renal function impairment eventually develops in more than 75% of cases. The need for renal biopsy is variable in lupus nephritis. Patients with acute renal insufficiency and an active nephritic sediment almost always have diffuse proliferative disease. In such cases, a histologic confirmation of the diagnosis is not necessary if there is clear clinical and serologic evidence for lupus. The main indication for renal biopsy is a less severe clinical presentation with mild proteinuria and/or hematuria, or nephrotic syndrome with a nonactive urine sediment. A repeat biopsy may be done for late progression of the disease to distinguish between "active" lupus, which may require an aggressive immunosuppressive therapy, and scarring of previous inflammatory injury.

Treatment

Treatment of lupus is dictated by the organ systems involved (e.g., arthralgias are treated with salicylates and nonsteroidal anti-inflammatory drugs [NSAIDs]). The optimal treatment of lupus nephritis varies with the histologic type and activity of the disease. Thus, lupus nephritis with only mesangial proliferation is the mildest form and is generally associated with a good renal prognosis and requires no further specific therapy. Aggressive therapy with high-dose steroids or cytotoxic agents, such as cyclophosphamide, is indicated primarily in patients with progressive renal failure: those with diffuse or severe focal proliferative GN and those with membranous lupus who have a rising serum creatinine concentration or nephrotic syndrome. Other studies have confirmed the predictive value of the severity of acute histologic changes like cellular proliferative GN and a moderate degree of irreversible chronic changes, such as interstitial fibrosis and tubular atrophy are at particular risk and may derive the greatest benefit from high-dose steroid or cytotoxic agents such as cyclophosphamide.

Prognosis

Relapse is primarily defined as renewed clinical activity and/or recurrence of renal lesions manifested by an active urine sediment (i.e., sediment containing red cell casts) that is often accompanied by increasing proteinuria and a rise in serum creatinine concentration. Clinical risk factors for progression include worsening renal function and increasing proteinuria before therapy and hypertension. Black patients are at additional risk for disease progression. An elevation in the titer of anti–double-stranded (native) DNA antibodies and a decrease in circulating complement levels are associated with a high likelihood of subsequent clinical relapse. Although plasma C3 and C4 levels tend to vary inversely with disease activity, there may be a prolonged reduction in C4 levels long after clinical remission has been induced. Disease exacerbation may also occur during or shortly after pregnancy, particularly in women whose renal disease is active at the time of conception. In this case, 22 to 50 mg oral prednisone is used successfully, although there is a risk of inducing or exacerbating hypertension. Cyclophosphamide should be avoided during pregnancy because possible effects on the fetus are unknown, but azathioprine can be given with relative safety if the white blood cell count is in the normal range.

Wegener's Granulomatosis

Wegener's granulomatosis is a primary form of systemic vasculitis affecting men and women with equal frequency. It begins typically in the upper and lower respiratory tracts with an initial infection of the paranasal sinuses or respiratory tract. This initial period can last from months to years before progression to a generalized vasculitis involving the kidneys and almost any other organ system.

Symptoms

Typically, the onset of the disease is gradual, which is also reflected in the significantly longer duration of illness between disease onset and renal biopsy. Renal insufficiency dominates the clinical picture; it is usually present at the time of hospitalization and is rapidly progressive. Blood pressure is normal in most cases or only slightly elevated. Common extrarenal complications include:

- Hearing loss
- Cosmetic and functional nasal deformities
- Cough with hemoptysis
- Tracheal stenosis

The chest radiograph may be highly abnormal, showing multiple dense shadows. In different studies, patient survival is currently more than 75% with a follow-up duration of 5 to 8 years.

Diagnosis

The diagnosis is suggested from the clinical and laboratory findings of the presence of circulating ANCA that are usually directed against proteinase 3 (cANCA) and myeloperoxidase (pANCA). Because a positive ANCA test alone is not sufficiently accurate, the diagnosis of Wegener's granulomatosis is generally confirmed by biopsy of a nasopharyngeal granuloma. Renal lesions occurring in this disease, however, cannot be distinguished from those of any forms of idiopathic rapidly progressive GN. If untreated, patients with cANCA may have a tendency to more active disease and more rapid progression than those with pANCA. Antiendothelial cell antibodies also have been described in patients with Wegener's granulomatosis. The urinalysis typically reveals an active urinary sediment similar to that found in acute GN: red cell and other cellular and granular casts and a mild proteinuria. If patients are already uremic or preuremic at the time of admission, it is usually because of tubulointerstitial alterations and not glomerular lesions.

Treatment

Early intervention with therapy is extremely important because tissue necrosis is difficult to reverse once it occurs. Renal failure severe enough to warrant dialysis treatment during the acute phase of the disease does not preclude a good initial response to immunosuppressive therapy. Cyclophosphamide is the most effective therapy and should be continued for 6 to 12 months after complete remission has been induced to minimize the risk of relapse. Cyclophosphamide is usually given orally in a dosage of 1.5 to 2 mg/kg/day, although a lower dosage of 1 mg/kg/day may be effective in the patient with relatively mild disease. Cyclophosphamide given intravenously every 2 or 3 months is effective; to minimize toxicity, azathioprine given orally is suitable. Although azathioprine is generally less effective as initial therapy, it is often sufficient to sustain a cyclophosphamide-induced remission. When compared with combined cyclophosphamide and prednisone, prednisone alone is associated with a lower remission rate, a higher relapse rate, and a higher mortality rate. At present, no clear optimal therapy emerges for persistent activity despite optimal cyclophosphamide dosing.

Risk factors for relapse include the previous or current use of corticosteroids alone, administration of azathioprine, or superimposed infections. Plasma ANCA titers usually parallel the course of the vasculitis, especially with cANCA. The disappearance of ANCA is almost always associated with clinical remission, and patients who maintain negative titers after therapy are at lower risk for clinical relapse. Therefore, it seems reasonable to monitor plasma ANCA titers at monthly intervals for the first year and to carefully follow those patients with a rise in titers for early signs of clinical relapse.

IgA Nephropathy

Idiopathic IgA nephropathy is a particular form of mesangioproliferative GN. IgA nephropathy is the most common form of immune complex nephritis, characterized by the mesangial deposition of predominantly immunoglobulin A (IgA). It is particularly prevalent in Asians and Caucasians, with an average patient age of 30 years. It is a relatively rare disease in African-Americans. Men are affected four times more frequently than women. Originally thought to be benign, long-term follow-up studies have shown a progression to end-stage renal disease (ESRD) in 20 to 40% of all patients. Although in some countries a familial incidence has been reported, IgA nephropathy is a sporadically occurring disease.

Symptoms

Respiratory tract infections immediately before disease onset are documented in one-third of patients. Recurrent hematuria is the typical presenting feature in children with IgA nephropathy. In adults, the disorder manifestations are highly variable. Some patients are asymptomatic. In a few cases, the illness begins gradually with isolated microscopic hematuria or is detected by mild proteinuria on routine physical examination. Patients may complain of flank pain during acute episodes, which usually indicates stretching of the renal capsules. In almost all instances, serum creatinine levels are at the upper end of the normal range, but blood pressure is in the normal range. Gross hematuria will eventually occur in 20 to 25% of these patients. Less than 10% of patients present with an acute GN picture characterized by edema, hypertension, renal insufficiency, and hematuria. In long-term studies, the development of chronic renal failure was observed in up to 25% of patients, especially older patients.

Diagnosis

Plasma IgA levels are elevated in 30 to 50% of patients, but this finding is not sufficiently specific to establish the diagnosis. Examination of the urinary sediment revealing deformed red blood cells indicates glomerular bleeding. Macroscopic hematuria is more common in children than in adults. Nevertheless, IgA nephropathy is diagnosed most frequently by renal biopsy.

Treatment

It is difficult to make definitive recommendations in the therapy of IgA nephropathy. No therapeutic regimen has been shown to clearly affect outcome in IgA nephropathy. Because macroscopic hematuria coincides with upper respiratory tract infections, eradication of septic foci in the oropharynx, including treatment with daily antibiotics and tonsillectomy to remove the site of recurrent infection, may be beneficial. Most attention has been focused on immunosuppressive drugs. In general, patients with a stable or very slowly progressive IgA nephropathy should not be treated with steroids. If corticosteroids are tried, only long-term therapy is likely to be effective.

REFERRAL

Patients with heavy proteinuria (≥ 3 g/24 hr) or hematuria associated with proteinuria and renal insufficiency must be referred to a nephrologist for thorough investigation and appropriate management. Patients with isolated hematuria without proteinuria and normal

KEY POINTS

- In office practice, proteinuria and microscopic hematuria may be common findings on urinalysis.

- Diagnostic serologic studies include anti-GBM antibody in Goodpasture's disease, dsDNA antibody in lupus nephritis, and cANCA in Wegener's granulomatosis.

- The typical form of postinfectious GN is acute poststreptococcal GN.

- Hypocomplementemia is a common accompaniment of postinfectious, lupus, and membranoproliferative GN.

- Total serum complement and C3 levels are required to determine if the nephritic process is active.

- Recovery of renal function to normal is a signal of reversal of the pathologic process.

- Abnormal urinalysis accompanied or preceded by systemic manifestations such as arthralgias, skin rash, or pleuropericarditis suggests lupus nephritis. ANA, dsDNA antibodies are essential. DNA level can be used to monitor the activity. Serum C3 and C4 levels are cheaper than DNA antibody for monitoring activity.

- The major aims of therapy in poststreptococcal GN are the control of blood pressure and treatment of volume overload. Furosemide orally or intravenously is the treatment of choice, providing prompt diuresis with reduction of blood pressure.

- For poststreptococcal infection, benzathine penicillin 1.2 million is adequate therapy.

renal function may be referred to an urologist for workup.

SUGGESTED READINGS

Abe S. The influence of pregnancy on long-term renal prognosis of IgA nephropathy. Clin Nephrol 1994;41: 61–64.

Andrassy K, Erb A, Koderisch J, et al. Wegener's granulomatosis with renal involvement: patient survival and correlations between initial renal function, renal histology, therapy and renal outcome. Clin Nephrol 1991;35: 139–147.

Austin HA, Boumpas DT, Vaughan EM, et al. Predicting renal outcomes in severe lupus nephritis: contributions of clinical and histologic data. Kidney Int 1994;45: 544–550.

Austin HA, Antonovych TT, MacKay K, et al. Membranous nephropathy. Ann Intern Med 1992;116:672–682.

Burstein DM, Korbet SM, Schwartz MM. Membranous glomerulonephritis and malignancy. Am J Kidney Dis 1993;22:5–10.

Burstein DM, Rodby RA. Membranoproliferative glomerulonephritis associated with hepatitis C virus infection. J Am Soc Nephrol 1993;4:1288–1293.

Cattran DC, Greenwood C, Ritchie S. Long-term benefits of angiotensin-converting enzyme inhibitor therapy in patients with severe immunoglobulin A nephropathy: a comparison to patients receiving treatment with other antihypertensive agents and to patients receiving no therapy. Am J Kidney Dis 1994;23:247–254.

Davda J, Peterson J, Weiner R, et al. Membranous glomerulonephritis in association with hepatitis C virus infection. Am J Kidney Dis 1993;22:452–455.

Donadio JV, Glassock RJ. Immunosuppressive drug therapy in lupus nephritis. Am J Kidney Dis 1993;21:239–250.

Glassock RJ. Intensive plasma exchange in crescentic glomerulonephritis: help or no help? Am J Kidney Dis 1992;20:270–275.

Glassock RJ. Natural history and treatment of primary proliferative glomerulonephritis. A review. Kidney Int 1984; 28:136–142.

Goodpasture EW. The significance of certain pulmonary lesions in relation to the etiology of influenza. Am J Med Sci 1919;158:863–870.

Gross WL. New developments in the treatment of systemic vasculitis. Curr Opin Rheumatol 1994;6:11–19.

Hoffman GS, Kerr GS, Leavitt RY, et al. Wegener's granulomatosis: an analysis of 158 patients. Ann Intern Med 1992;116:488–498.

Hoffman GS, Leavitt RY, Fleisher TA, et al. Treatment of Wegener's granulomatosis with intermittent high-dose intravenous cyclophosphamide. Am J Med 1990;89: 403–410.

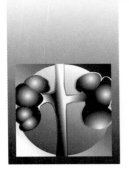

CHAPTER 18

Cystic Disease of the Kidney

Anil Agarwal
P. George John

BACKGROUND

Renal cysts are epithelium-lined spaces filled with fluid or debris arising from the renal parenchyma (i.e., cortex or medulla). The cyst epithelium resembles that part of the kidney from which it originates. Cysts enlarge as a result of a variety of factors, including growth factors and accumulation of secretions, and are accommodated by the normal renal tissue. The cysts cause distortion of the renal parenchyma and result in loss of renal function.

Renal cysts can be inherited or acquired and may be associated with developmental abnormalities. The cysts can arise in the cortex, the medulla, or both, and can be solitary or multiple, unilateral or bilateral.

A simple classification of cystic diseases of the kidney is presented in Table 18.1. The characteristic features of various cystic diseases of the kidney are presented in Table 18.2. In this chapter, the more common types of renal cysts, including simple cysts, autosomal-dominant

| TABLE 18.1 | Cystic Diseases of the Kidney |

Simple cysts
Hereditary cystic diseases
   Autosomal dominant polycystic kidney disease
   Autosomal recessive polycystic kidney disease
   Tuberous sclerosis
   von Hippel-Lindau syndrome
Medullary cysts
   Medullary cystic disease
   Medullary sponge kidney
Acquired cystic kidney disease
Miscellaneous cystic diseases
   Cystic renal dysplasia
   Multilocular cyst
   Pyelocalyceal cyst
   Hilar cyst
   Perinephric pseudocyst
   Renal lymphangiomatosis

polycystic kidney disease, autosomal-recessive polycystic kidney disease, and medullary cystic disease, will be discussed in detail. Less common types of renal cysts, such as acquired cystic kidney disease and medullary sponge kidney, will be discussed briefly.

SIMPLE RENAL CYSTS

Simple renal cysts are the most common cystic disorder of the kidneys. The incidence of simple cysts increases with age; approximately 50% of the population older than age 50 is likely to have simple renal cysts. **Simple cysts are not inherited and do not affect renal function.**

   Simple cysts vary in size from 0.4 cm to 4.0 cm, but are commonly less than 2.0 cm and typically solitary; however, they sometimes occur in multiples. The cavity of a simple cyst is usually unilocular and contains fluid with a composition similar to that of plasma. The thin cyst wall can become thick and calcified as a result of recurrent infections.

Symptoms

Simple cysts are usually asymptomatic and are most commonly detected as an incidental finding on imaging with ultrasound or CT scan done for unrelated problems. Rarely, they can present as an abdominal mass. Hematuria is rare in simple cysts and should raise a suspicion of renal cell carcinoma. Cyst infection is uncommon and may cause fever, flank pain, pyuria, and leukocytosis. The cysts may occasionally give rise to renin-dependent hypertension.

Diagnosis

The diagnosis of simple cysts is made by imaging with renal ultrasound or abdominal CT scan (done using contrast materials unless their use is contraindicated). The radiologic criteria for the diagnosis of simple cyst include the presence of thin wall, homogeneous attenuation (near water density, without debris) and smooth interface with surrounding parenchyma. An atypical-appearing cyst should almost always be differentiated from a malignant cyst on the basis of CT scan, ultrasound, or fluid characteristics on aspiration. The differential findings are presented in Table 18.3. Cysts that remain indeterminate on diagnosis will require surgical exploration.

Treatment

Asymptomatic cysts need periodic follow-up. A large cyst may require aspiration and alcohol instillation to sclerose the cavity. Cysts containing more than 500 mL of fluid should be drained surgically. Cyst infection should be differentiated from renal abscess and treated with antibiotics that have high lipid solubility and a high pKa (see ADPKD section). If associated with calyceal obstruction, an infected cyst requires aspiration or surgical removal. Occasionally, hypertension caused by compression of intrarenal blood vessels will improve after decompression of the cyst.

   Because approximately 2 to 4% of patients can have both a simple cyst and a tumor in the same kidney, the cysts should be followed periodically with CT scan.

HEREDITARY CYSTIC DISEASES

The most common type of hereditary cystic kidney disease is autosomal-dominant polycystic kidney disease (ADPKD), which should be differentiated from the other less common types of polycystic kidney disease called autosomal-recessive polycystic kidney disease (ARPKD), and also from the even less common tuberous sclerosis (TS) and von Hippel-Lindau disease.

Autosomal-Dominant Polycystic Kidney Disease (ADPKD)

Pathophysiology

ADPKD is the most common hereditary disease in the United States, affecting approximately one-half million people. It is more common than cystic fibrosis, sickle cell disease, hemophilia, and muscular dystrophy. ADPKD is the cause of end-stage renal disease (ESRD) in approximately 7% of patients on hemodialysis and in 5 to 10% of renal transplant recipients.

   The genetic defect for the most common type of the disease (i.e., ADPKD1) is located on chromosome 16, and is found in 85 to 90% of all ADPKD patients.

TABLE 18.2

Characteristic Features of Cystic Diseases of the Kidney

	Inheritance	Bilaterality	Salt-wasting	Hematuria	ESRD	Cancer	Incidence/Age of Presentation	Diagnosis	Associated Features
Autosomal-dominant polycystic kidney disease	AD	Present	Uncommon, mild	Present	Follows (10% of all ESRD)	No more common than general population	1:1000 4th–5th decade	CT	Cysts of liver, pancreas, spleen, and thyroid; AAA, berry aneurysm, MVP, diverticuli
Autosomal-recessive polycystic kidney disease	AR	Present	Present	Present	Present	Absent	1:6–14000 Early (varies)	US, liver biopsy	Hepatic fibrosis, lung, hypoplasia, AAA, berry aneurysm, Ehlers-Danlos syndrome
Acquired cystic kidney disease	Absent	Present	Present	Present	Precedes	High incidence renal cell	Common after 5 years of dialysis	CT	Absent
Medullary sponge kidney	Absent	Present 70%	Present	Present	Absent	Absent	1:5000 4th–5th decade	IVP	Hemihypertrophy of body
Medullary cystic disease	AD and AR	Present	Present Severe	Absent	Present	Absent	Rare 1st–2nd decade	IVP, renal biopsy	Absent
Tuberous sclerosis	AD	Present	Doubtful	Present	Rare	Varies	Rare	CT, angiography	Hamartomas, seizures
Simple cysts	Absent	Varies	Absent	Varies	Absent	Absent	Common, rare in children	US, CT	Absent
von Hippel-Lindau disease	AD	Present	Absent	Absent	Absent	Present Common	Rare 3rd–4th decade	CT	Retinal and cerebellar hemangioblastoma, pancreatic (ca) & cysts, pheochromocytoma

ESRD, end-stage renal disease; AD, autosomal-dominant; CT, computed tomography; AAA, abdominal aortic aneurysm; MVP, mitral valve prolapse; AR, autosomal-recessive; US, ultrasound; IVP, intravenous pyelogram; ca, cancer.

TABLE 18.3 Differentiation of Simple Cyst from Malignancy (By Contrast–enhanced CT or US)

Cyst Characteristic	Simple Cyst	Malignancy
CT scan		
Cyst wall	Thin	Thick
Attenuation	Homogeneous (near water density)	Heterogeneous, may be solid
Contrast enhancement	No	Yes
Interface with surroundings	Smooth	Irregular
Calcification	Usually none, or peripheral	Central
US		
Echogenicity	Echolucent	Echogenic
Aspiration		
Cyst fluid	Straw-colored, clear	Dark or bloody, elevated lipids and cholesterol
Cytology	No atypical cells on microscopy	Malignant cells on microscopy

CT, computed tomography; US, ultrasound.

The other type (ADPKD2) is caused by an abnormality on chromosome 4 and is present in 10 to 15% of patients with the disease. The genetic defect seems to alter cell growth, secretion, and matrix formation. There is also evidence of accelerated apoptosis (i.e., programmed cell death).

ADPKD involves both kidneys. Kidney enlargement may be minimal to massive, unequal on both sides, and tends to be more common in males than in females. The individual cysts can be 2 to 10 cm in diameter and are distributed throughout the cortex and medulla, distorting the structure of the kidney. Approximately two-thirds of the cysts contain fluid resembling proximal tubular fluid, which is iso-osmotic to plasma and has a high sodium concentration. These are called "nongradient cysts." The remaining one-third of the cysts arise from distal tubules and contain a hyperosmolar fluid with low sodium concentration and are called "gradient cysts."

Renal concentrating ability is usually impaired. Renal cell carcinoma is no more common in ADPKD patients than in the general population, although renal adenoma is more common.

The pathologic examination of the kidneys shows an enlarged kidney with distortion of the parenchyma and collecting system caused by cysts of variable sizes, with intervening normal kidney. There may be associated nephrosclerosis, infection, hemorrhage, or calculus formation.

ADPKD is a systemic disease that involves other organs (Table 18.4). Liver cysts are typically demonstrable on CT scan of the liver, but liver function im-

TABLE 18.4 Manifestations of ADPKD

Renal	Polycystic kidney disease
	Adenoma
	Stones
Extrarenal	
Cardiovascular	Hypertension
	Valvular regurgitation
	Mitral valve prolapse
	Intracranial aneurysms
Gastrointestinal	Hepatic cysts
	Rarely cholangiocarcinoma, congenital hepatic fibrosis
	Pancreatic cysts
	Colonic diverticuli
Miscellaneous cysts	Ovarian
	Seminal vesicle, epididymis
	Arachnoid
	Pineal
	Spleen
Musculoskeletal	Hernia formation

pairment and portal hypertension that are observed in patients with ARPKD do not occur in patients with ADPKD. The cysts can also be found in the pancreas and spleen, and, rarely, in the thyroid, ovary, endometrium, seminal vesicle, and epididymis. Colonic diverticulosis frequently accompanies ADPKD but appears to be more common in those patients treated with intermittent hemodialysis. Intracranial aneurysms (berry aneurysm) are reported in up to 50% of patients and are responsible for approximately 10% of deaths. However, recent studies using angiographic techniques refute the previously reported high incidence of intracranial aneurysms in ADPKD. Approximately 6% of patients with berry aneurysm have ADPKD. Hypertension occurs in approximately 30% of children, in 60% of adults with chronic renal insufficiency, and in 80% of patients on dialysis with ADPKD. There is an increased incidence of aneurysm of the thoracic and abdominal aorta, valvular regurgitation of all four cardiac valves, and mitral valve prolapse.

Symptoms

The disease affects all races and occurs equally in males and females. Because of the usual clinical presentation in the fourth or fifth decade of life, it was previously called adult polycystic kidney disease; however, the disease can present at any age, including childhood. The mean age of onset of symptoms, diagnosis, and death is 41 years, 47 years, and 52 years, respectively. Evidence of the disease increases with age: almost 50% of patients will have some symptoms at age 60, and 100% will have symptoms at 80 to 90 years of age. Approximately 60% of patients with ADPKD have a positive family history, and almost all family members follow a similar pattern of the disease process.

Thus, a patient with ADPKD may typically present in the following ways:

- Family screening of a known patient with ADPKD
- Flank pain (30%), caused by infection in a cyst, rupture of cysts, bleeding in cysts, or stones
- Hematuria (25–30%), microscopic or gross
- Presence of abdominal mass (renal or hepatic) in approximately 20% of patients (this is almost always associated with abnormal renal function)
- Recurrent urinary tract infection (UTI) (30%)
- Hypertension
- Renal insufficiency with mild proteinuria, impaired sodium conservation, and unusually mild anemia relative to the degree of renal insufficiency
- Extrarenal manifestations such as aneurysmal symptoms, subarachnoid hemorrhage, colonic diverticulosis, mitral valve prolapse, and abdominal aortic aneurysm

The complications of ADPKD include:

- Cyst infection
- UTI

- Cyst rupture
- Hematuria
- Intractable pain
- Upper urinary tract obstruction caused by an abdominal mass
- Nephrolithiasis
- Renal tumors
- Malignant hypertension
- Subarachnoid hemorrhage
- Malnutrition caused by abdominal distension
- Liver failure (rare)

Diagnosis

The diagnosis of ADPKD depends on the finding of bilaterally enlarged kidneys with diffuse distribution of cysts in both kidneys and a positive family history (in most cases) with or without extrarenal manifestations. Renal ultrasound can detect the presence of cysts in more than 95% of patients without exposing them to radiation and is easier to do in children who cannot remain still for CT scan or MRI. However, either technique can miss small cysts and is operator dependent. Moreover, approximately 11 to 17% of individuals with ADPKD1 under age 30 may show normal findings on kidney ultrasound. Abdominal CT scan, using contrast materials, can detect large and small cysts with high sensitivity, cysts in other organs, and also differentiate between solid and cystic masses. CT scan is currently the recommended test for diagnosing ADPKD. Intravenous pyelography (IVP) shows the presence of deformed renal structure and a stretched out calyceal system. Nuclear renal scan can estimate renal function for each kidney. These techniques lack sensitivity, however. Although gene linkage analysis can identify the disease in almost 99% of patients, it is more cumbersome and expensive, requires testing of at least two family members, and does not provide any anatomic or functional information.

ADPKD should also be differentiated from multiple simple cysts, which are uncommon in children and lack family history. The kidneys are normal-sized and the cysts are generally unilateral with nondiffuse distribution. However, simple cysts can also be bilateral. Simple cysts show no evidence of extrarenal involvement and, most importantly, renal function remains intact during follow-up periods. In doubtful cases, gene linkage analysis can be helpful.

Treatment

The therapeutic options basically aim for preservation of renal function and treatment of complications.

Summary of Diagnosis: ADPKD

- Approximately 60% of patients with polycystic kidney disease have a positive family history.
- Patients with ADPKD have an increased incidence of aneurysm of the thoracic and abdominal aorta, valvular regurgitation of all four heart valves, and mitral valve prolapse. Berry aneurysm is rare; previous reports of a high incidence of berry aneurysm in ADPKD patients could not be substantiated.
- Simple cysts are usually asymptomatic and present as an incidental finding on ultrasound imaging of the kidneys.
- ADPKD makes up 5 to 10% of the dialysis population.
- ADPKD usually causes moderate to massive enlargement of the kidneys.
- Gross hematuria, recurrent UTI, and increased abdominal girth are common presenting features.
- Colonic diverticulosis, mitral valve prolapse, and abdominal aortic aneurysm are uncommon accompaniments of ADPKD.
- Kidney ultrasound is the simple technique to make a diagnosis of ADPKD. CT scan confirms the diagnosis by showing cysts in the kidneys and in the liver.
- The incidence of renal stones is higher in ADPKD than in the general population.
- Approximately half of patients with ADPKD progress to ESRD requiring dialysis by age 60. Nephrectomy is recommended in patients with recurrent UTI.

The following guidelines may be used to delay progression of renal failure:

- Intensive management of hypertension is important because it is one of the bad prognostic factors. Treatments include sympathetic inhibitor, alpha blockers, or calcium channel blockers. Angiotensin-converting enzyme (ACE) inhibitors should be used with caution in the presence of impaired renal function, especially in patients with large cysts, where they may precipitate acute renal failure. Sodium volume depletion, diuretic use, and cyst hemorrhage can further predispose the patient to ACE-inhibitor-induced acute renal failure.

- Diuretics should be used with caution to avoid hypokalemia, which has been proposed as a factor in spontaneous renal cyst development.
- All nephrotoxic agents should be avoided as much as possible.
- Patient participation in activities and sports that can result in abdominal trauma should be avoided to prevent injury to kidneys and, consequently, rupture of cysts.
- Unnecessary instrumentation, primarily bladder or urethral catheterization, of the urinary tract should be avoided.
- The role of dietary restriction of protein, phosphate, and caffeine is currently not established in delaying progression of renal failure or mitigating cyst enlargement. Similarly, the role of cyst decompression as a means of preserving renal function is not yet established.

Nephrectomy is an extreme treatment measure and should be reserved for patients with intractable hemorrhage, intractable pain, severely infected cysts, malignancy, obstruction caused by calculi, or pretransplant preparation to avoid recurrent UTI, hemorrhage, or to make space for the allograft. Nephrectomy may be associated with inadvertent adrenalectomy during surgery and requires lifelong steroid replacement. This should be kept in mind when a patient develops signs and symptoms of adrenal insufficiency in the postoperative period. Cyst decompression has been thought to be associated with worsening renal function based on past experience, but recently it has been resurrected as treatment for intractable pain when cysts are more than 3 cm in diameter. Slight worsening of renal function after surgery may be noted.

Treatment of Complications

Hematuria   Bed rest, analgesics, and hydration are usually adequate for managing of intrarenal bleeding and hematuria. If bleeding is persistent and severe, requiring transfusion of more than 5 or 6 units of packed red blood cells in 24 hours, renal angiography is recommended. Intra-arterial injection of Gelfoam has been used successfully to stop bleeding during angiography.

Infections   Most infections occur in females and are usually caused by Gram-negative organisms. The infection can be a simple UTI, parenchymal infection, or cyst infection. Cyst infection should be suspected when there is renal tenderness associated with negative urine culture, with or without positive blood culture, and when usual antibiotic treatment of UTI fails. The possibility of renal stones should be considered, especially in case of recurrent infections. All UTI in patients with ADPKD should be treated aggressively.

If there is clinical suspicion for parenchymal or cyst infection, antibiotics with high lipid solubility and a high pKa should be used, which can achieve higher antibiotic concentrations in the cyst fluid than those with lower solubility.

These antibiotics include:

- Trimethoprim-sulphamethoxazole
- Ciprofloxacin
- Erythromycin
- Clindamycin
- Tetracycline
- Chloramphenicol

Surgical drainage may occasionally be necessary. Nephrectomy is recommended in patients with recurrent UTI and when all treatment options fail.

Preventive measures include routine hygiene, avoidance of invasive urologic procedures, and removal of any stones. Prolonged use of oral antibiotics may be necessary at times.

Nephrolithiasis Approximately 20% of patients with ADPKD develop calcium oxalate or uric acid stones in the urinary tract. Treatment and prevention include general measures such as hydration to improve urinary flow, citrate supplementation (with potassium citrate) for hypocitraturia, and thiazide diuretics for hypercalciuria. Allopurinol can be used in the presence of hyperuricemia and/or hyperuricosuria. Stones that are too large to pass spontaneously have to be removed by using extracorporeal shock wave lithotripsy or percutaneous nephrolithotomy.

ESRD Approximately 45 to 50% of patients with ADPKD progress to ESRD by the age of 60 years. Factors predicting poor renal outcome include:

- ADPKD1 gene
- Male sex
- Black race
- Sickle hemoglobin in black patients
- Early age at diagnosis
- Large kidneys
- Hypertension
- Recurrent UTI
- Recurrent gross hematuria
- Moderate proteinuria (> 2 gm every 24 hr)

Dialysis can be instituted in these patients as usual. ESRD in ADPKD is associated with a lower erythro-

poietin requirement because of its production by the renal cysts. Survival of patients with ESRD resulting from ADPKD is better than that of patients of comparable age with ESRD caused by glomerulonephritis, but the risk of osteodystrophy, diverticular disease, and subarachnoid hemorrhage is higher. The course may also be complicated by peritonitis, infections, and hernias. The cysts may decrease in size. Continuous ambulatory peritoneal dialysis (CAPD) is not very successful in these patients.

Renal transplantation from cadaver donors (rather than from relatives because of the possibility of genetic polycystic disease) is successful in this group with usual graft survival (90% 1-year survival). Pretransplant nephrectomy may be required when the patient experiences recurrent infections, pain, bleeding, stones, neoplasm, inferior vena cava compression, and extremely large kidney size leading to distressing abdominal symptoms or technological difficulties.

Intracranial aneurysms Berry aneurysms are present in approximately 5% of patients with ADPKD and tend to cluster in families. Approximately 9% of patients with ADPKD die of subarachnoid hemorrhage. Because not all patients have aneurysms and not all patients who have aneurysms have complications, it is not cost-effective to screen all patients with ADPKD. Only those patients with aneurysm symptoms (such as bursting headache, transient neurologic symptoms, blurred vision, focal neurologic deficit, etc.), with a family history of berry aneurysm, and those involved in high-risk occupations (e.g., airline pilot) should undergo screening with cerebral arteriography. However, cerebral arteriography causes a higher morbidity rate because of the use of contrast materials. Asymptomatic patients with a previous history of aneurysm rupture can be followed noninvasively by periodic contrast-enhanced CT or with MRI. In the presence of advanced renal insufficiency (serum creatinine concentration ≥ 3.5 mg/dL), the diagnostic modality should avoid use of contrast medium.

Aneurysms greater or equal to 10 mm in size should be removed; those between 6 mm and 9 mm should be followed every year, and those 5 mm or less should be followed every 1 to 2 years noninvasively. Blood pressure control is especially important in patients with intracranial aneurysms to prevent rupture of aneurysms and intracranial hemorrhage.

Hepatic cysts Liver cysts are rare in children and uncommon before age 30, but thereafter increase in incidence to 75% or higher, even to 90% among patients whose lives have been sustained by renal replacement therapy. Liver cysts are more common in females than in males and increase in incidence and size with pregnancy. Large liver cysts are also more common in females and are accompanied by pain. However, liver cysts rarely cause abnormality in liver function, which, if present, should prompt a search for another cause. Hepatic cysts can occasionally become infected and may require percutaneous aspiration and sclerosing therapy for a solitary cyst. Multiple infected liver cysts may require partial resection of the liver.

Prognosis

When the glomerular filtration rate starts decreasing significantly, the rate of loss of renal function is usually fixed each year. This results in a linear decline in the absence of another complication. A doubling of serum creatinine concentration can be expected approximately every 36 months in uncomplicated cases.

Screening

Screening for ADPKD in an asymptomatic individual with a positive family history of ADPKD or cerebral aneurysm should be done only after 18 years of age. An informed consent should be taken because a positive diagnosis can result in difficulty finding medical and life insurance, aside from the psychological trauma. The benefits of diagnosis are better management, prevention of complications, and family planning.

Renal ultrasonography is a cost-effective method for screening but may result in a significant number of false–negatives in young patients, and it is operator-dependent. A contrast-enhanced CT scan is more sensitive, with almost 100% sensitivity in individuals older than 30 years. This method can be used to detect patients suspected of having false–negative results with ultrasonography. Gene linkage analysis can detect patients who still remain negative but have a high likelihood of the disease.

Prevention

Appropriate screening within the family of patients with ADPKD and genetic counseling can prevent disease transmission.

Autosomal-Recessive Polycystic Kidney Disease (ARPKD)

ARPKD is a rare disorder inherited recessively with a defect on chromosome 6. Thus, parents are not affected and occurrence in siblings is variable.

Renal involvement is bilateral. The kidneys are large initially but later decrease in size as a result of fibrosis. Liver dysfunction (without cysts) is associated with renal involvement and helps in differentiating this disease from ADPKD.

Pathologically, the renal cysts originate from collecting ducts and are small in size. These are arranged radially with no intervening normal renal parenchyma (which is the case in ADPKD). There may be poor development of intrahepatic bile ducts (Caroli's disease) with variable amounts of fibrosis.

Symptoms

ARPKD may present in the perinatal period, in early childhood, or in early adulthood. Occurrence in the perinatal period is associated with high mortality because of the presence of pulmonary hypoplasia. Children with this disease who survive the first month of life have a more than 75% chance of surviving beyond 15 years of age.

In early life, the presentation is dominated by features of liver disease. Hepatic cysts are uncommon, but symptoms result from hepatic fibrosis and portal hypertension. The hepatic fibrosis and portal hypertension may be responsible for causing gastrointestinal bleeding, hepatosplenomegaly, and hypersplenism. The severity of liver involvement is inversely proportional to the degree of renal involvement. With increasing age, symptoms of renal involvement become prominent, resulting in the following signs and symptoms:

- Abdominal mass
- Failure to thrive
- Early hypertension
- Recurrent UTIs
- Renal osteodystrophy

Renal failure gradually sets in by adolescence. At times, berry aneurysms, aortic aneurysms of the thoracic and abdominal aorta, and Ehlers-Danlos syndrome may be associated with ARPKD.

Diagnosis

Ultrasonography is the test of choice for ARPKD and demonstrates enlarged kidneys of smooth appearance with increased echogenicity. Normal ultrasound may not exclude the diagnosis. Contrast CT scan may show the presence of persistent nephrogram. Absence of a family history (by demonstrating a normal ultrasound in parents older than 30 years), evidence of liver disease with absence of liver cysts and absence of other manifestations of ADPKD help in confirming the diagnosis of ARPKD.

Treatment

There is no good treatment for the neonatal presentation of this disease with pulmonary hypoplasia. Patients who survive gradually develop chronic renal failure and liver disease. Hypertension should be treated aggressively. UTIs must be treated promptly, and invasive urologic procedures should be avoided.

Dialysis and transplantation are good options for treating renal failure, but liver failure increases the risk of complications. Portal hypertension can be managed by shunting procedures, and hypersplenism may require splenectomy. Simultaneous liver and kidney transplantation is also an option.

Screening

Ultrasonography is used for screening in utero and will demonstrate the presence of the disease after the gestational age of 24 weeks. Oligohydramnios (i.e., less than 300 mL of amniotic fluid at term) may also be detected at times.

Tuberous Sclerosis

TS is an autosomal-dominant disorder with a frequency of approximately 1 in 10,000 individuals. The genetic defect is located on chromosomes 9 and 16, close to the ADPKD1 gene. It is a systemic disorder that can affect skin, brain, bone, liver, lungs, heart, and kidney.

Symptoms

Clinical manifestations of TS include epilepsy, mental retardation, and skin abnormalities—especially adenoma sebaceum and ash-leaf spots. Angiomyolipomas of the kidneys, present in 40 to 50% of patients, with the presence of renal cysts in 15 to 20% of those patients, signify the presence of TS. Hypertension and renal insufficiency are common. Renal failure is the most common cause of death after age 30 in this group of patients. Rarely, it may be associated with renal cell carcinoma.

Diagnosis

The diagnosis is based on typical clinical features, including family history and findings on the examination of skin and retina. The retinal examination may show phakomas of the retina (i.e., looks like a retinal tumor). The diagnosis can be confirmed by ultrasonography, CT scan, and angiography.

Treatment

There is no specific treatment, and renal failure is treated in the usual manner. Genetic counseling may help in preventing disease transmission.

von Hippel-Lindau Disease

von Hippel-Lindau disease is an uncommon disorder affecting 1 in 36,000 live births. It is inherited in autosomal-dominant fashion with the genetic defect on chromosome 3 (close to the defect for renal cell carcinoma).

Symptoms

von Hippel-Lindau disease usually presents in the third or fourth decade of life with central nervous system or visual complaints. Renal cysts are common (in up to 76% of cases), and tumors can occur in association with cerebellar, spinal, and retinal hemangioblastomas. The renal cysts are multiple (in up to 75% of patients) and are irregularly distributed. In 38 to 55% of cases, renal cell carcinoma can develop; they are multicentric in up to 60% of patients. The cancer develops in the fourth or fifth decade and is responsible for 20 to 50% of deaths in this group. Other manifestations include:

- Pancreatic cysts
- Islet cell carcinoma
- Pheochromocytoma (may be bilateral)
- Epididymal masses

Diagnosis

CT scan is the diagnostic modality of choice and includes imaging of brain and abdomen.

Treatment

There is no specific treatment for von Hippel-Lindau disease. The complications are treated in the usual manner (e.g., treatment of renal cell carcinoma or islet cell carcinoma). Family screening and genetic counseling are recommended because of the increased cancer risk.

Medullary Cystic Disease (MCD)

MCD is a rare disorder that is mainly transmitted in an autosomal-recessive (85%) and autosomal-dominant (15%) pattern. The entity is also known as cystic medullary complex. It is called renal-retinal dysplasia when associated with retinitis pigmentosa, retinal degeneration, and pigmentary optic atrophy in association with genetic defect on chromosome 2p. The cystic medullary complex accounts for 1 to 5% of ESRD in the general population, and for 10 to 20% of ESRD in early childhood.

Pathologic examination of the kidney shows approximately 8 to 10 mm cysts at the corticomedullary junction and in the medulla. Tubular basement membrane is abnormal with associated interstitial infiltrate and fibrosis.

Symptoms

The autosomal-recessive form of medullary cystic complex usually occurs in childhood (juvenile nephronophthisis). The common symptoms are polydipsia, polyuria and enuresis, probably related to loss of renal concentrating ability, and profound renal sodium wasting. These patients are especially prone to pre-renal failure. Growth retardation and renal insufficiency are concomitant features of MCD. The rate of progression is relatively slow with a doubling time for serum creatinine concentration of approximately 3 years. This results in renal failure, usually by age 13. Anemia is unusually severe and is out of proportion to the degree of renal insufficiency. Renal osteodystrophy is also severe. Hypertension is uncommon or is mild when present, and hematuria is rare. The disease may occasionally present later in life. The autosomal-dominant form presents in early adulthood and causes renal failure by 60 years of age.

The disease may occasionally be associated with hepatic fibrosis, retinal dysplasia, hyperuricemia, and gout. Skeletal and central nervous system defects are seen occasionally. Cysts in other organs or cerebral aneurysms are not seen in this disease.

Diagnosis

The presence of renal disease at an early age in association with family history of renal disease, mild hypertension, and severe anemia are the clues to the presence of cystic medullary complex. Urine sediment may be bland in approximately 30% of patients. The diagnosis can be made by contrast-enhanced CT scan, which shows medullary cysts of small size and smooth kidneys. IVP may show accumulation of contrast in tubules or may be completely normal. IVP should be avoided in patients with impaired renal function. Ultrasound usually does not detect any cysts in the kidneys. Renal biopsy may occasionally be necessary for diagnosis. The patient's eyes should be checked to exclude any abnormalities.

Treatment

There is no specific treatment for this disease. Because of excessive sodium wasting, it is unnecessary to restrict dietary sodium intake, and sodium supplementation to maintain blood pressure may actually be required. There is no specific treatment for anemia. The usual management of ESRD can be done with dialysis or transplantation with increased erythropoietin requirement. Severity of osteodystrophy caused by secondary hyperparathyroidism may complicate the management of patients on dialysis or after transplantation. Because of the hereditary nature of MCD, evidence of renal disease should be carefully investigated in related donors.

Prevention

Genetic counseling with family planning can decrease the frequency of this disease.

Medullary Sponge Kidney (MSK)

MSK is a more common disease affecting approximately 1 in 5,000 individuals in the general population. Some clinicians consider it to be a developmental anomaly, but patients with familial autosomal-dominant inheritance have been seen. Hemihypertrophy of the body may occur with this condition. MSK disease is characterized by the presence of dilated collecting ducts in renal papillae bilaterally within normal-sized kidneys.

Symptoms

MSK affects both sexes and is bilateral in 75% and unilateral in 25% of patients. The disease is usually asymptomatic in the absence of complications and is associated with normal renal function. Mild impairment of concentrating ability and acidification of urine may occur, causing high fractional excretion of sodium, metabolic acidosis, and hypercalciuria. Type I (distal) renal tubular acidosis may cause formation of calcium phosphate stones. Patients may present with symptoms resulting from urolithiasis in 50 to 60% of cases. The stones form within the ectatic collecting ducts. Calcification is usually not symmetric on both sides, which helps to differentiate this condition from calcification associated with primary hyperparathyroidism and renal tubular acidosis. Hyperparathyroidism may be associated with MSK. Twenty to thirty percent of patients may also present with recurrent UTI. Recurrent hematuria occurs in 10 to 20% of patients. The prognosis is good in the absence of complications. Recurrent infections or urolithiasis may complicate the course of MSK.

Diagnosis

IVP is the test of choice for diagnosis of MSK. The findings include normal to slightly enlarged kidneys with dilated medullary collecting tubules forming brush-like patterns in renal papillae, referred to as "bouquets of flowers" or "bunches of grapes". These tubules fill with contrast material before calyceal opacification and then persist. The filled tubules fail to fill on retrograde pyelogram.

Ultrasonography and CT scan help in further diagnosis of stones, abscess, or tumors. Renal tumors may need to be excluded with the help of CT scan. Other diseases that need to be differentiated from MSK include calyceal diverticuli, papillary necrosis, renal tuberculosis, and other causes of nephrocalcinosis. The MCD complex can be differentiated on the basis of absence of family history, presence of hematuria, UTIs, urinary obstruction, calculi, and absence of renal failure.

Treatment

Patients with stone formation should be advised to keep a urine output of more than 2 liters. Thiazide diuretics can help in decreasing hypercalciuria. If there is evidence of absorptive hypercalciuria (i.e., increased GI absorption of calcium), oral phosphates may help in decreasing absorption. The patient may require additional management of stones by urologic interventions.

Renal infections may require appropriate antibiotic therapy for prolonged periods. An abscess may require surgical drainage, and recurrent lithiasis in a particular location may require partial nephrectomy. Periodic urinalysis, urine culture, and renal function tests are recommended for crystalluria and infection. Patients should be informed about the benign nature of the disease.

Acquired Cystic Kidney Disease (ACKD)

Development of cysts in previously noncystic kidneys is not uncommon. Approximately 40 to 100% of patients undergoing long-term hemodialysis develop cysts. Patients on peritoneal dialysis also develop cysts, but less frequently. In a different series, 7 to 22% of patients with long-term chronic renal insufficiency developed cysts. Cyst development can occur in native kidneys as well as in failed transplant kidneys. Risk factors for the development of cysts include:

- Male sex
- Black race
- Long duration of chronic renal failure
- Renal insufficiency
- Long-term hemodialysis

The cysts occasionally regress after successful renal transplantation.

Cysts in ACKD are bilateral, with a minimum of five cysts in each kidney required for the diagnosis. The cysts arise from proximal, distal, and collecting tubules. Cyst fluid is usually clear but can be hemorrhagic and contains high concentrations of sodium and creatinine.

Symptoms

Acquired cysts are usually asymptomatic and may be an incidental finding on imaging studies done for some other reason. Occasionally, the cysts can cause hematuria or retroperitoneal hemorrhage. A palpable mass, fever, or renal colic may also be present. Erythrocytosis, hypercalcemia, and hypoglycemia have been reported in rare cases.

The course of ACKD may be complicated by the occurrence of adenoma or adenocarcinoma, which are more common with large cysts. Indeed, there is an increased incidence of renal malignancies (5–15%) in patients with large cysts. The malignancies may also be complicated by metastasis, and there may be matrix-stone formation.

Diagnosis

Contrast-enhanced CT scan is the diagnostic method of choice. It shows bilateral cysts, usually in the small kidneys. Ultrasonography can be used when radiocontrast materials are contraindicated (i.e., contrast allergy). Gadolinium-enhanced MRI is useful when CT is indeterminate.

Treatment

Cysts smaller than 3 cm can generally be followed by annual CT scan. Larger cysts can be aspirated and cytology done to rule out malignancy. Radical nephrectomy is usually done for large cysts because of the possibility of malignant development. Any questionable cysts should be removed before renal transplantation. As stated earlier, smaller cysts can occasionally regress after a successful renal transplantation. Bleeding in or around the cyst can usually be treated with bed rest, analgesics, and supportive treatment. Persistent bleeding may require arteriographic embolization.

Screening

Screening for ACKD in all dialysis patients is controversial because of a low cost–benefit ratio. Some experts recommend periodic (yearly or every 2 years) re-screening after 3 years of dialysis. The differential

diagnosis of three major types of renal cysts—
ADPKD, ACKD, and simple cysts—can be found at a
glance in Table 18.5.

REFERRAL

Simple Renal Cysts

The patient with an atypical-appearing cyst and persistent hematuria or abnormal renal function should be referred to a nephrologist for consultation. For recurrent or persistent infection despite adequate medical therapy, the patient should be evaluated by a urologist or a nephrologist.

ADPKD

Patients with ADPKD should be referred to a nephrologist if there is evidence of renal dysfunction, moderate proteinuria, difficulty controlling hypertension, or any other complications. Surgical referral may be needed in patients who have indications for surgery (as

---

KEY POINTS

- Simple renal cysts are the most common type of renal cystic disease. The incidence increases with age. Approximately 50% of the population older than 50 years is likely to have one or more renal cysts. Simple cysts are not inherited and do not affect renal function.

- Evidence of ADPKD increases with age. Almost 50% of patients will have symptoms of the disease at age 60, and 100% by 80 to 90 years of age.

- ADPKD or polycystic kidney disease in general is the most common type of symptomatic renal cystic disease in the adult population.

- Renal cell carcinoma is no more common in ADPKD patients than in the general population.

- Approximately 40 to 100% of patients undergoing long-term hemodialysis develop renal cysts (ACKD).

- ACKD is usually asymptomatic except for an increased incidence of renal malignancies (adenocarcinoma), an incidence that is much higher than in the general population.

- Simple renal cyst is the most common cystic disorder of the kidneys. Approximately 50% of the population older than 50 years is likely to have one or more renal cysts.

- Renal infection should be treated with lipophilic antibiotics, including Bactrim, ciprofloxacin, erythromycin, clindamycin, and chloramphenicol.

TABLE 18.5	Kidney Cysts at a Glance	
ADPKD	**ACKD**	**Simple Cyst**
Hereditary: autosomal-dominant	Acquired	Spontaneous/acquired
Both kidneys	Both kidneys	One or both kidneys
Liver, pancreas cysts, aneurysms	No concomitant cyst formation, no concomitant aneurysm	No concomitant cyst formation or aneurysm formation
Causes renal failure	Follows renal failure	Normal renal function
Complications: infections, bleeding	Bleeding, malignancy	Benign
Incidental diagnosis	Screening studies	Incidental diagnosis

ADPKD, autosomal-dominant polycystic kidney disease; ACKD, acquired cystic kidney disease.

mentioned earlier in the text), such as intractable hemorrhage, intractable pain, severely infected cysts, malignancy, etc.

ARPKD

The presence of renal dysfunction and hepatic dysfunction in early life with an absence of family history should prompt referral to a nephrologist and a hepatologist for aggressive treatment of complications and evaluation for transplantation.

MSK

Patients with MSK should be referred to a nephrologist or an urologist.

COMMONLY ASKED QUESTIONS

What is ADPKD?

ADPKD is a common hereditary disorder characterized by multiple fluid-filled cavities, called cysts, in both the kidneys. The cysts can occur in other organs as well, such as the liver, pancreas, and spleen. There may be abnormalities of the blood vessels in the brain, called aneurysms.

How does one get ADPKD?

The disease is caused by an abnormality of chromosome 16 in most patients and by an abnormality of chromosome 4 in a small number of patients. It is transmitted from the parents in most instances but can also occur as a result of a mutation. There is a 50% risk of inheriting the disease from one affected parent, none if the parents are unaffected.

What are the symptoms of ADPKD?

The patient can have renal failure, hypertension, infection, blood in the urine, or flank pain. Occasionally, there may be other symptoms caused by cysts in other organs. The patients are occasionally diagnosed after bleeding from an aneurysm in the brain.

How is ADPKD diagnosed?

The diagnosis depends on a demonstration of the presence of cysts in both kidneys, which are large in size, with the help of ultrasound or CT scan. However, there may be false–negatives, especially before the age of 30. In doubtful cases, genetic defect can be detected by linkage analysis from blood, but it is more expensive and cumbersome.

What are the consequences of having ADPKD?

Fifty to sixty percent of patients who have ADPKD develop renal failure and require dialysis treatment to sustain life. However, approximately 50% of patients have reasonably preserved renal function at the age of 70 years and do not require dialysis. Hypertension worsens renal failure and expedites the development of ESRD. Other common complications include recurrent UTI, cyst infection, flank pain, blood in the urine, and, occasionally, stone

formation. Currently, no scientific evidence suggests an increased frequency of renal cancer in these patients.

How is ADPKD treated?

There is no specific treatment for ADPKD. The renal failure and end-stage renal disease are treated in the usual fashion with dialysis and transplantation. Episodes of infection should be promptly treated. Blood pressure should be controlled aggressively to prevent stroke and slow progression of renal failure.

Are there any specific restrictions?

The patients should avoid activities that could cause trauma to the abdomen. All invasive urologic procedures should be avoided. Currently, no evidence suggests any benefit from protein or caffeine restriction.

Can other family members be screened for the presence of ADPKD?

Family members older than 18 years can be tested after an informed consent, especially if they have hypertension or renal failure. The presence of cysts in the kidneys can be detected by ultrasonography or CT scan. It is not necessary to look for aneurysms in the brain unless symptoms suggest their presence or the person has a high-risk occupation that may harm the patient as well as others.

How can it be prevented?

Genetic counseling for persons affected by ADPKD can help in making the decision to have children and in determining the risks involved. Because of a 50% chance of the disease occurring in children, the decision is difficult. Once pregnant, patients with ADPKD should have close follow-up, including periodic blood pressure measurement and urine examination. There may be an increased risk of premature delivery in these patients.

What is ARPKD?

ARPKD is also inherited but has a 25% chance of occurring in children. The parents are usually not affected. The disease causes renal failure in early life.

SUGGESTED READINGS

Gabow PA, Ikle DW, Holmes JH. Polycystic kidney disease: prospective analysis of nonazotemic patients and family members. Ann Intern Med 1984;101: 238–247.

Grantham JJ, Gabow PA. Polycystic kidney disease. In: Schrier RW, Gottschalk CW, eds. Diseases of the Kidney. 4th ed. Boston: Little, Brown, 1988: 583–615.

Parfrey PS, Bear JC, Morgan J, et al. The diagnosis and prognosis of autosomal-dominant polycystic kidney disease. N Engl J Med 1990;323:1085–1090.

Welling LW, Grantham JJ. Cystic and developmental diseases of the kidney. In: Brenner BM, ed. The Kidney. 5th ed. Philadelphia: Saunders, 1996:1828–1863.

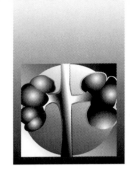

19
CHAPTER

Nephrolithiasis

Daniel Bloch
N. Stanley Nahman Jr.

BACKGROUND

Nephrolithiasis is a common clinical problem accounting for extensive patient morbidity. Symptomatic nephrolithiasis may account for up to 10 of every 1,000 hospital admissions. Ten percent or more of North Americans will experience a kidney stone by the age of 70. The disease has a four-to-one gender preponderance in males. The majority of kidney stones recur within 10 years. Therefore, any attempt to decrease the morbidity, expense, and loss of productivity for such a large percentage of the population will have significant impact on patient health and associated medical costs.

The medical management of patients with nephrolithiasis is based on the chemical composition of the stone or, in the absence of material from the stone for analysis, 24-hour urinary chemistries. The majority of kidney stones are composed of calcium oxalate

(75%), struvite (10-20%), uric acid (5-10%), calcium phosphate (5%), and cystine (less than 1%). A small proportion of kidney stones consist of rare substances including xanthine, allopurinol metabolites, or triamterene.

PATHOPHYSIOLOGY

Nephrolithiasis results from urinary precipitation of specific stone-forming components (Table 19.1). Crystal precipitation and stone propagation may result from urinary supersaturation with the offending agents, from nidus formation from other urinary components (heterogenous nucleation), or be the result of a lack of inhibitors of stone formation (Table 19.2).

Calcium Oxalate Stones

As outlined above, calcium oxalate stones may result from supersaturation of the urine with calcium or oxalate, from nidus formation from elevated urinary uric acid levels, or from a decrease in urinary citrate, an inhibitor of stone formation. Approximately 70% of patients with documented calcium oxalate stones have demonstrable biochemical abnormalities in urine, whereas up to 30% of patients may have completely normal urine chemistries. Serum chemistries and parathyroid hormone (PTH) level and 1,25 $(OH)_2$ vitamin D$_3$ levels are normal in the majority of patients who form stones.

Uric Acid Stones

Uric acid stones result primarily from supersaturation of the urine with uric acid. In addition, acidic urine promotes uric acid precipitation and stone formation. Thus, patients with hyperuricosuria and low urinary pH are at increased risk for developing uric acid stones.

Struvite Stones

Struvite stones or infection stones result from precipitation of magnesium salts in the presence of an alkaline urine and elevated urinary ammonia levels. Elevated urinary ammonia levels result from infection with bacteria containing the urea-degrading enzyme urease. *Proteus* species are the classic organisms associated with this condition. Most patients with struvite stones have anatomically abnormal urinary tracts that allow for colonization and infection with the appropriate bacterial pathogen. The development of struvite stones leads to recurrent obstruction, urinary stasis, and increased bacterial growth. This vicious cycle promotes the development of very large struvite stones. Struvite stones that fill the renal calices and renal pelvis are termed staghorn calculi. In this

Causes of Abnormal Urine Chemisty Predisposing to Nephrolithiasis	TABLE 19.1

Abnormality	Associated Conditions or Risk Factors
Hypercalciuria	Hypercalcemia
	Calcium ingestion (antacids)
	Renal leak
	Familial hypercalciuria
Hyperoxaluria	Inborn lack of metabolism regulation
	Enteric hyperoxaluria
	Megadose of vitamin C
	Iced tea, chocolate
Hyperuricosuria	Inborn lack of metabolism regulation
	Purine gluttony
	Medications (probenecid)
Hypocitraturia	Renal tubular acidosis
	Chronic diarrhea
	Hypokalemia
Alkaline urine	Renal tubular acidosis
	Carbonic anhydrase inhibitors
	Increased urinary ammonia levels

Pathophysiology and Associated Risk Factors for Development of Kidney Stones

Stone Type	Pathophysiology	Clinical Risk Factors
Calcium oxalate	Supersaturation	Hypercalciuria
		Hyperoxaluria
	Heterogenous nucleation	Hyperuricosuria
	Lack of inhibitors	Hypocitraturia
Uric acid	Supersaturation	Hyperuricosuria
	Acid urine	
Struvite	Infection	Urease-containing pathogens
		Anatomic abnormalities
	Alkaline urine	Elevated urinary ammonia concentrations
Calcium phosphate	Supersaturation	Hypercalciuria
	Lack of inhibitors	Hypocitraturia
	Alkaline urine	Renal tubular acidosis
Cystine	Supersaturation	Faulty transport of cystine
	Acid urine	

disease, stones can never be eradicated until the urinary tract is sterilized and all anatomic defects corrected.

Calcium Phosphate Stones

Calcium phosphate stones may result from urinary calcium supersaturation with persistent alkaluria. Calcium phosphate stones may form from hypocitraturia. Patients with persistently alkaline urine associated with struvite stones, renal tubular acidosis, or the administration of carbonic anhydrase inhibitors (i.e., acetazolamide in the therapy of glaucoma) are particularly susceptible to the development of calcium phosphate stones. Therapy is directed at correcting the hypercalciuria and urinary acidification defect.

Cystine Stones

Cystine stones result from an inherited disorder of amino acid transport mechanisms in the proximal tubule. Of the divalent amino acids, cystine may form insoluble dimers and present as cystine stones. This outcome results from urinary supersaturation. Acid urine decreases cystine solubility and also promotes precipitation. In extreme cases, cystine stones can calcify and form into staghorn calculi, which may be evident on supine abdominal or pelvic radiographs.

ASSOCIATED SYSTEMIC DISEASES

Diseases associated with the development of nephrolithiasis result primarily from supersaturation of the urine with precursors of stone development, and include:

- Gout (hyperuricosuria leading to uric acid stones)
- Granulomatous disease (hypercalciuria leading to calcium oxalate stones)
- Renal tubular acidification defects (alkaline urine leading to calcium phosphate precipitation or hypo-citraturia promoting calcium oxalate stones)
- Parathyroid disease (hypercalciuria leading to calcium-containing stones)
- Chronic diarrhea (hypocitraturia causing calcium oxalate stones, or uric acid stones resulting from volume depletion and metabolic acidosis)

Steatorrhea associated with ileal disease also results in secondary hyperoxaluria and is a major cause of calcium oxalate stones. Finally, excess ingestion of oxalate precursors (iced tea, chocolate, or vitamin C) induces hyperoxaluria and promotes development of calcium oxalate stones.

UNCOMMON CAUSES OF KIDNEY STONES

Several rare components have been associated with the development of nephrolithiasis, including:

- Xanthine
- Allopurinol metabolites
- Triamterene, a component of commonly used potassium-sparing diuretics

Stones that result from these rare components do so as a result of urinary supersaturation of the offending agent. Although extremely uncommon, they should be considered a cause of nephrolithiasis when a patient is using these drugs.

SYMPTOMS

Patients with symptomatic nephrolithiasis present with signs and symptoms of partial or complete urinary tract obstruction. Obstruction manifests as pain, hematuria, and, if complicated by infection, with fever. Acute oliguric or anuric renal failure may supervene.

The pain from nephrolithiasis results from irritation or dilatation of the distal urinary tract. If a stone is lodged in the ureter, the pain may be aggravated by peristaltic activity. The pain is typically severe and colicky in nature. The pain may be limited to the ipsilateral flank or radiate into the abdomen, pelvis, or groin. There may be referred testicular or labial pain or bladder irritability when stones obstruct the ureterovesicular junction.

On physical examination, patients with renal colic are frequently in moderate distress because of the pain. Nausea and vomiting may accompany the acute episode. Palpation and percussion of the flank may reproduce or intensify the symptoms, as may palpation of the abdomen. Microscopic or macroscopic hematuria may be present on urinalysis. In patients with associated infection (i.e., struvite stones), pyuria may be present. If obstruction is chronic, hydronephrosis will develop and result in renal parenchymal destruction and enlargement of the kidneys. If pyelonephritis complicates the obstruction, leukocyte casts may be present in the urine. Urinary crystals may be seen in patients with calcium oxalate stones, struvite stones, or cystine stones.

DIAGNOSIS

Acute Renal Colic

The clinical assessment of a patient suspected of acutely passing a kidney stone is based on an anatomic assessment of the urinary tract, including the location of the stone (when possible) and careful attention to the presence of partial or complete obstruction of the urinary tract. Abdominal films, with the patient in the supine position, are the first step in defining the presence, composition, and anatomic location of a suspected stone. Calcium-containing stones (calcium oxalate, calcium phosphate, struvite, or calcified cystine stones) present as radiopaque objects in the kidney, ureter, or bladder. Calcified phleboliths should not be confused with calcified stones.

Patients with renal colic and supine abdominal radiographs lacking calcified lesions may be symptomatic from radiolucent stones or urinary obstruction. Radi-olucent stones can result from uric acid or noncalcified cystine, xanthine, allopurinol metabolites, or triamterene. Radiolucent objects in the urinary tract can be attributed to a blood clot or sloughed renal papillae. Demonstrating the presence of radiolucent objects may require imaging studies, such as renal ultrasonography, intravenous or retrograde urography, or CT scan.

Renal ultrasonography and nonenhanced CT scan are adequate studies to exclude the presence of obstruction and may give clues to the anatomic location of a suspected stone. In addition, neither study requires the administration of intravenous contrast, which is nephrotoxic and can cause acute renal failure in selected patients.

Intravenous contrast material may induce acute renal failure in up to 27% of patients with abnormal renal function. The percentage of patients developing contrast-induced renal insufficiency is nearly 50% if both renal insufficiency and diabetes are present. If nonionic contrast is used, the incidence of renal failure in these high-risk groups is decreased by approximately 15%. Thus, the administration of ionic or nonionic contrast remains a significant risk factor for inducing acute renal failure in patients with diabetes and/or underlying renal insufficiency. The indiscriminate use of intravenous contrast in these groups should be discouraged. The use of intravenous hydration, furosemide, or mannitol may help decrease the risk of kidney failure when contrast studies are absolutely indicated. Intravenous urography provides excellent imaging of the excretory anatomy but carries the risk of acute renal failure in susceptible patients. In patients at high risk for contrast-induced renal insufficiency, retrograde urography may be used to define the anatomy.

Stone Analysis and Biochemical Evaluation

The diagnosis of nephrolithiasis is based on recovery of a stone from the urine or inferred from typical clinical signs and symptoms and associated abnormal urine chemistries.

Biochemical analysis of a kidney stone is based on spontaneously passed samples or on fragments recovered following lithotripsy or urologic intervention. The patient should be instructed to strain all urine passed during an acute episode, saving any solid material that may be passed with the urine. Likewise, in those patients referred for urologic evaluation, all recovered stone fragments should be analyzed.

When the chemical composition of a stone is known, evaluation of serum and urine chemistries may be indicated to guide therapy. However, it has been suggested that no additional diagnostic studies are necessary in patients suffering a single, uncomplicated bout of nephrolithiasis from a "calcium-containing" (presumably calcium oxalate) kidney stone. The rationale for this approach was derived by comparing the risk of recurrence with the relative risks of therapy over the ensuing 10 years. This work did not investigate "non-calcium oxalate" forms of nephrolithiasis, nor was consideration given to the role of hypocitraturia in mediating the development of calcium-containing stones. Recent reports suggest that metabolic evaluation of patients with nephrolithiasis may be advantageous to both patient health and medical costs.

It is the authors' practice to do basic blood and urine testing in all patients with a first kidney stone and in patients with suspected renal colic, but, lacking a stone evaluation, the goal is to define treatable causes.

The mainstay in evaluating the etiology of nephrolithiasis is an assessment of urine chemistries. A 24-hour urine collection, to assure complete collection (normal 24-hour urinary creatinine excretion equal to 20 mg/kg for males and 10 mg/kg for females), measures urinary excretion of the following:

- Creatinine
- Sodium
- Calcium
- Uric acid
- Oxalate
- Citrate

Increased urinary sodium excretion results from high dietary sodium intake and represents a reversible cause of hypercalciuria. A urinary cystine assessment should be done in patients who have acid urine and radiolucent stones with normal serum uric acid concentrations because these features are indicative of cystine stones. In addition, serum electrolytes, BUN, calcium, and phosphorous are assessed to exclude the presence of hypercalcemia, hyperuricemia, renal failure, or other unexpected electrolyte abnormalities. Serum PTH and vitamin D levels are also drawn if hypercalcemia is observed.

Differential Diagnosis

The presentation of typical renal colic, positive radiograph results, and recovery of the stone makes the diagnosis of nephrolithiasis straightforward. However, clinicians are frequently confronted with patients who present with typical signs and symptoms of nephrolithiasis but the presence of a stone is never confirmed. For these patients, a detailed evaluation of the abdomen and pelvis is indicated to exclude visceral, vascular, neurologic, musculoskeletal, or gynecologic sources of the pain.

Recurrent flank pain and hematuria with an otherwise negative evaluation finding may occur in patients with isolated hypercalciuria, the loin-pain hematuria

Summary of Diagnosis

- Approximately 70% of patients with documented calcium oxalate stones have demonstrable biochemical abnormalities in urine consisting of hypercalciuria, hyperuricosuria, and hyperoxaluria.
- Bilateral renal stones may present with acute oliguric or anuric renal failure. Flank pain with radiation to the groin is the typical presentation.
- Intravenous pyelogram and kidney ultrasound are adequate studies to confirm diagnosis. CT scan is rarely necessary.

syndrome (IgA nephropathy), glomerulonephritis, or factitious hematuria in a patient seeking secondary gain. Nephrology referral may be useful in helping to distinguish among these syndromes.

TREATMENT

Management of an Acute Event

Conservative management of acute nephrolithiasis consists of pain control until the stone passes. In the absence of obstruction or associated infection, outpatient management is possible. All urine should be strained and any solid material passed sent for analysis. Stones that do not pass within 48 hours necessitate lithotripsy or urologic intervention.

Hospital admission is indicated in patients requiring parenteral analgesics, in those with intractable nausea and vomiting, in those with an inability to ingest oral medication or fluids, or in any patient with obstructive or infectious complications. When indicated, appropriate cultures and urologic consultation should be obtained.

The end point of acute management of nephrolithiasis is spontaneous passage of the stone. The majority of ureteral stones less than 5 mm in diameter pass spontaneously. Larger stones, or stones that fail to progress toward passage, necessitate lithotripsy and/or urologic intervention.

Extracorporeal shock-wave lithotripsy (ESWL) successfully disrupts 49 to 88% of stones that remain lodged in the kidney or proximal ureter and are 2 cm or less in diameter. Larger stones, stones in the distal ureter, or stones composed of calcium oxalate monohydrate may require multiple treatments, urologic manipulation before ESWL, or endoscopic lithotripsy. Obesity (weight over 300 lb) may decrease the success of ESWL because of limitations in imaging the stone.

Finally, because of the risk of overwhelming postoperative sepsis, ESWL should be used with caution in patients with struvite stones and urinary tract infection.

Metabolic Evaluation and Therapy

Following the acute event, future therapeutic decisions can be made based on stone analysis and/or the results of the blood and urinary evaluations. In most cases, the urinary chemistry will correlate with the stone analysis. The therapeutic approach for each of these conditions is presented in the sections following and is summarized in Table 19.3.

Calcium Oxalate Stones

Calcium oxalate stones may result from urinary supersaturation, heterogenous nucleation, lack of inhibitors, or be idiopathic in origin.

Supersaturation with calcium or oxalate   Therapy of hypercalciuria from secondary causes is directed at the underlying disease. Familial hypercalciuria, renal tubular calciuria, or idiopathic hypercalciuria can be corrected with thiazide diuretics. Hyperoxaluria resulting from secondary causes can be treated by correcting the underlying source of the oxalate (i.e., dietary indiscretion). Enteric hyperoxaluria in patients with small bowel disease may require reevaluation and therapy of the underlying disorder. Calcium supplements can be given to these patients to decrease oxalate absorption from the intestine and thereby reduce the severity of

hyperoxaluria. Patients who have undergone intestinal bypass procedures for weight control may require reoperation if complications of stones (recurrent obstruction and/or infection) threaten renal function.

Nidus formation   Heterogenous nucleation from hyperuricosuria provides the nidus for calcium oxalate precipitation and, thus, promotes the development of calcium oxalate stones. Hyperuricosuria may be treated with allopurinol in affected patients.

Hypocitraturia   Low urine citrate levels in patients with hypocitraturia can be reversed with potassium citrate or potassium bicarbonate.

Idiopathic   In approximately 30% of patients with calcium oxalate stones, all blood and urinary evaluations will be normal. In this setting, management is conservative and includes encouraging the patient to increase fluid intake to maintain urinary volumes of at least 3 liters daily. In particularly difficult-to-control stone formation, empiric thiazide diuretics with or without allopurinol may be of therapeutic benefit. In idiopathic hyperoxaluria, pyridoxine (vitamin B6) given in doses of 50 to 150 mg daily may help to reduce the recurrence of oxalate stone formation.

Uric Acid Stones

Uric acid stones result from hyperuricosuria and persistently acid urine. Allopurinol corrects hyperuricosuria

Diagnostic and Therapeutic Approach to Nephrolithiasis		**TABLE 19.3**
Stone Type	**Associated Clinical Abnormality**	**Treatment Approach**
Calcium oxalate	Hypercalciuria, secondary causes	Treat the cause
	Familial, renal leak, or idiopathic	Hydrochlorothiazide
	Secondary hyperoxaluria	Treat recognizable causes
	Idiopathic hyperoxaluria	Pyridoxine (vitamine B6)
	Hyperuricosuria	Allopurinol
	Hypocitraturia	Potassium citrate
Uric acid	Hyperuricosuria	Allopurinol
	Acid urine	Acetazolamide at bedtime
Struvite	Bacterial infection	Antibiotics
	Anatomic abnormalities	Correct abnormality if possible
	Alkaline urine	Eradicate bacteria, acidify if indicated
Calcium phosphate	Hypercalciuria	Hydrochlorothiazide
	Alkaline urine	Correct acidification defect
	Hypocitraturia	Potassium citrate
Cystine	Cystinuria	Penicillamine to chelate cystine
	Acid urine	Acetazolamide

KEY POINTS

- The majority of kidney stones are composed of calcium oxalate (75–80%).

- Almost all renal stones are radiopaque. Uric acid renal stones per se are radiolucent but as a result of secondary deposit of calcium can become radiopaque.

- Serum calcium and phosphate, serum PTH, and 1,25(OH)2 vitamin D3 levels are normal in the majority of patients who form stones.

- Struvite stones (staghorn calculi) tend to develop in patients with anatomically abnormal urinary tracts, allowing for colo-nization and recurrent infection with *Proteus* organisms.

- Hospital admission is required for treatment of pain. Stones that do not pass within 48 hours require lithotripsy or urologic intervention.

- Patients who form recurrent, idiopathic stones are treated with hydrochloro-thiazide and allopurinol. Bicitra may be helpful.

- Penicillamine is the recommended treatment for patients who form cystine stones.

and combined with administration of acetazolamide at bedtime will alkalinize the urine and minimize precipitation of uric acid and uric acid stone formation.

Struvite Stones

Struvite stones result from anatomic abnormalities, persistent infection with urea-splitting organisms, and an alkaline urine. Therapy is directed at removing the stones, correcting the anatomic defect, and sterilizing the urine with appropriate antibiotics.

Calcium Phosphate Stones

Calcium phosphate stones may result from hypercalciuria and/or hypocitraturia and should be treated as for struvite stones. In drug-induced forms of renal tubular acidosis (i.e., acetazolamide administration), stopping the offending agent is indicated.

Cystine Stones

Cystine stones result from cystine supersaturation of the urine and are promoted by an acid urine. Hypocitraturia may also complicate the clinical presentation. Initial therapy is directed at correcting the low urinary pH with acetazolamide or potassium citrate if hypocitraturia accompanies the condition. Penicillamine can be used if these initial approaches are unsuccessful.

REFERRAL

Patients with urinary tract obstruction or retained stone fragments require urologic referral. Therapeutic options include cystoscopic procedures and/or lithotripsy to relieve obstruction and/or remove retained fragments.

Patients who do not respond to conservative manipulation of urinary chemical disturbances, those with more than one abnormality, or patients with ab-normal renal function may benefit from referral to a nephrologist.

COMMONLY ASKED QUESTIONS

Do kidney stones lead to kidney failure?
Not unless renal parenchymal damage has occurred from recurrent obstruction, infection, or repeated urologic procedures.

Can kidney stones be cured?
When correctable causes can be identified, the incidence of stone-forming events clearly declines. Compliance with the medical prescription is essential. In patients with idiopathic calcium oxalate stones, increasing urinary output to 3 liters per day is recommended. Empirically, thiazide diuretics with or without allopurinol have been reported to decrease the number of stone-forming events in this setting.

SUGGESTED READINGS

Bleyer A, Agus Z. Approach to nephrolithiasis. The Kidney 1992;25(2):1–10.

Coe F, Parks J, Asplin J. The pathogenesis and treatment of kidney stones. N Engl J Med 1992;327:1141–1152.

Grasso M, Loisides P, Beaghler M, et al. The case for primary endoscopic management of upper urinary tract calculi: I. A critical review of 121 extracorporeal shock-wave lithotripsy failures. Urology 1995;45:363–371.

Parks J, Coe F. The financial effects of kidney stone prevention. Kidney Int 1996;50:1706–1712.

Rudnick M, Goldfarb S, Wexler L, et al. Nephrotoxicity of ionic and nonionic contrast media in 1,196 patients: a randomized trial. Kidney Int 1995;47:254–261.

Silver J, Rubinger D, Friedlaender MM, et al. Sodium-dependent idiopathic hypercalciuria in renal stone formers. Lancet 1983;2:484–486.

Uribarri J, Oh M, Carroll H. The first kidney stone. Ann Intern Med 1989;111:1006–1009.

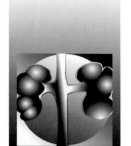

CHAPTER 20

Urinary Tract Infection

P. George John

BACKGROUND

Physiology

The urinary tract consists of two kidneys in the lumbar region; the ureters, which drain the urine from the kidneys into the urinary bladder; the bladder, which functions as a reservoir for urine; and the urethra, which drains the urine out of the body. In females, the urethra is short, and bacteria can easily migrate into the bladder from the urethra. In males, the prostate surrounds the proximal urethra, and enlargement of the prostate can cause urinary obstruction and urinary infection.

The urinary bladder consists of a detrusor muscle, which is supplied by the parasympathetic nerve from the sacral segments. The internal sphincter is supplied by the sympathetic nerves from the lower thoracic and lumbar region. The external sphincter is supplied by the pudendal nerve and is under voluntary control.

When there is dysfunction of the nervous system supply to the bladder, evacuation of urine is impaired, leading to urinary retention and infection.

Pathophysiology

Urinary tract infection (UTI) is one of the most commonly encountered conditions in the office, hospital, and extended care facility. UTI is more common in women than in men and is reported by more than 50% of adult women. UTI is a common complication of pregnancy, diabetes mellitus, and neurologic conditions that interfere with the urine flow. UTI also is a leading cause of Gram-negative sepsis. The frequency of UTI is 1 to 2% among newborns, and male newborns are more commonly affected than are female newborns. However, after the first year of life, UTI is predominant in females.

Micro-organisms that cause UTI are listed in Table 20.1. Nearly 90% of community-acquired UTI is

TABLE 20.1	Organisms That Cause Urinary Tract Infections

Escherichia coli[a]
Klebsiella sp.
Enterobacter sp.
Proteus sp.
Enterococcus sp.
Group B streptococcus[b]
Staphylococcus saprophyticus[c]
Pseudomonas sp.
Fungi
Viruses
Mycobacterium tuberculosis

[a]Causes approximately 85% of first episodes of urinary tract infections.
[b]Occurs primarily in newborns.
[c]Occurs primarily in females.

caused by *Escherichia coli*. *E. coli* is responsible for 50% of hospital-acquired infections; *Pseudomonas aeruginosa, Proteus, Klebsiella, Serratia, Enterobacter,* and *Enterococcus* cause the rest of hospital-acquired infections. *Staphylococcus saprophyticus* accounts for 10% of UTI in sexually active young women.

Group B streptococcus infection occurs mainly in newborns. Occasionally, yeast can cause UTI. Gram-positive organisms are cultured in 30% of elderly men with UTI, whereas Enterobacteriaceae (*E. coli, Klebsiella, Proteus*) is seen in 90% of women with UTI. *Candida* infection occurs in diabetics, in patients on long-term antibiotics, and in patients undergoing long-term catheterization. Resistance to multiple antibiotics is common in UTI.

Pathogenesis

Studies on the pathogenicity of UTI caused by E. coli have produced several important observations:

- Serologic classification of *E. coli* by cell wall (O) antigens was essential in defining the pattern of recurrent infections and their response to antimicrobial therapy, the role of introital and periurethral colonization in the pathogenesis of UTI in women, and the differences among strains that cause UTI in young girls.
- Most recurrent infections are caused by reinfection with a new serotype of *E. coli* or a new species, not to relapse caused by the original infecting organism.
- The amount of capsular (K) antigen and pili in the infecting strain seems to be important in determining virulence.

UTI is most often an ascending infection. Susceptible individuals are colonized with Gram-negative bacteria. Susceptibility may be genetic because women who do not secrete blood-group antigens are overrepresented among those with recurrent infections. Urethral epithelial cells from these women have specific *E. coli*–binding glycolipids, which are absent in those who secrete blood-group antigens. The shorter urethra in females is also a factor in the frequency of recurrent UTI in women. Sexual intercourse and use of the vaginal diaphragm increase the risk of UTI. UTI, especially pyelonephritis, can be caused by hematogenous spread.

Signs and Symptoms

UTI can be asymptomatic. When signs do occur, lower tract symptoms include:

- Dysuria
- Frequency
- Urgency
- Suprapubic pain

Upper UTI (pyelonephritis) presents with:

- Fever
- Chills
- Nausea
- Vomiting
- Flank pain

In infants and in the elderly, symptoms may be nonspecific. Hyperthermia or hypothermia, lethargy, poor feeding, prolonged hyperbilirubinemia, and vomiting may be symptoms of UTI in the neonatal period. Older children may present with abdominal pain, nausea, vomiting, fever, and chills. In the elderly, the presenting manifestations could be a change in mental status, unexplained fever, hypotension, shock, or new-onset incontinence.

Diagnosis

Proper diagnosis of UTI is extremely important. UTI is occasionally missed and sometimes misdiagnosed. Physical examination may reveal lumbar or suprapubic tenderness. Rectal and pelvic examination may also aid in the diagnosis. Examination of the urine is critical. Bagged urine in children and regular voided urine in females may be misleading; a midstream, clean-catch specimen is considered satisfactory.

The criteria for diagnosis is the presence of 20 or more bacteria and 10 or more leukocytes in a high-power field in a centrifuged specimen. The leukocyte esterase measurement correlates with the leukocyte count. The nitrate reduction test is specific but not very sensitive.

The standard of bacterial infection is greater than 100,000 colonies of bacteria grown in a cultured midstream clean-catch urine specimen. Recent studies in women with typical symptoms of UTI showed that urine cultures by suprapubic aspiration or urethral catheterization have less than 10^5 colony-forming units per milliliter. Normally, specimens obtained by catheterization or suprapubic aspiration should have no growth. Even a midstream clean-catch urine specimen with 50,000 colonies of a single organism may suggest UTI, especially with characteristic symptoms and 20 or more bacteria and 10 or more leukocytes per high-power field. More than one type of organism in a culture is usually a sign of contamination or superinfection. In an extremely sick patient, it may be advisable to take two separate cultures to confirm the organism. **Urine should be plated as soon as possible. Delay could cause false–positive or false–negative results.** If there is delay in plating, urine should be kept at 4°F.

Differential Diagnosis

Differential diagnosis includes vaginal infection, sexually transmitted disease, prostatitis, and urethral syndrome.

Dysuria and frequency in the absence of significant bacteriuria is called urethral syndrome and is usually caused by *Chlamydia*. Infection is most often localized by the clinical evaluation; antibody-coated bacteria is not reliable, and invasive procedures such as ureteral catheterization are unnecessary.

Indications for workup (Table 20.2) include:

- First infection in the neonatal period
- Two or more infections in girls
- UTIs in young males

Indications for Imaging Studies in Patients with Urinary Tract Infection — **TABLE 20.2**

Infection in a newborn
Recurrent infection occurring in childhood
Two or more infections in adult females
One infection in adult males
Elevated creatinine level
History of urinary calculi
Neurologic bladder dysfunction
Persistent hematuria
Previous genitourinary surgery
Prolonged fever after initiation of antibiotic therapy
Relapsing infection
Urea-splitting organisms
Unusual causative organism

- Unusual organisms
- Prolonged fever after initiation of therapy

The usual suggested workup for evaluation of the urinary tract is kidney ultrasound and bladder and voiding cystourethrography. Intravenous pyelography may be used instead of renal ultrasound. Radionuclide cystography can aid in the evaluation of the lower urinary tract with less radiation to the patient.

Summary of Diagnosis

- UTI is more common in women than in men; more than 50% of adult women report to physicians for UTI one or more times.
- Nearly 90% of community-acquired UTI is caused by *E. coli*.
- Most recurrent infections are caused by reinfection with a new serotype of *E. coli* or a new species, not by infection with the same organism.
- The criteria for diagnosis is the presence of 20 or more bacteria and 10 or more leukocytes in centrifuged urine when examined under high power.
- The standard of bacterial infection is greater than 100,000 colonies of bacteria grown in a cultured midstream clean-catch urine sample.
- Strong indications for workup for UTI include recurrent UTI in girls, even one episode of UTI in young males, and recurrent UTI in elderly men.
- The suggested workup for evaluation of the urinary tract is kidney ultrasound and bladder and voiding cystourethrography.
- Lower UTI symptoms are mainly those of cystitis and urethritis, such as dysuria, frequency, urgency, and suprapubic pain.
- Upper UTI (pyelonephritis) signs and symptoms include fever, chills, nausea, vomiting, and other systemic symptoms.

TREATMENT

Tables 20.3 and 20.4 list treatment regimens and dosages, respectively, for UTI. Women presenting with typical symptoms, urine with increased leukocytes and bacteriuria, and a positive nitrate reduction test result may be treated with a 3-day course of antibiotics, even without culture or follow-up. Many studies have shown

TABLE 20.3   Treatment Regimens for Bacterial Urinary Tract Infections

Condition	Characteristic Pathogens in Urine Culture	Recommended Treatment
Acute uncomplicated cystitis	E. coli, S. saprophyticus, P. mirabilis, Klebsiella	3-day regimen: oral trimethoprim-sulfamethoxazole, nitrofurantoin, norfloxacin, ciprofloxacin, ofloxacin
Diabetes, recent urinary tract infection, symptoms lasting more than 7 days, age more than 65 yrs		Consider 7-day regimen: oral trimethoprim-sulfamethoxazole, nitrofurantoin, norfloxacin, ciprofloxacin, ofloxacin
Pregnancy		Consider 7-day regimen: oral amoxicillin, macrocrystalline nitrofurantoin, cefpodoxime proxetil, trimethoprim-sulfamethoxazole
Acute uncomplicated pyelonephritis in women	E. coli, P. mirabilis, K. pneumoniae, S. saprophyticus	Oral trimethoprim-sulfamethoxazole, nitrofurantoin, norfloxacin, ciprofloxacin, ofloxacin, for 10–14 days
Moderate to severe symptoms: fever, nausea, or vomiting; positive blood culture	E. coli, P. mirabilis, K. pneumoniae	Parenteral trimethoprim-sulfamethoxazole, ceftriaxone, ciprofloxacin, ofloxacin, or gentamicin (with or without ampicillin) until fever remits; then oral amoxicillin, a cephalosporin, or trimethoprim-sulfamethoxazole for 14 days
Complicated urinary tract infection, without fever or nausea or vomiting; negative blood culture	E. coli, Proteus, Klebsiella, Pseudomonas, Serratia, Enterococcus, Staphylococcus	Oral norfloxacin, ciprofloxacin, ofloxacin, lomefloxacin, or enoxacin for 10–14 days
Complicated urinary tract infection, with nausea or vomiting	E. coli, Proteus, Klebsiella, Pseudomonas, Serratia, Enterococcus, Staphylococcus	Parenteral ampicillin and gentamicin, ciprofloxacin, or ofloxacin; ceftriaxone and aztreoman; ticarcillin-clavulanate or imipenem-cilastatin until fever remits; then oral trimethoprim-sulfamethoxazole, norfloxacin, ciprofloxacin, ofloxacin, lomefloxacin, or enoxacin for 14–21 days

that a 3-day regimen with most antimicrobial agents appears optimal, with efficacy comparable to a 7-day treatment regimen and with fewer side effects and lower cost. Single-dose therapy is associated with a lower cure rate and increased recurrences.

Approximately 30% of the bacterial strains causing UTI are resistant to amoxicillin, 5% are resistant to sulfonamides, and 15% are resistant to nitrofurantoin. In general, trimethoprim-sulfamethoxazole is the optimal drug for empiric treatment. Fluoroquinolone can

| Treatment and Dosage for Urinary Tract Infection | | TABLE 20.4 |

Diagnosis	Oral Regimens	Dosage
Cystitis	Trimethoprim-sulfamethoxazole	160–800 mg/12 hr
	Trimethoprim	100 mg/12 hr
	Norfloxacin	400 mg/12 hr
	Ciprofloxacin	250 mg/12 hr[a, b]
	Ofloxacin	200 mg/12 hr[a, b]
	Lomefloxacin	400 mg/daily
	Enoxacin	400 mg/12 hr[a, b]
	Macrocrystalline nitrofurantoin	100 mg/q.i.d.
	Amoxicillin	250 mg/8 hr
	Cefpodoxime proxetil	100 mg/12 hr
Pyelonephritis and complicated urinary tract infection	Trimethoprim-sulfamethoxazole	160–800 mg/12 hr
	Norfloxacin	400 mg/12 hr[a]
	Ciprofloxacin	500 mg/12 hr[a, b]
	Ofloxacin	200–300 mg/12 hr[a, b]
	Lomefloxacin	400 mg/daily
	Enoxacin	400 mg/12 hr[a]
	Amoxicillin	500 mg/8 hr
	Cefpodoxime proxetil	200 mg/12 hr
	Parenteral Regimens	
	Trimethoprim-sulfamethoxazole	160–800 mg/12 hr
	Ciprofloxacin	200–400 mg/12 hr[a, b]
	Ofloxacin	200–400 mg/12 hr[a, b]
	Gentamicin	1 mg/kg body weight/8 hr[a, b]
	Ceftriaxone	1–2 g/daily
	Ampicillin	1 g/6 hr
	Imipenem-cilastatin	250–500 mg/6–8 hr
	Ticarcillin-clavulanate	3.2 g/8 hr[a]
	Aztreonam	1 g/8–12 hr[a, b]

[a]The treatments listed are those to be prescribed before the etiologic agent is known; they can be modified once the agent has been identified. The recommendations are the authors' and are limited to drugs currently approved by the Food and Drug Administration, although not all the regimens listed are approved for these indications. Fluoroquinolones should not be used in pregnant patients. Trimethoprim-sulfamethoxazole, although not approved for use in pregnant patients, has been widely used in women. Gentamicin should be used with caution in pregnant patients because of its possible toxicity to eighth nerve development in the fetus.
[b]Dosage adjustment is necessary in patients with impaired renal function.

be used in patients with recurrent infections, in those who experience treatment failure, and in those who are allergic to sulfonamides. Nitrofurantoin also can be used in these situations, but there is a 15 to 20% resistance rate and increased recurrence. Complicated UTI occurs in patients with a functional abnormality or metabolic problems; these patients should be treated for 7 to 10 days.

As stated earlier, most recurrent infections are reinfections; however, the occasional patient may have an anatomic or functional abnormality of the urinary tract. Urologic workup for a functional or anatomic abnormality may be necessary in a small number of patients.

Recurrent infections in women may be treated with continuous prophylaxis, postcoital prophylaxis, and patient-initiated treatment, for which the patient is given a prescription for an appropriate antibiotic and takes a 3-day course at the onset of symptoms. Antibiotic prophylaxis and topical estrogen may be useful in postmenopausal women. The agent of choice for prophylaxis is trimethoprim-sulfamethoxazole or nitrofurantoin.

Management of asymptomatic bacteriuria is controversial. Many authorities feel that the bacteria in asymptomatic bacteriuria are not virulent and may not cause UTI; however, asymptomatic bacteriuria in pregnancy should be treated.

PREVENTION

The patient should be educated about the pathogenesis of UTI. If there is a correctable cause, it should be eliminated. Women with recurrent UTI should be advised to void before and after sexual intercourse and may be given continuous prophylaxis with trimethoprim-sulfamethoxazole or nitrofurantoin, if allergic to sulfa. Low-dose prophylaxis is reported to have a good effect in the prevention of UTI.

The care of an indwelling catheter is extremely important in preventing UTI. The drainage should have a closed system, with the collecting bag positioned below the level of the bladder. Treatment of the meatus with antibiotics is not known to have any great effect on the incidence of UTI. Prophylactic treatment is not indicated.

REFERRAL

Referral to a urologist is indicated if there is congenital or acquired obstruction or significant vesicoureteral reflux. A perinephric abscess may need surgery. Obstruction caused by an enlarged prostate gland, a cystocele, or a rectocele needs surgical treatment.

COMMONLY ASKED QUESTIONS

Why do women get frequent urinary tract infections?
Women have a shorter urethra than men. Vaginal colonization with bacteria thus make them more prone to infections. Mechanical or neurologic problems that impair drainage also predispose them to infections.

Does a UTI cause permanent kidney damage?
One or two episodes of UTI do not cause kidney damage. Recurrent UTI can cause kidney damage through back-drainage of infected urine into the kidneys.

SUGGESTED READINGS
Forland M. Urinary tract infection. Postgrad Med 1993; 93(5):71–74, 77–78, 84–86.

Johnson JR, Stamm WE. Diagnosis and treatment of urinary tract infection. Infect Dis Clin North Am 1987;1:773–791.

Pappas PG. Diagnosis and management of urinary tract infection. Med Clin North Am 1991;75:339–357.

Shapiro ED. Infections of the urinary tract. In: Burg FD, Ingelfinger JR, Wald ER, et al., eds. Gellis and Kagan's Current Pediatric Therapy. Philadelphia: Saunders, 1996.

Shortliffe LM. Management of urinary tract infections in children without urinary tract abnormalities. Urol Clin North Am 1995;22(1):67–73.

Wilke ME, Almond MK, Mason FP. Diagnosis and management of urinary tract infection in adults. Br Med J 1992;305:1137–1141.

KEY POINTS

- UTI is a leading cause of Gram-negative sepsis.
- Group B streptococcus infection occurs mainly in newborns.
- *Enterobacter* species (*E. coli, Klebsiella, Proteus*) are the cause of 90% of UTI in women.
- *Pseudomonas* UTI is common among hospitalized patients, in those patients on long-term antibiotics, and in those with an indwelling catheter. Rarely, *Candida* infection occurs in these individuals.
- More than one type of organism in a culture is usually a sign of contamination or superinfection.
- Dysuria and frequency in the absence of significant pyuria and bacteriuria is called urethral syndrome and is caused by *Chlamydia*.
- Trimethoprim-sulfamethoxazole or nitrofurantoin is the drug of choice for prophylaxis.
- Single-dose therapy is associated with a lower cure rate and increased recurrences.
- Fluoroquinolone may be used in recurrent infections.
- Recurrent UTI in women may be treated with continuous prophylaxis, postcoital prophylaxis, and patient-initiated treatment.
- Complicated UTI occurs in patients with anatomic or functional abnormalities, and they should be treated for 7 to 10 days initially, then intermittently on a long-term basis unless the cause of the UTI is removed.

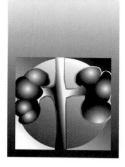

CHAPTER 21

Management of Renal Transplant Patients

Todd E. Pesavento
Michael E. Falkenhain

BACKGROUND

Transplantation has advanced rapidly in the last decade. It has changed from being considered a rare, lifesaving miracle to a procedure that is just as miraculous and lifesaving but is now performed on a daily basis. Advances in molecular biology and pharmacology have improved the survival of transplanted organs. Older patients and patients with more complicated medical conditions are now receiving transplants with long-term success. The success of transplantation, coupled with the effects of managed care, allow patients to receive most of their posttransplant medical care away from the transplant center and in the convenience of their local medical community.

The interaction between donor organ and recipient requires life-long immunosuppressive therapy, causing unique concerns about patient care. The short- and long-term complications that occur in renal transplant recipients will be discussed in this chapter, along with an introduction to the various types of immunosuppressive agents commonly used.

GRAFT AND PATIENT SURVIVAL

The goals of kidney transplantation are to improve the quality of life, maintain a functioning allograft throughout a patient's life, and improve mortality in the patient with end-stage renal disease (ESRD). Great strides have been made toward achieving these goals in the last 15 years. Evidence shows that transplantation improves the quality of life for the patient with ESRD.

Short-term graft survival has improved dramatically (Fig. 21.1), to the point that 1-year graft survival now exceeds 80%.

Graft loss 1 year posttransplantation occurs for two reasons: through death of a patient with a functioning transplant and from chronic transplant nephropathy. Within 7 years of transplant, patients have approximately a 25% chance of dying and a 25% chance of graft loss. Although overall mortality is improved with transplant compared with dialysis, there is hope that both patient and graft survival will improve as health professionals learn more about the causes of patient mortality and graft loss. And even though infections account for many deaths in the early transplant period, cardiovascular disease remains a major cause of patient death in the early, but especially late, transplant period.

ORGAN AVAILABILITY

Organ availability is the limiting factor in providing a transplant for patients with ESRD. The number of cadaveric organs transplanted has remained fairly constant while the number of patients waiting for a transplant has increased tremendously. Currently, more than 30,000 patients are waiting for a kidney transplant. Organs of living, related donors are being safely used and make up an increasing percentage of the transplants performed. More recently, organs of living, unrelated donors, such as a spouse, have been used with success that exceeds that of cadaveric transplantation and approaches living, related transplantation.

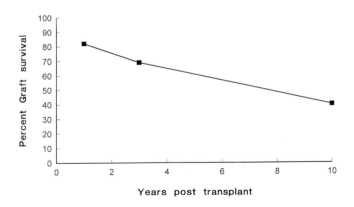

FIGURE 21.1.

Long-term allograft survival after kidney transplantation. Short-term kidney allograft survival commonly exceeds 80% because of new immunosuppressive agents. Long-term transplant survival, however, continues to decline. Summary of data from the United Network for Organ Sharing (UNOS) based on over 35,000 cadaveric transplants done between 1987 and 1993 in the United States. (Adapted from Terasaki PI, Cecka JM, eds. Clinical Transplants, 1994. Published by UCLA Tissue Typing Laboratory.)

IMMUNOSUPPRESSIVE AGENTS

The immunology of transplantation is a rapidly expanding field that has resulted in the development of numerous new immunosuppressive agents. Before 1984, most transplant centers employed only corticosteroids and azathioprine. Since 1984, most centers have used cyclosporine (CsA) in either double therapy (CsA with corticosteroids) or triple therapy (CsA with corticosteroids and azathioprine). Subsequently, monoclonal antibody therapy has been introduced, and, recently, a new purine antagonist, mycophenolate mofetil, has been approved and is gaining widespread use. The wider array of immunosuppressive agents may complicate management of the transplant patient, but hopefully the more numerous options offered will improve both short- and long-term outcomes. Because of the changing spectrum of immunosuppressive agents available, there will no longer be a standard immunosuppressive regimen that is used exclusively.

Glucocorticoids

Glucocorticoids are useful in maintenance therapy as well as in the treatment of acute rejection. Most transplant centers use 1 to 2 mg/kg at the time of transplantation, tapering to 0.1 to 0.2 mg/kg by 6 months posttransplant. An increase in the steroid dosage followed by tapering is often first-line therapy for an acute rejection episode. Further weaning from a typical maintenance dose of 10 mg/day remains controversial. Some centers have routinely placed patients on steroid regimens of alternate-day dosing or attempt complete steroid withdrawal. Data on the effects of steroid withdrawal are still being gathered, but it appears that maintenance with CsA alone or CsA and azathioprine without glucocorticoids is associated with an unacceptable rate of acute rejection and with a higher incidence of chronic graft loss. Whether newer immunosuppressive regimens will allow for steroid withdrawal remains to be seen.

Efforts to avoid the use of glucocorticoids have arisen because their use may cause or participate in the adverse effects of chronic steroid therapy. These adverse effects include:

- Cataract formation
- Osteopenia
- Avascular necrosis of the hip
- Hypercholesterolemia
- Hypertension
- Skin fragility
- Increased susceptibility to infection
- Posttransplant diabetes mellitus

Many of these effects are dose-dependent; as such, maintenance therapy is often as low as 10 mg/day of prednisone. Complications of steroid therapy are discussed in more detail later in this chapter.

Some commonly used medications may affect steroid metabolism. Phenytoin increases glucocorticoid metabolism, creating a need to increase the dosage of prednisone by 1.5 to 2 times the usual amount. Phenobarbital and cimetidine may also increase glucocorticoid metabolism.

Azathioprine

Azathioprine continues to play a role in maintenance immunotherapy despite the advent of newer immunosuppressive agents. In patients treated with the combination of corticosteroids and azathioprine but not CsA, short-term graft survival is worse and the incidence of acute rejection is higher compared with patients treated with a regimen containing CsA. However, long-term graft survival does not differ whether CsA is added to the regimen. Even in this era of newer immunosuppressive drugs, azathioprine will likely continue to play an important role in transplantation. Currently, many centers continue to use azathioprine in triple therapy regimens at doses of 1 to 2 mg/kg/day.

Azathioprine is well-tolerated by the patient. Long-term use has been associated with an increased incidence of cutaneous warts, bone marrow suppression, and malignancy. Liver function tests should be done every 6 months to seek evidence of azathioprine-induced hepatic dysfunction. A dropping white blood cell (WBC) count should signal a reduction in dosage, a search for other inciting medications, or a concomitant viral infection.

Allopurinol decreases the ability of the patient to metabolize azathioprine. Therefore, this combination should be used with caution and the dosage of azathioprine reduced by half when deemed necessary. More information on this combination of drugs is presented later in the chapter.

Cyclosporine

CsA became widely available in 1983 and immediately improved short-term graft survival rates. CsA acts by binding to an intracellular protein, cyclophilin, which eventually results in the decreased production of interleukin-2, a substance seemingly central to the prevention of acute rejection. CsA has helped the transplant recipient achieve 1-year graft survival rates approaching 90%. CsA continues to be a mainstay of most maintenance immunosuppressive regimens. The pharmacokinetics of CsA demonstrate marked variability in drug absorption and even individual variations in serum levels. This problem has been ameliorated with the introduction of a newer formulation of CsA that provides more consistent serum levels. Most centers prefer to start CsA at the time of transplant or in the early posttransplant period at a dose of 8 to 10 mg/kg. Within 1 year, the dose is usually tapered to a maintenance regimen of 3 to 5 mg/kg/day, generally in two divided doses. CsA serum levels can vary greatly, depending on the method used to measure the drug and on overall transplant function. However, within the first year, 12-hour trough levels of 200 to 400 ng/mL and long-term maintenance at 100 to 300 ng/mL are reasonable. If intravenous CsA is deemed necessary, one-third of the oral dosage is used to provide equivalent activity.

Adverse Effects

CsA is generally well-tolerated by patients, but it does have an adverse effect profile that includes acute renal failure (ARF), neurotoxicity, hypertension, hyperlipidemia, hyperkalemia, and perhaps long-term nephrotoxicity.

Acute renal failure   CsA, through afferent vasoconstriction, can cause hemodynamically mediated ARF that is readily reversible on temporary discontinuation of the medication or with a reduction in dosage. Because of this tendency of CsA to cause afferent vasoconstriction, transplant patients taking nonsteroidal anti-inflammatory drugs (NSAIDs) are at high risk for ARF. Likewise, the transplant patient on CsA is susceptible to deterioration in renal function secondary to volume depletion.

Hypertension   CsA has increased the incidence of hypertension seen in the posttransplant setting. Afferent vasoconstriction leads to excessive sodium reabsorp-

tion, resulting in volume expansion. Thus, the hypertension may be volume-mediated, secondary to increased peripheral vasoconstriction, or a combination of both. The increased blood pressure seen posttransplant is multifactorial, as discussed below.

Chronic nephropathy   Acute, reversible renal failure associated with CsA has been well accepted. More controversial is whether CsA contributes to chronic transplant nephropathy. Clinicians generally agree that CsA promotes interstitial fibrosis and a chronic arteriolaropathy. These chronic changes seem to be more severe in the innervated kidney (as seen in heart or liver transplant patients) as opposed to the renal transplant kidney, which is denervated. Although there is no consensus regarding chronic CsA nephrotoxicity, most agree that, for a subset of patients with chronic transplant nephropathy, CsA is the cause. Because of the potential for chronic transplant nephropathy, some centers have withdrawn CsA in patients more than 6 months to 1 year posttransplant. Whether the risk/benefit ratio favors late CsA withdrawal remains unknown; however, most centers do not routinely withdraw CsA.

Other adverse effects of CsA include:

- Resting tremor
- Gum hyperplasia
- Hirsutism

CsA also contributes to posttransplant diabetes and hyperlipidemia.

Drug Interactions

Various drug interactions with CsA are outlined in Table 21.1. Most interactions are caused by alteration of CsA metabolism. CsA is hepatically metabolized through the cytochrome P-450 3A system. Therefore, other drugs that are metabolized via this pathway

TABLE 21.1   Medication Interactions with Cyclosporine/Effects on CsA Metabolism

Increase CsA Levels	Decrease CsA Levels	No Effect on CsA Metabolism
Danazol	Carbamazepine	Beta blockers
Diltiazem	Phenobarbital	Clonidine
Erythromycin	Phenytoin	Digoxin
Fluconazole	Rifampin	Diuretics
Ketoconazole		H-2 receptor antagonists
Metoclopramide		Nifedipine and Isradipine
Verapamil		Isradipine
		Penicillin
		Cephalosporin antibiotics

CsA, cyclosporine.

would be expected to alter CsA metabolism. It is important to emphasize that many drugs interact with CsA, and Table 21.1 is not meant to be comprehensive. Drugs that are structurally similar, such as the erythromycin (macrolide) group and the antifungal antibiotics, often have the same effect on CsA metabolism. Most transplant physicians prefer to use medications that do not interfere with CsA to avoid precipitating either toxicity or acute rejection. When prescribing a new medication in a patient receiving CsA, it is best to consult a drug information reference, a pharmacist, or the transplant center.

Hepatic hydroxymethylglutaryl coenzyme A (HMG CoA)-reductase inhibitors have been reported to cause rhabdomyolysis when given in conjunction with CsA. It is the authors' practice to use HMG CoA-reductase inhibitors at lower doses and periodically follow serum creatine phosphokinase (CPK) levels if there is a need to increase the dosage. Because the incidence of rhabdomyolysis seems to be higher with lovastatin than with HMG CoA, lovastatin is generally not recommended in patients receiving CsA.

Tacrolimus (FK-506)

Tacrolimus is chemically and structurally distinct from CsA but shares many of the immunosuppressive properties and adverse effects. It was initially used extensively at the University of Pittsburgh in liver transplant recipients but is now used in most transplant centers to varying degrees in both hepatic and renal allografts.

Tacrolimus is derived from the fungus *Streptomyces tsukubaensis* and is a macrolide antibiotic. It binds to an intracellular protein, FK binding protein, which eventually results in the decreased production of interleukin-2, which appears to be central in preventing acute organ rejection. Tacrolimus is highly lipophilic and well absorbed from the gastrointestinal tract. Absorption is not altered by food but may be altered by aluminum or magnesium antacids. Intravenous tacrolimus can be highly toxic and is not recommended; in hospitalized patients, it can be administered through a nasogastric tube because it is generally well absorbed.

A general dosing guideline for tacrolimus is 0.1 mg/kg twice daily. Desired 12-hour trough levels are 10 to 20 ng/mL in the first 6 months posttransplant, with levels of 5 to 10 ng/mL in long-term stable patients.

Adverse Effects

Tacrolimus shares many of the adverse effects seen in patients receiving CsA. An important difference seen with tacrolimus is the development of neurologic complications. Patients are more likely to exhibit tremors, headache, and insomnia but also occasionally experience seizures, psychosis, or encephalopathy. These adverse effects appear to be dose-related; thus, lower doses are now being employed.

Other important adverse effects of tacrolimus include nephrotoxicity, hyperkalemia, gastrointestinal intolerance, and hypertension. Glucose intolerance and overt diabetes mellitus certainly can occur with tacrolimus, as is also seen in CsA-treated patients. They occur more commonly with tacrolimus but may be related to the concomitant use of steroids.

Gum hyperplasia and hirsutism, which can cause substantial morbidity, occur less frequently with tacrolimus than with CsA. Patients with these conditions may benefit from conversion to tacrolimus.

Drug Interactions

Tacrolimus is hepatically metabolized through the cytochrome P-450 system. As such, agents that would be expected to alter CsA metabolism (Table 21.1) can also affect metabolism of tacrolimus, although this agent has not been studied as intensively as CsA.

OKT3 and Antithymocyte Globulin

OKT3 and antithymocyte globulin are monoclonal and polyclonal antibody agents, respectively, that act against T cells. These extremely potent agents are often used in the initial days after the transplant and to treat acute rejection episodes. Infections (typically viral) and, less commonly, malignancies (typically lymphomas) are important complications associated with these medications.

EARLY TRANSPLANT COMPLICATIONS (WITHIN FIRST 6 MONTHS)

Potential problems within the first year posttransplant include acute rejection, technical problems, and infections. Hypertension is a common problem and will be dealt with later in this chapter.

Acute Rejection

Preventing or limiting acute rejection has been the goal of transplant centers since the early period of transplantation. Acute rejection most often occurs in the first 6 months posttransplant. If not quickly identified and treated, acute rejection will result in graft loss. The impact of acute rejection is further revealed in correlative studies of long-term graft survival. The absence of an acute rejection episode is the strongest predictor of prolonged graft survival.

With standard double- or triple-immunosuppressive therapy, the incidence of acute rejection is approximately 40 to 50%. With newer immunosuppressive regimens, the incidence has been reduced to 20% or less. Whether the decreased incidence of acute rejection correlates to better long-term graft survival is yet to be determined.

Because of the importance of early identification and treatment of acute rejection, diligent surveillance during the first year is mandatory. At the authors' institution, blood work is obtained three times per week. If the serum creatinine increases by 25%, the patient's CsA or tacrolimus dosage is withheld or reduced and a repeat creatinine measurement obtained within 24 hours. If the serum creatinine does not return to baseline in a specified period, a transplant biopsy (following a renal ultrasound to rule out obstruction) to assess for acute rejection is done. Not all centers routinely perform transplant kidney biopsies to assess for rejection, preferring instead to use clinical criteria or nuclear medicine scans. When acute rejection is identified, patients often receive high doses of corticosteroids, which are tapered off after a period. The use of OKT3 to treat acute rejection varies from center to center—some employ it frequently, while others reserve this therapy only for those rejection episodes not responsive to high doses of corticosteroids (pulse therapy).

Frequent use of high doses of corticosteroids, followed by tapering, increases the likelihood of cortico-steroid-induced adverse effects, including infections. Thus, even the successful reversal of an acute rejection may result in irreversibly decreasing renal mass and in placing the patient at increased risk for adverse effects from immunosuppressive therapy.

Technical Problems

Figure 21.2 shows the standard anatomy of the transplanted kidney. The kidney is usually placed extraperitoneally in the iliac fossa, with the ureter connected to the native bladder and the external iliac vessels used as the blood supply. Because of the location of the kidney, the authors recommend avoiding the femoral artery and femoral vein on the ipsilateral side of the graft when placing lines or catheters or when obtaining blood samples.

Technical complications are rare but can include:

- Failure of the bladder and ureteral anastomosis, resulting in a "leak" of urine outside the bladder
- Obstructive uropathy secondary to a lymphocele, atonic bladder, or ureteral ischemia
- Arterial stenosis at the anastomosis of the transplant renal artery and the native external iliac artery
- Renal artery or vein thrombosis

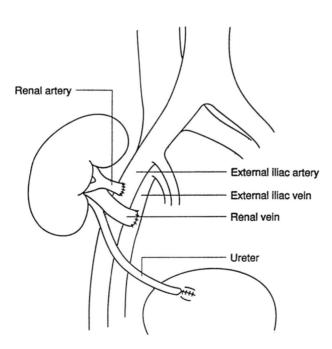

FIGURE 21.2.
Anatomy in renal transplantation. In renal transplantation, the transplanted kidney is placed extraperitoneally in the iliac fossa. Note that the native kidneys and ureters are left intact.

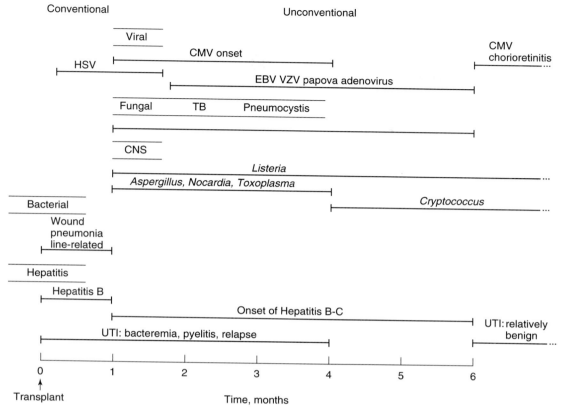

Conventional   Unconventional

FIGURE 21.3.

Timetable of the occurrence of infections in renal transplant recipients. After renal transplantation, common bacterial infections occur in the first month posttransplant. Opportunistic infections, including cytomegalovirus, occur during months 2 through 6. Long-term, typical routine
bacterial and viral infections commonly occur in stable patients, while opportunistic infections
occur in unstable patients with graft dysfunction. *HSV*, herpes simplex virus; *CMV*, cytomegalovirus; *EBV*, Epstein-Barr virus; *VZV*, varicella-zoster virus; *TB*, tuberculosis; *CNS*, central nervous
system; *UTI*, urinary tract infection. (Reprinted with permission from Rubin RH. Infectious disease
complications of renal transplantation. Kidney Int 1993;44:221-236.)

Most technical problems are identified early posttransplant. Wound infections, intra-abdominal abscesses,
and pulmonary emboli are also potential posttransplant
complications.

Infectious complications, an important complication in the early stages of transplant, are discussed later.
Also refer to Figure 21.3 and Table 21.2 for evaluation
of infections.

EARLY OR LATE COMPLICATIONS

Hypertension

Hypertension is one of the most common complications affecting recipients of solid organ transplantation. The overall prevalence varies according to the type

of organ transplanted and the age of the recipient. In
adult recipients of a kidney transplant, 55% develop hypertension. The incidence increases to between 65 and
75% in pediatric renal transplant recipients and to more
than 80% in patients receiving a heart transplant. Ninety
percent of all renal transplant recipients will require at
least one antihypertensive agent during the first year
posttransplant. Because hypertension is so common after
transplantation, its etiology so complex and multifactorial, and its occurrence common in patients who were
normotensive before transplant, it is frequently termed
posttransplant hypertension. The management of posttransplant hypertension has received increased attention
recently because of the strong correlation of hypertension and allograft failure and cardiovascular death.

TABLE 21.2	General Guidelines: Evaluation of Fever in a Transplant Patient

Identify the length of time from the transplant date or time from most recent acute rejection episode. Refer to Fig. 21.3 for help in identifying infections likely to occur.

Perform thorough history and physical examination with close attention paid to urinary symptoms.

An exhaustive search for opportunistic infections is unnecessary unless warranted by history, examination, or routine laboratory studies because stable, long-term transplant patients typically have routine viral or bacterial infections (UTIs, pneumonia, or "the flu").

Aminoglycoside antibiotics should be used only when clearly indicated and avoided if other suitable alternatives exist. They should not, however, be withheld in cases of life-threatening infections.

UTI, urinary tract infection.

Despite the complex and multifactorial nature of posttransplant hypertension, the pathogenesis of this disease has been well studied, and many of the inciting factors have been elucidated. This is in distinction to "essential hypertension," which affects 90% of hypertensive patients in the general population. In the general population, despite exhaustive research no single factor has convincingly been shown to cause hypertension, although considerable progress has been made.

Some of the causes of posttransplant hypertension are:

- Medications
- Function of the allograft
- Vasculature of the recipient

Medications

Corticosteroids are used extensively in transplantation; they cause sodium retention and may provide excess substrate for angiotensin. The hypertensive effect of corticosteroids generally is dose related, and low dose, long-term maintenance therapy is generally not a major cause of hypertension. In contrast, CsA and tacrolimus can cause hypertension in the short and long term. CsA promotes excessive sodium reabsorption and additionally induces selectively afferent arteriole vasoconstriction. CsA also causes stimulation of sympathetic nervous activity. These latter effects can lead to further sodium retention. Recent evidence suggests hypertension caused by CsA may also involve endothelin. There is little evidence that mycophenolate mofetil or azathioprine contributes to the elevated blood pressure seen posttransplant.

Function of the Allograft

Impaired renal allograft function and chronic rejection are the most important causes of posttransplant hypertension. Impaired renal function can lead to elevated renin production with activation of the angiotensin

system. Additionally, impaired excretory function leads to further sodium retention, volume expansion, and elevated renal vascular resistance. The native kidneys can also contribute to hypertension, and in cases of severe hypertension without other causes, bilateral native nephrectomy has been useful.

Vasculature of the Recipient

Vascular causes of hypertension generally reflect chronic small- and medium-vessel renal disease. There is no specific therapy in this situation. Large-vessel renal artery stenosis may account for 5 to 10% of posttransplant hypertension. Most patients present 6 to 12 months after transplantation and have severe, refractory hypertension. Diagnosis is generally made by angiography; however, advances in Doppler ultrasound make this a useful modality. Percutaneous angioplasty is generally successful, although bypass surgery is necessary in some cases.

Treatment of posttransplant hypertension requires examination of the inciting factors. Dietary sodium restriction, less than 150 mEq/day, is essential and should be the initial approach. No uniform regimen of medications is used; however, calcium channel blockers (CCBs) are considered the agents of choice by some individuals. CCBs preferentially dilate the afferent arteriole and thus may reduce vasoconstriction caused by CsA. Dihydropyridine CCBs, such as nifedipine or isradipine, do not significantly interfere with CsA metabolism, while nicardipine and nondihydropyridine CCBs, such as verapamil and diltiazem, cause substantial elevations in CsA levels (Table 21.1). For this reason, the authors typically initiate therapy with a dihydropyridine CCB. Because posttransplant hypertension is often salt-sensitive, loop diuretics are often employed. These should be used cautiously because volume depletion may exacerbate CsA toxicity, leading to impaired renal function. Other agents, including centrally acting alpha agonists (clonidine), beta blockers, and vasodilators, including minoxidil, are useful alternatives.

Angiotensin-converting enzyme (ACE) inhibitors deserve special mention, because in the authors' experience they are useful but must be used cautiously in the posttransplant patient. Because of the reversible (CsA-induced) or irreversible (chronic transplant nephropathy) vascular disease that is often present posttransplant, ACE inhibitors have the potential of decreasing the glomerular filtration rate. If used, serum creatinine and potassium concentrations must be checked frequently and the patient advised that if dehydration occurs (e.g., viral gastroenteritis), the ACE inhibitor should be withheld. The authors advise against the use of NSAIDs in the posttransplant setting, and this is especially true if the patient is receiving an ACE inhibitor.

HYPERLIPIDEMIA

Transplant patients frequently develop increased total cholesterol concentration, with an excess of the low-density lipoprotein (LDL) fraction, as well as increased triglycerides levels. Causes include:

- Diet
- Corticosteroids as well as CsA and tacrolimus
- Antihypertensive therapy
- Obesity

Because 55% of deaths in patients with functioning transplants are cardiovascular related, aggressive treatment of hyperlipidemia is warranted.

Dietary therapy should be the initial step in treatment but even in compliant patients is rarely successful. Initial drug therapy should be with HMG CoA-reductase inhibitors. Low dosages should be employed and, when used with CsA, may cause rhabdomyolysis. In patients with hypertriglyceridemia, fibrates such as gemfibrozil may be effective. Fibrates may also cause myopathy and should not be used concomitantly with an HMG CoA-reductase inhibitor and CsA. Bile acid resins may inhibit CsA metabolism and should be used cautiously.

LATE TRANSPLANT COMPLICATIONS

Bone Disease

Most patients who receive a renal transplant have underlying renal osteodystrophy. Lack of the active form of vitamin D leading to secondary hyperparathyroidism is the most prevalent form of renal osteodystrophy and, in the majority of patients, resolves within

1 year posttransplant. The resolution is difficult to document because corticosteroid therapy also leads to a secondary hyperparathyroidism. Although transplantation often improves renal dysfunction, allowing for adequate 1,25 vitamin D_3 levels, corticosteroids provide a new etiology for a secondary hyperparathyroidism. Therapy with calcium carbonate (650 mg between meals) along with low-dose 1,25 vitamin D_3 replacement therapy is indicated to counteract the effects of steroid-induced secondary hyperparathyroid bone disease.

Every posttransplant patient should have a yearly parathyroid hormone (PTH) evaluation. If the PTH is elevated, vitamin D therapy should be continued. There is controversy regarding the optimal target level of PTH before discontinuing vitamin D therapy. Some experts feel that vitamin D therapy should not be administered unless the PTH is three to four times normal to avoid producing adynamic bone disease.

In addition to secondary hyperparathyroidism, corticosteroids also produce osteopenia. The major loss of bone mass occurs within 6 months to 1 year posttransplant. The prevention of corticosteroid-induced bone loss has not been fully studied; however, early evidence suggests that bisphosphonate therapy may be indicated. Further studies on the safety and efficacy of bisphosphonate are ongoing. Hormonal replacement therapy is indicated for its bone mass-sparing effects. In males, testosterone levels should be checked, and, if found to be low, replacement therapy is recommended. Postmenopausal women are urged to consider estrogen replacement therapy. In the patient who has suffered a low impact fracture, posttransplant bone densitometry and bisphosphonate therapy are usually indicated.

Weight control and regular exercise should be encouraged as a way of preserving bone mass. The risk for steroid-induced osteopenia occurs regardless of gender or race.

Avascular necrosis of the hip occurs in approximately 5% of the renal transplant population. In any patient who complains of hip pain posttransplant, a high index of suspicion with prompt radiologic imaging (MRI) and orthopaedic referral is advised.

Posttransplant Diabetes

The development of diabetes posttransplant occurs in approximately 10% of kidney transplant recipients. The causes are multifactorial, with the following variables playing a role:

- Weight gain
- Age of the allograft recipient

- Immunosuppressive drugs used
- Race of the recipient
- Family history of maturity-onset diabetes

Prednisone is thought to play the central role in posttransplant diabetes because of its effect on lipid and carbohydrate metabolism. However, prednisone is not the sole contributor, as evidenced by trials of steroid withdrawal in which a large percentage of patients have persistent diabetes despite complete steroid removal. Tacrolimus and CsA are both reported to be diabetogenic and may cause a state of relative insulin resistance. The combination of prednisone and tacrolimus or CsA may be more diabetogenic than either therapy alone.

Treatment of posttransplant diabetes is similar to the therapy for the nontransplant diabetic patient. A weight-reducing diet combined with a structured exercise program cannot be overemphasized as the first mode of therapy. Oral hypoglycemic agents are useful, and insulin is required in 50% of those affected.

Chronic Transplant Rejection

Chronic rejection is a major cause of graft loss in long-term organ transplantation. It is not a single disease but a heterogenous condition with a multitude of causes that eventually lead to graft loss. There is currently no specific treatment for chronic transplant rejection, and increasing immunosuppressive therapy does not have any beneficial effect. Most patients develop hypertension, proteinuria, and slowly progressive renal insufficiency. Some patients may develop nephrotic syndrome. Aggressive control of blood pressure and dietary sodium restriction may halt renal insufficiency and alleviate edema.

Malignancy

One of the most devastating adverse effects of chronic immunosuppressive therapy is the increased incidence of malignancy. The renal transplant recipient is especially prone to develop squamous cell carcinoma of the skin, and, in females, carcinomas of the cervix, vulva, and perineum. They are also at increased risk of developing non-Hodgkin lymphomas and Kaposi's sarcoma. An increased incidence of other solid tumors, including cancer of the lung, breast, or prostate, has not been documented.

The risk of developing a malignancy is approximately 15% in the first 10 years posttransplant and 40 to 65% by 20 years posttransplant. The Australian Tumor Data Registry shows the total incidence of all cancers to be 64% at 20 years posttransplant; the majority (57%) are skin-related cancers. Squamous cell and basal cell carcinomas are common and necessitate that all posttransplant patients use protective sunscreens and undergo careful skin examinations with prompt biopsy when a suspicious lesion is identified. Besides frequent skin examinations, a high index of suspicion with routine cancer screening guidelines is advised. Women are especially urged to undergo yearly gynecologic examinations, given the increased incidence of vulvar and cervical malignancies.

Cardiovascular Disease

Transplant patients, like the general population, have significant morbidity and mortality from cardiovascular disease. Many risk factors are obvious, for example, age, tobacco use, family history, diabetes, hypertension, and hyperlipidemia. Other factors may be more insidious: preexisting left ventricular hypertrophy, prior rejection episodes, and cumulative doses of corticosteroids.

When cardiovascular disease is suspected, the evaluation should proceed as for a nontransplant patient with attempts to modify all cardiovascular risk factors. If coronary angiography is deemed necessary, the authors recommend prehydration and withholding the dose of CsA the day before and the day of the angiography.

Gout

Renal transplant patients have approximately a 10% incidence of gouty arthritis, while asymptomatic hyperuricemia is seen in 55% of CsA-treated patients. Causes include impaired renal function with the inability to excrete uric acid, CsA, which promotes uric acid retention, and the concomitant use of diuretics.

Treatment generally consists of colchicine during acute attacks. NSAIDs are avoided because they may lead to ARF. Cautious use of allopurinol to prevent future attacks is initiated during the quiescent period. Azathioprine metabolism is prolonged by allopurinol, and when both are used concurrently, the dosage of azathioprine must be reduced, usually by one-half. Allopurinol does not interfere with the metabolism of mycophenolate mofetil and thus no dosage adjustment is necessary.

Posttransplant Erythrocytosis

Posttransplant erythrocytosis is a condition unique to kidney transplantation. It can be defined as the development of a hematocrit greater than 52% in the absence of secondary causes such as volume depletion, diuretic use, or tobacco use (smoker's polycythemia).

Approximately 10 to 15% of patients will manifest this condition, usually within the first 1 to 2 years posttransplant. They usually have excellent allograft function. The etiology of posttransplant erythrocytosis is unknown.

Measurement of erythropoietin (EPO) levels can be highly variable and have been either unmeasurable or elevated. Given this, the authors do not measure EPO levels because it is unrewarding and expensive. Because this condition usually does not spontaneously remit, prolonged treatment is generally required. Until recently, recurrent therapeutic phlebotomy was the standard treatment. Others have advocated the use of theophylline. Recently, the use of ACE inhibitors has been shown to be extremely effective and is now considered standard therapy. Typically, very low doses of enalapril, 2.5 mg daily, have been efficacious. A response is often seen in 6 weeks, and the condition often recurs on cessation of the drug.

INFECTIOUS COMPLICATIONS

The evaluation of a fever in a transplant patient can be daunting but if approached in a systematic and logical manner will frequently lead to the correct diagnosis without an extensive workup. It is important to remember that, because of the immunosuppression, transplant patients may not manifest a fever, and a slight elevation in the CBC count may be explained by the effect of steroids. Because of these limitations, a thorough history and physical examination become exceedingly important.

One of the most useful approaches in the evaluation of any infection in a transplant patient is to identify the elapsed time from the date of the transplant. Many opportunistic infections can be restricted to certain groups of patients, making this evaluation even easier. Figure 21.3 summarizes infections that are common at different time periods posttransplant. It is useful to consider three distinct time periods:

- First Month Posttransplant
- One to Six Months Posttransplant
- Beyond Six Months Posttransplant

First Month Posttransplant

This may be the period that is most straightforward in the evaluation of infectious complications. Most infections are caused by the same organisms and type of infection that nonimmunosuppressed patients would contract. Usual infections would be wound infections, urinary tract infections (UTIs), indwelling intravenous line infections, or pneumonia. Opportunistic infections during this time period are unusual, and antibiotic coverage should be aimed at typical causative organisms.

Of special importance is the development of a UTI. These are frequently caused by the same organisms that lead to UTI in the general population. However, these organisms are associated with a high incidence of bacteremia, pyelonephritis, and rate of relapse when treated with a conventional course of antibiotics. Initial intravenous antibiotics followed by a prolonged course of appropriate oral antibiotics are important management guidelines.

One to Six Months Posttransplant

This time period is one of unusual, opportunistic infections. Cytomegalovirus (CMV) is the most important cause of infections during this period and alone accounts for two-thirds of posttransplant febrile episodes. In addition to causing CMV infection, this virus can itself lead to further immunosuppression, which can allow the manifestation of more severe infections such as *Aspergillus fumigatus*, *Listeria monocytogenes*, and *Pneumocystis carinii*.

Beyond Six Months Posttransplant

In this period, patients can be divided into two general categories: those with well-functioning allografts being treated with low-dose maintenance immunosuppressive therapy (approximately 75% of patients) and those either with poor allograft function or having received large doses of potent immunosuppressive drugs because of rejection episodes. The former group develops infections as would the general population (i.e., uncomplicated UTIs, pneumococcal pneumonia, influenza, etc.). The latter group is at high risk for serious opportunistic infections such as *Cryptococcus neoformans*, *Nocardia asteroides*, *Listeria monocytogenes*, and *Pneumocystis carinii*. Chronic viral hepatitis (hepatitis B or C) may lead to either cirrhosis or hepatocellular carcinoma. Additionally, viral-induced malignancies (lymphoproliferative disorders or squamous cell carcinomas) can be manifested.

Most transplant patients have previously been exposed to CMV and experience symptoms either within the first few months after undergoing transplantation or after the treatment of acute rejection, especially if they have received either OKT3 or antithymocyte globulin. A typical presentation commonly includes fever, often with rigors and in a daily relapsing pattern. Also typical are leukopenia and elevated liver enzymes and, less commonly, gastrointestinal ulcers (gastric or colonic) or pneumonia.

Diagnosis is often made on clinical grounds and supported by viral culture from the buffy coat, serology, or by demonstrating viremia using polymerase chain reaction (PCR). Treatment generally consists of intravenous ganciclovir for 7 to 14 days. An oral formulation of ganciclovir has been recently marketed but has not been widely used thus far.

PREGNANCY

One of the benefits of a successful kidney transplant is the ability of women to become pregnant. Because of the effect of uremia, many women on dialysis and some with advanced renal insufficiency stop ovulating. These endocrinologic abnormalities can be rapidly reversed with the correction of the uremic state after a kidney transplant. The result is there have been more than 2000 pregnancies in kidney transplant recipients.

Pregnancy in a transplant patient places the women in the category of a "high-risk pregnancy." Transplant patients frequently have hypertension and, even with allografts with excellent function, they experience moderate renal impairment. Because of the impairment there is a high rate of preeclampsia, premature delivery, decreased spontaneous delivery, and a high number of cesarean section deliveries. The child may be small for gestational age or have low birth weight.

Women contemplating pregnancy should be advised of a waiting period of 1 to 3 years posttransplant before becoming pregnant. They should demonstrate stable renal function with average serum creatinine concentrations less than 2 mg/dL. In addition, blood pressure should be normal or under adequate control with therapy. The patient should be taking only maintenance doses of immunosuppressive therapy. If all the criteria are satisfied before conception takes place, the birth of a healthy baby is highly likely.

Exposure of Fetus to Cyclosporine

Despite the greater risk of premature delivery and low birth weight, the incidence of newborn complications or malformations is not increased in women taking CsA. Prednisone and azathioprine also appear to be safe treatments during pregnancy. Of importance, mycophenolate mofetil has been associated with abnormalities in animals and should be avoided in women planning to become or who are pregnant. The authors' approach in women with stable renal function is to replace mycophenolate mofetil with azathioprine.

Similar to women, men have fathered children safely and without an increased rate of birth defects when treated with standard doses of prednisone, azathioprine, and CsA.

Effect of Pregnancy on Allograft

In women with stable renal function before pregnancy, there appears to be no adverse effect on the allograft. Acute rejection and graft loss have been reported, typically in patients with preexisting or unstable graft dysfunction. Given this, at least 2 years should have passed since the transplant or the last rejection episode to minimize risk to the allograft. CsA levels also need to be closely monitored to ensure they do not decline. Lastly, a rising serum creatinine during pregnancy is distinctly abnormal and demands prompt investigation.

In summary, all pregnancies in transplant patients should be considered high risk. Consultation and close follow-up with the transplant center is required during, and preferably before, the pregnancy. Despite higher rates of preeclampsia and low birth weight, there does not appear to be an increase in birth defects.

IMMUNIZATIONS

Transplant patients are susceptible to a number of infectious complications previously discussed. With the exception of live polio virus, immunizations that already exist for the nontransplant patient can be safely and successfully administered to transplant patients. The general principle regarding immunizations is that transplant patients should receive the same course of injections that the general population receives. Neither transplant recipients nor their household members should receive the live polio virus. They should receive the inactivated vaccine to prevent the development of polio.

Transplant patients are at increased risk for influenza and should be immunized annually. There is a theoretic risk of inciting acute rejection because of the induced immune state. The authors therefore do not administer the influenza vaccine in patients transplanted less than 6 months previously or who have suffered an episode of acute rejection in the preceding 6 months.

LIVING KIDNEY DONORS

The use of living kidney donors, both genetically related and unrelated (usually spouses), has continued to expand across the United States caused in large part by the continued shortage of organ donors and the superior results obtained with live donors. Living donors now account for at least one-fourth of all kidney transplants. As such, it is increasingly likely that primary care physicians will be caring for at least one or more of these living organ donors.

Although kidney donors are almost always evaluated at transplant centers, some general guidelines may be useful to know. Donors are screened to exclude any systemic disease such as diabetes, cardiopulmonary or liver disease, or malignancy. Heavy emphasis is placed on ensuring donors are normotensive and have normal renal function.

After patients have donated their kidney, they can be expected to live normal lives. They do experience a minor reduction in their renal function and develop abnormal proteinuria (greater than 150 mg/day). They may also develop hypertension, although it is typically mild. Some patients have developed ESRD, but these patients may have developed superimposed conditions, had poorly controlled hypertension, or had poor medical follow-up.

Table 21.3 lists some general guidelines in the care of kidney donors. If hypertension develops, any effective agent may be used to return the systolic pressure to less than 130 mm Hg. There is a rational basis for using either ACE inhibitors or angiotensin-receptor antagonists because these reduce hyperfiltration.

General Guidelines: Long-term Care of the Kidney Donor	TABLE 21.3

Annual evaluation of renal function
Serum creatinine, 24-hour urine creatinine clearance, and protein
At least annual monitoring of blood pressure
Aggressive control of hypertension; keep systolic BP <130
Prompt treatment of urinary tract infections, especially in females
Prompt use of intravenous antibiotics in cases of pyelonephritis
Avoid long-term nephrotoxic medications
Refer to a nephrologist in cases of declining renal function: proteinuria >500 mg/day, difficult-to-control hypertension, abrupt deterioration of renal function

KEY POINTS

- Graft loss after 1 year of transplantation occurs because of death with a functioning graft, chronic rejection, or recurrence of the native disease.

- Triple immunosuppressive therapy consisting of CsA, corticosteroids, and azathioprine is most commonly used.

- Glucocorticoids are useful in maintenance therapy, as well as in the form of pulse therapy in the treatment of acute rejection.

- Phenytoin increases glucocorticoid metabolism, necessitating an increase in the dosage of corticosteroid by 1.5 to 2 times the usual dose.

- Phenobarbital and cimetidine may also increase glucocorticoid metabolism.

- Allopurinol decreases the metabolism of azathioprine. Allopurinol is risky in transplant patients treated with azathioprine.

- Hyperuricemia and/or gout is a complication of CsA therapy; allopurinol is helpful. If allopurinol is prescribed, the dosage of azathioprine will be reduced by 50%.

- Although the transplanted kidney helps to cause involution of parathyroid hyperplasia, corticosteroids provide a new etiology for a secondary hyperparathyroidism.

- If PTH levels are elevated, vitamin D therapy should be continued.

- Avascular necrosis of the hip occurs in approximately 5% of the renal transplant population. Complaint of persistent hip pain in transplant patients is highly suspicious of avascular necrosis and warrants an MRI of the hip and referral to an orthopaedic surgeon.

- CsA use and chronic rejection are the most important causes of posttransplant hypertension.

- Large-vessel renal artery stenosis may account for 5 to 10% of posttransplant hypertension. Most patients present 6 to 12 months after transplantation and have severe, refractory hypertension.

- Vigilant watch should be made for cutaneous and mucocutaneous malignancy and lymphoma. Any suspicious skin lesion should be biopsied.

- Regular pelvic examinations are essential in females.

- The incidence of coronary artery disease is high. Blood pressure, glucose, and cholesterol should be kept under adequate control.

SUGGESTED READINGS

Curtis JJ. Hypertension and kidney transplantation. Curr Opin Nephrol Hypertens 1992;1:100–105.

Ferguson RM, Henry ML. Renal transplantation. In: Greenfield LJ, ed. Surgery Scientific Principles and Practice. Philadelphia: JB Lippincott Company, 199:516–524.

Rubin R. Infectious disease complications of renal transplantation. Kidney Int 1993;44:221–236.

Suthanthiran M, Strom T. Renal transplantation (Review article). N Engl J Med 1994;331(6):365–375.

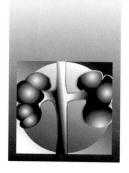

CHAPTER 22

Drug Dosing and Toxicities in Renal Failure

Shiv K. Seth

Julie Beck Kendle

BACKGROUND

The comprehensive care of patients with end-stage renal disease (ESRD) and renal insufficiency involves not only the treatment of renal disease and its complications but also the appropriate management of concomitant disorders. Regardless the condition being treated, medical management is complicated by renal impairment, which frequently warrants dosage adjust-ment of medications. Changes in drug absorption, distribution, metabolism, and excretion must be considered in the therapeutic management of patients with impaired renal function or ESRD. The purpose of this chapter is to give general guidelines for appropriate dosage adjustment of medications in patients with impaired renal function. Basic principles of estimating renal function and a summary of drug pharmacokinetics, pharmacodynamics, interactions, and toxicities are also presented.

Medication regimens in this patient population are often complex. For example, the average dialysis patient receives more than eight different medications each day. To minimize drug interactions and simplify drug regimens, the clinician should try to individualize drug therapy and, if possible, use one drug to treat several conditions. An angiotensin-converting enzyme inhibitor can be used for hypertension and congestive heart failure, a beta blocker for hypertension and angina. This approach minimizes the number of drugs a patient takes and therefore may improve compliance and decrease the risk of drug interactions.

ESTIMATION OF GLOMERULAR FILTRATION RATE (GFR)

Generally, the decision to adjust the dosage of a given drug in a patient with renal insufficiency depends on the level of kidney function and on the extent of renal elimination. The primary measure of renal function is GFR. For purposes of drug dosing, the GFR is approximately equivalent to creatinine clearance (C_{cr}). It is therefore necessary to measure C_{cr} to appropriately adjust drug dosage. If it is difficult to measure C_{cr}, its value may be estimated using one of several formulas developed for this purpose. The most commonly used method is the Cockcroft-Gault equation as shown here:

$$C_{cr} \text{ (mL/min)} = \frac{[140 - \text{age (years)}] \times \text{IBW (kg)}}{\text{SCr (mg/dL)} \times 72}$$

$$(\times\ 0.85 \text{ if female})$$

where C_{cr} is creatinine clearance in milliliters per minute and SCr is serum creatinine in milligrams per deciliter. An ideal body weight (IBW) should be used if a patient is greater than 120% of his or her ideal body weight. For obese patients, the IBW is 50 kg plus 2.3 kg for each inch in height over five feet (for men) or 45.5 kg plus 2.3 kg for each inch over five feet (for women).

Any estimation of C_{cr} is most accurate when renal function is stable. Any method of estimation may be inaccurate if the GFR is changing. It is important to note that C_{cr} estimates from the Cockcroft-Gault equation do not accurately reflect GFR in patients with severe renal failure. As GFR declines, a larger percentage of creatinine is secreted rather than filtered; thus, the C_{cr} from the Cockcroft-Gault equation will overestimate the true GFR. Although the 24-hour C_{cr} is also of limited value in this setting, it may give a more accurate

estimate than the Cockcroft-Gault equation of GFR in patients with moderate renal impairment. The 24-hour C_{cr} is calculated from the following equation:

$$C_{cr} \text{ (mL/min)} = \frac{UV}{P}$$

U = urinary creatinine from 24-hour collection (mg/dL)
V = volume of urine in mL/min from 24-hour collection (24 h = 1440 min)
P = plasma creatinine (mg/dL)

Dosage adjustment is not necessarily as simple as a reduction in dosage proportional to the reduction in GFR because a 24-hour C_{cr} will still overestimate GFR (increased urinary creatinine caused by hypersecretion will increase the numerator of the above equation). Other factors such as altered volume of distribution and protein binding, as well as the presence of active or toxic metabolites, may also play a role. Failure to reduce the dosage may lead to serious complications as a result of the accumulation of these substances.

PHARMACOKINETICS AND PHARMACODYNAMICS

Drugs are eliminated from the body via two major pathways: hepatic metabolism and renal elimination. The extent to which each process occurs varies with the drug being eliminated; however, the two processes are not distinct. Many drugs metabolized by the liver are converted to active or toxic metabolites that subsequently must be eliminated by the kidney. Thus, the role of renal function may be very important even if a drug is primarily metabolized by the liver. Drugs that are excreted unconverted in the urine may be freely filtered by the glomerulus, actively secreted, reabsorbed by the tubules, or eliminated by a combination of these processes. Each process may be affected to a different extent in various types of renal disease. In addition, a few drugs such as insulin and imipenem may be metabolized by enzyme systems located in the kidney. Regardless the mechanism of drug elimination, renal failure can adversely affect the efficiency of drug removal and therefore has a direct impact in prescription of drug regimens.

Although renal failure has the potential to influence all aspects of drug pharmacokinetics and pharmacodynamics, a few specific parameters are more directly affected than others. Some of these parameters are:

- Bioavailability
- Half-life
- Protein binding
- Volume of distribution

Bioavailability

Drug bioavailability is defined as the rate at which a drug enters the central circulation. Intravenously administered drugs enter the venous circulation directly and have the most rapid onset of action. The absorption rate of orally administered drugs depends on pH, gastric motility, and first-pass metabolism by the liver (as the oral drug is absorbed directly into the portal circulation and must immediately pass through the liver). Gastrointestinal symptoms of nausea, vomiting, diarrhea, and edema of the gut are common in renal patients and may prevent or delay oral absorption of many drugs. Motility disturbances such as gastroparesis are especially common in diabetic renal patients and may also cause a delay in absorption of many drugs.

Gastric pH can also directly influence enteral drug absorption. For example, with a rising BUN, gastric pH is increased because of enhanced ammonia production from gastric urease. The increase in gastric pH may hinder the absorption of a number of medications. An acidic environment is required for the conversion of ferrous iron to ferric iron, the form necessary for absorption. Thus, patients with renal insufficiency and increased gastric pH may have impaired ability to absorb iron. Antacids also increase the pH of the stomach and delay the absorption of certain drugs, such as ciprofloxacin. Therefore, administration of these two drugs should be separated by at least two hours to prevent malabsorption of ciprofloxacin. The multivalent ions contained in antacids can also delay the absorption of several drugs, such as digoxin, quinidine, and phenytoin. Additionally, it has been shown that the absorption of a simple sugar, D-xylose, is delayed in renal patients, meaning that carbohydrate absorption may generally be impaired.

Drug absorption can also be compromised by concomitantly administered drugs. Lipid-binding agents, such as cholestyramine and colestipol, can bind levothyroxine, digoxin, warfarin, and phenytoin and significantly reduce their therapeutic efficacy. Similarly, antacids like calcium acetate, aluminum hydroxide, and sucralfate can bind to these drugs and delay or decrease their absorption. Finally, the administration of enteral nutrition supplements can decrease the bioavailability of drugs such as phenytoin.

Elimination Coefficient and Half-life

The elimination coefficient (k_e) is a measure of the amount of drug eliminated from the body per unit of time. Most drugs are eliminated via concentration-dependent mechanisms, and k_e can be determined from a plot of the log of drug concentration versus time.

The estimated slope is the k_e for the drug. Usually, k_e has little variability among normal individuals; however, it tends to decrease significantly in patients with renal disease. In patients with renal disease, drugs that are excreted mostly unchanged by the kidney are subject to the greatest decrease in k_e.

The half-life of a drug is determined from the k_e value because the two are inversely proportional. As drug clearance decreases, the half-life increases, extending the period of time the drug remains in the body. Clinically, this necessitates decreasing the total daily dose of the drug. The decision to decrease the dose, increase the dosing interval, or both, is often arbitrary, although issues such as cost and patient compliance may influence the decision. For some medications, drug-specific characteristics such as desired plasma concentrations (i.e., the aminoglycoside antibiotics) also play a role in determining appropriate specific drug dosages.

Protein Binding

Many drugs used in renal failure patients are reversibly bound to plasma or tissue proteins. Proteins act as a reservoir or storage site for these drugs. Generally, the unbound or free drug is responsible for the pharmacologic action of the drug at the receptor site. Acidic drugs, like warfarin, are bound mainly to albumin; basic drugs like lidocaine, propranolol, and disopyramide bind to α-acid glycoprotein in the serum. Other drugs, such as cyclosporine (CsA), are bound to lipoproteins.

Tissue binding plays an important role in the action of digoxin. The portion of drug that is bound to protein is pharmacologically inactive. The protein binding of acidic drugs is generally decreased in uremia. Basic drugs, for the most part, are not affected. Examples of these drugs are found in Table 22.1.

The binding of drugs to serum proteins is influenced by the number of available sites on the protein, the affinity of the drug for the protein, and the potential displacement and/or inhibition of binding by endogenous acidic inhibitors, which accumulate in renal disease. When a drug is displaced from its binding site, it is available for pharmacologic effect, metabolism, or redistribution to other tissue sites. Examples of drugs that are highly protein-bound include:

- Phenytoin (90%)
- Tolbutamide (99%)
- Warfarin (99%)

Any drug or disease state that displaces these drugs can cause an increase in their pharmacologic effect. In the case of phenytoin, the total "therapeutic" range in normal individuals is 10 to 20 mg/L. Because 90% of

TABLE 22.1   Acidic and Basic Drugs

Protein Binding

Acidic Drugs	Basic Drugs
Cefazolin	Amphotericin B
Cefoxitin	Bepridil
Ceftriaxone	Clonazepam
Cloxacillin	Clonidine[a]
Diazoxide	Clorazepate
Dicloxacillin	Disopyramide[a]
Diflunisal	Fluoxetine
Doxycycline	Ketoconazole
Methotrexate	Morphine
Moxalactam	Prazosin
Pentobarbital	Propafenone
Phenytoin	
Salicylate	
Sulfamethoxazole	
Valproic acid	
Warfarin	

[a]Protein binding has been reported to increase in renal failure, although this is clinically insignificant.

the drug is protein bound, the percentage of drug available for physiologic action (the free fraction) is only 10%. This results in a therapeutic level of free fraction of 1 to 2 mg/L. In ESRD, the free fraction of phenytoin is increased to approximately 20% as a result of both drug displacement and decreased albumin levels. This causes the volume of distribution for phenytoin to increase, resulting in a lower total drug concentration in these patients. Although a total serum concentration of 5 to 10 mg/L might at first appear to be subtherapeutic (the normal therapeutic range is 10 to 20 mg/L), after considering the decreased protein binding in renal patients, the free concentration remains within the therapeutic range (20% of 5–10 mg/L).

Volume of Distribution

Apparent volume of distribution is defined as an amount of drug distributed throughout the body divided by plasma concentration of drug at equilibrium. This is not an anatomic space but a mathematical concept designed to define a therapeutic drug concentration. Water-soluble drugs (aminoglycosides) or highly protein-bound drugs (phenytoin), which are restricted to the extracellular fluid space, have small volumes of distribution. In comparison, drugs that are lipid soluble (CsA) or widely tissue bound (digoxin) throughout the body exhibit large volumes of distribution. Renal insufficiency alters the volume of distribution of many drugs, resulting in higher or lower plasma concentrations. Edema and ascites tend to increase the volume of

distribution of water-soluble drugs, whereas dehydration decreases it.

Perhaps the most clinically significant example of the impact of altered volume of distribution is digoxin. Because of its decreased volume of distribution, lower loading doses must be used to avoid toxicity. Furthermore, when dosing the aminoglycosides, if the volume of distribution is increased, the total serum concentration may appear lower, even though the half-life of the drug may be prolonged. This results in the need for a higher individual dose given less frequently.

METABOLISM

Most drugs are metabolized by the liver. Renal disease reduces the activity of the enzymes involved in this biotransformation. Generally, oxidation, reduction, and hydrolysis reactions are affected more than glucuronidation, sulfation, and glycemic conjugation. The hydrolysis of peptides and esters is substantially reduced.

The metabolism of drugs can result in toxic or inactive metabolites. Because most metabolites are water soluble and excreted by the kidney, renal failure can result in accumulation of these metabolites. Eventually, these accumulated metabolites may lead to drug toxicity as a result of potentiation of the parent compound. For example, oxypurinol, a metabolite of allopurinol, is pharmacologically active and contributes to the effect of the parent compound. The total dose of allopurinol can, therefore, be reduced in ESRD patients secondary to accumulation of the active metabolite. N-acetylprocainamide (NAPA), the major metabolite of procainamide, also accumulates in renal failure. Because NAPA possesses antiarrhythmic activity both similar to and, possibly, separate from procainamide, routine drug level monitoring for both procainamide and NAPA may be helpful in patients with renal failure. Similarly, glyburide, an oral sulfonylurea, is completely metabolized by the liver, and, although the metabolites are only mildly active (0.25% to 2.5%), the accumulation of these compounds over time in patients with renal failure can lead to pronounced hypoglycemia. Analgesics such as codeine, morphine, and hydromorphone are metabolized to compounds that have greater analgesic activity than the parent drug. These agents accumulate in patients with renal failure and are not readily dialyzed. Their accumulation may lead to excessive sedation and possibly respiratory failure.

Alternatively, a metabolite can have toxicities that are independent of the parent drug. For example, normeperidine has a central nervous system (CNS) stimulant effect that may induce grand mal seizures, while the parent drug (meperidine) is an analgesic and CNS sedative. Table 22.2 lists drugs that have active or toxic metabolites in renal failure patients. The table does not

Parent Drug	Pharmacologic Action	Metabolite	Comments
Acebutolol	B_1-selective blocker	Diacetolol	Metabolite is equipotent
Acetohexamide	Hypoglycemic agent	Hydroxyhexamide	Metabolite is active and the hypoglycemic effect may be prolonged
Acetaminophen	Analgesic	Conjugated metabolites	Can accumulate and may be toxic in renal failure patients
Allopurinol	Xanthine oxidase inhibitor	Oxypurinol	Metabolite is responsible for primary action of the drug
Bupropion	Antidepressant	Hydroxybupropion	Metabolite is half as potent as parent drug
Buspirone	Anxiolytic agent	Several metabolites	May contribute to longer action of drug
Cefotaxime	Antibiotic	Desacetyl cefotaxime	One-quarter to one-tenth as active as parent drug
Chlorpropamide	Antidiabetic agent	Hydroxymetabolite	Activity similar to parent in vitro
Codeine	Analgesic	Norcodeine, morphine-6-glucuronide	May be responsible for prolonged narcotic effect in renal failure patients
Diazepam	Tranquilizer	Desmethyldiazepam	Metabolite is active and can accumulate
Diltiazem	Calcium channel blocker	Demethylation products	Active metabolite is half as potent as parent drug
Enalapril	ACE inhibitor	Enalaprilat	Metabolite is more active than parent compound
Encainide	Antiarrhythmic	O-dimethyl encainide (ODE), 3-methoxy-o-dimethylencainide (MODE)	Metabolites are active
Imipramine	Antidepressant	N-monodemethylated metabolite	Half as active as parent drug
Glyburide	Hypoglycemic agent	Hydroxymetabolite	Hypoglycemic effect of metabolite may be cumulative in renal failure patients
Meperidine	Analgesic	Normeperidine	Metabolite is less active as an analgesic, but can cause CNS stimulation leading to seizures
Methyldopa	Antihypertensive agent	Methyldopamono-O-sulfate	Metabolite may accumulate, leading to prolonged hypotension
Minoxidil	Antihypertensive agent	Conjugated glucuronides	Less active than parent compound
Morphine	Analgesic	Morphine-6-glucuronide	May be more active than parent drug; accumulation may lead to prolonged narcotic effect
Primidone	Anticonvulsant	Phenylethyl-malonamide, phenobarbital	Metabolite can potentiate parent drug, causing toxicity
Procainamide	Antiarrhythmic agent	N-acetyl-procainamide	Metabolite is potent antiarrhythmic
Propoxyphene	Analgesic agent	Norpropoxyphene	Metabolite has less CNS depressant activity, but more local anesthetic activity
Sodium nitroprusside	Antihypertensive agent	Thiocyanate	Metabolite is toxic
Sulfonamides	Antibiotic	N-acetylsulfonamide	Inactive metabolite, but may be toxic in renal failure patients

include pro-drugs, which are formulated to be metabolized into active compounds. In the examples given in this table, most of the active metabolites have some pharmacologic activity and have the potential to accumulate in renal insufficiency. Information on the effect of hemodialysis on drug metabolites is not readily available. Furthermore, because the removal of any substance by dialysis is dependent on the length of dialysis, flow rate, and type of dialysis membrane, much variability occurs. For this reason, the authors have chosen not to include this information in the table. The reader should consult the original drug monograph or the manufacturer for information of this type.

Drugs actively secreted by the tubules (ampicillin, cephalexin, penicillins) can be substantially altered in tubulointerstitial renal disease. Drug interactions by agents that impair the secretion of these compounds in the proximal tubule may increase drug levels in patients with renal insufficiency. For example, probenecid decreases proximal tubular secretion of methotrexate and penicillins, resulting in increased blood levels of the latter two agents. Similarly, quinidine reduces the renal and biliary clearance of digoxin by 30 to 40%, thereby increasing digoxin levels.

Tubular reabsorption of a drug may be passive and depends on the pH and pKa of the drug. Nonionized drugs are absorbed more readily than are ionized molecules. Weakly acidic drugs (nonionized) will be reabsorbed from acidic urine, whereas basic drugs (ionized) will be excreted in acidic urine. In an alkaline urine, the opposite will occur. For example, administration of sodium bicarbonate to increase urinary pH is associated with increased clearance of salicylates. These can result in lower salicylate levels that could be detrimental in the treatment of inflammatory conditions but may be desirable in the treatment of salicylate overdose.

DRUG DOSAGE ADJUSTMENT IN RENAL FAILURE

Determining a patient's appropriate drug dosage regimen depends on volume of distribution, k_e, half-life, and other important pharmacokinetic parameters. However, for clinical purposes, the following tables will summarize suggested dosing adjustments. Table 22.3 illustrates the dosage adjustments recommended for drugs with significant (50 to 90%) renal elimination. These drugs will have extensively prolonged half-lives in renal failure patients, and their total daily dosage must often be decreased by more than 50% to prevent toxicity. It is not possible to include every drug that needs adjustment; therefore, only commonly used drugs are included in this table. Table 22.4 includes drugs whose major route of elimination is nonrenal and, therefore,

may need only minor or no dosage adjustment in renal failure.

DRUG-INDUCED NEPHROTOXICITY

A few of the commonly used drugs that cause nephrotoxicity are discussed in this section:

- Aminoglycosides
- ACE Inhibitors
- Amphotericin B
- NSAIDs
- Cisplatin
- CsA
- Radiographic Contrast Media
- Drug-induced Crystal Formation and Nephrolithiasis

Aminoglycosides

The primary mechanism of aminoglycoside-induced nephrotoxicity involves damage to the proximal renal tubule. Although the exact mechanism has not been fully elucidated, aminoglycosides appear to bind to renal cell membrane phospholipids, destabilizing the cell membrane and ultimately leading to dysregulation of transport mechanisms and cell necrosis. This can result in potassium and magnesium wasting and loss of concentrating ability. In addition, some evidence suggests that aminoglycosides prevent cell protein synthesis in renal cells in a manner similar to that of bacterial cells. Aminoglycosides concentrate within the cortex of the kidney. Although renal dysfunction usually manifests itself several days after the antibiotic is started, microscopic changes in the renal brush border are sometimes detectable after the first dose.

Nephrotoxicity is generally related to the duration of therapy and manifests itself after 8 to 10 days. Acute renal failure (ARF) from aminoglycoside therapy is typically nonoliguric and is usually reversible on stopping the medication. Therapeutic drug monitoring can decrease the likelihood of nephrotoxicity and ototoxicity. Peak serum concentrations generally should fall in the range of 6 to 8 mg/L (or μg/mL) for gentamicin and tobramycin and 15 to 25 mg/L for amikacin. Recommended trough concentrations for gentamicin and tobramycin are less than 2 mg/L, and for amikacin less than 7 mg/L. Desirable levels for netilmicin have not been established. Even though the serum levels may be maintained within these ranges, renal toxicity may still occur, and BUN and serum creatinine should be monitored daily.

In dialysis patients, nephrotoxicity is no longer a concern, but ototoxicity remains a potential complication. As peak gentamicin or tobramycin serum concentrations approach greater than 6 mg/L (or μg/mL),

Drug	Normal Dose: $C_{cr} > 50$ mL/min	Renal Impairment: $C_{cr} = 10–50$ mL/min	Renal Failure: $C_{cr} < 10$ mL/min
Acyclovir IV	5 mg/kg Q 8 hr	5 mg/kg Q 12–24 hr	2.5 mg/kg Q 24 hr
Acyclovir PO	200–800 mg Q 4 hr	Dose Q 8 hr	Dose Q 12 hr
Allopurinol	300 mg QD	200 mg QD	100 mg QD
Amoxicillin	250–500 mg Q 8 hr	Dose Q 12 hr	Dose Q 24 hr
Ampicillin IV	1–2 g Q 4–6 hr	1–1.5 g Q 6 hr	1 g Q 8–12 hr
Ampicillin PO	250–500 mg Q 6 hr	Dose Q 8–12 hr	Dose Q 12 hr
Atenolol	50–100 mg QD	Decrease 50% and titrate	Decrease 50% and titrate
Cefazolin	1–2 g Q 8 hr	0.5–1.5 g Q 12 hr	0.5–1 g Q 24 hr
Cefotetan	1–2 g Q 12 hr	1–2 g Q 24 hr	0.5–1 g Q 24 hr
Cefoxitin	1–2 g Q 6–8 hr	1–2 g Q 12–24 hr	0.5–1 g Q 24 hr
Ceftazidime	1–2 g Q 8 hr	1 g Q 12–24 hr	0.5 g Q 24 hr
Ceftibuten	400 mg Q 24 hr	Decrease dose 50%	Decrease dose 75%
Cefuroxime	0.75–1.5 g Q 6–8 hr	1 g Q 12 hr	0.5–1 g Q 24 hr
Cephradine	250–500 mg Q 6 hr	250–500 mg Q 12 hr	250–500 mg Q 24 hr
Cimetidine	PO: 400 mg Q 12 hr; IV: 300 mg Q 8 hr	Decrease dose 25%	Decrease dose 50%
Ciprofloxacin	PO: 250–750 mg Q 12 hr; IV: 400 mg Q 12 hr	Decrease dose 25%	Decrease dose 50%
Digoxin PO	0.125–0.25 mg QD	0.125 QD	0.125 QOD
Digoxin IV	0.1–0.2 mg QD	0.1 QD	0.1 QOD
Enalapril	Titrate	Titrate	Titrate
Ethambutol	15 mg/kg Q 24 hr	7.5–10 mg/kg Q 24 hr	5 mg/kg Q 24 hr
Fluconazole	100–200 mg Q 24 hr	50–200 mg Q 24 hr	100 mg Q 24 hr
Foscarnet	Consult dose chart in package literature	Consult dose chart in package literature	Consult dose chart in package literature
Ganciclovir IV	> 80 mL/min: 5 mg/kg Q 12 hr; 50–80 mL/min: 2.5 mg/kg Q 12 hr	1.25–2.5 mg/kg Q 24 hr	1.25 mg/kg Q 24 hr
Ganciclovir PO	1000 mg Q 8 hr or 500 mg 6 times daily	500–1000 mg QD	500 mg 3 times weekly
Imipenem	5–10 mg/kg Q 6–8 hr	5–10 mg/kg Q 8–12 hr	5–10 mg/kg Q 12–24 hr
Lamivudine	150 mg BID	Consult dose chart in package literature	Consult dose chart in package literature
Lithium	TDM[a]	Decrease dose 25–50%	Decrease dose 75%
Meperidine	Titrate	Titrate cautiously	DO NOT USE
Methotrexate	Titrate	Titrate	Titrate
Nadolol	Titrate	Decrease dose 50% and titrate	Decrease dose 50% and titrate
Penicillin G	2–3 million unit Q 4 hr	Dose (million unit/day) = $3.2 + C_{cr}/7$	Dose (million unit/day) = $3.2 + C_{cr}/7$
Piperacillin	50 mg/kg Q 6 hr		
Procainamide	0.5–1.5 g Q 4–6 hr TDM[a]	100% Q 6–12 hr TDM[a]	100% Q 12–24 hr TDM[a]
Ranitidine	PO: 300 mg Q HS; IV: 50 mg Q 6–8 hr	Decrease dose 25%	Decrease dose 50%
Sotalol	80 mg BID	Dose Q 24–48 hr	Individualize dose
Stavudine	30–40 mg BID	15–20 mg Q 12–24 hr	Insufficient data
Sulfamethoxazole	0.5–1.0 g Q 6 hr	Q 12–24 hr	Q 24 hr
Vancomycin	TDM[a]	TDM[a]	TDM[a]
Zalcitabine	0.75 mg Q 8 hr	0.75 mg Q 12 hr	0.75 mg Q 24 hr

[a]TDM = Therapeutic Drug Monitoring suggested.
Q, every; QD, every day; PO, by mouth; IV, intravenous; QOD, every other day; BID, twice daily; HS, at bedtime.

TABLE 22.4	Drugs Requiring Minimal or No Adjustment in Renal Failure

Cefoperazone
Clindamycin
Cyclosporine
Erythromycin
Ibuprofen
Indomethacin
Ketoconazole
Labetalol
Lidocaine
Metronidazole
Nafcillin
Nifedipine
Pentamidine
Phenobarbitol
Phenytoin
Propranolol

the risk of ototoxicity increases. Ototoxicity may manifest as ringing in the ears, tremor, loss of balance, ataxia, and potentially irreversible loss of hearing. Because therapeutic drug monitoring is the only modality available to potentially decrease the risk of aminoglycoside toxicities, alternative agents should be considered in patients at significant risk for renal failure (e.g., the elderly, patients with preexisting renal disease, diabetics). Table 22.5 gives general guidelines for initiating aminoglycoside dosing in patients with impaired renal function who are on dialysis. Note that the dosing interval, rather than the dose itself, must be adjusted.

Angiotensin-Converting Enzyme (ACE) Inhibitors

The use of ACE inhibitors has been associated with reversible nonoliguric ARF. This is particularly common in patients with bilateral large-vessel renal artery stenosis or in patients with fixed small-vessel disease (i.e., nephrosclerosis). Patients with low cardiac output and decreased effective circulating volume may have a decrease in renal perfusion. Low renal perfusion leads to compensatory activation of the renin-angiotensin system to maintain adequate renal blood flow. ACE inhibitors inhibit this compensatory mechanism and may cause a profound decrease in perfusion pressure and renal blood flow, resulting in ARF.

Amphotericin B

The mechanism of amphotericin B nephrotoxicity has been less well elucidated than that for ACE inhibitors,

although two proposed mechanisms exist. Amphotericin B may bind to the renal tubule cells, causing an alteration in membrane permeability and resulting in direct cellular toxicity, similar to the aminoglycosides. The other proposed mechanism involves the stimulation of the tubuloglomerular feedback system by amphotericin B, resulting in vasoconstriction and a drop in GFR. Nephrotoxicity is a common adverse effect of amphotericin B and may occur in up to 90% of patients. It is usually reversible on discontinuation, with adequate hydration, although permanent renal damage sometimes occurs.

Because amphotericin B remains the only treatment option in certain fungal infections, research into methods of preventing nephrotoxicity has been popular. One proposed method is "sodium loading." The infusion of 0.9% sodium chloride solution prior to amphotericin B has been shown to prevent nephrotoxicity in some patients, although few well-designed studies exist. This approach, however, is not warranted in patients sensitive to sodium loading, such as those with congestive heart failure, underlying renal insufficiency, nephrotic syndrome, or liver disease.

Amphotericin B in a lipid complex has been developed to minimize nephrotoxicity. In this formulation, the amphotericin B is encased in a phospholipid emulsion. It is thought that this protects the renal cells from direct contact with amphotericin B. Numerous reports of decreased nephrotoxicity have been seen with this formulation, but the antifungal efficacy has been questioned because less amphotericin B is available for contact with the fungus cells. Additionally, adverse effects are associated with phospholipid, such as cardiopulmonary toxicity and elevated cholesterol and triglycerides. All lipid formulations of amphotericin B are significantly more expensive than the colloidal forms. For these reasons, the lipid preparations should be used judiciously. In cases in which amphotericin B is the only therapeutic option and the risk of nephrotoxicity is high (as in patients with underlying renal dysfunction, elderly patients, and those with a history of nephrotoxicity secondary to amphotericin B), the use of liposomal amphotericin B may be justified.

Nonsteroidal Anti-Inflammatory Agents (NSAIDs)

NSAIDs commonly induce a form of pre-renal ARF by inhibiting prostaglandin formation necessary for vasodilation and maintenance of renal blood flow. All NSAIDs have been implicated in causing renal insufficiency.

In particular, pre-renal ARF from NSAIDs occurs when renal prostaglandin production is increased to

| Aminoglycoside Dosing in Patients with Renal Failure[a] | | | | **TABLE 22.5** |
Drug	Loading Dose (mg/kg)	Maintenance Dose (mg/kg) (C_{cr} 10–50 mL/min)	Maintenance Dose (mg/kg) (C_{cr} < 10 mL/min)	Maintenance Dose (mg/kg) Hemodialysis
Amikacin	7.5 mg/kg	5–7.5 mg/kg Q 12–48 hr	5–7.5 mg/kg Q 48–72 hr	5 mg/kg after each dialysis
Gentamicin	1.5–2 mg/kg	1–1.5 mg/kg Q 12–48 hr	1–1.5 mg/kg Q 48–72 hr	1–1.5 mg/kg after each dialysis
Tobramycin	1.5–2 mg/kg	1–1.5 mg/kg Q 12–48 hr	1–1.5 mg/kg Q 48–72 hr	1–1.5 mg/kg after each dialysis

[a]TDM should be conducted with all these agents after the third maintenance dose and adjusted accordingly. Q, every.

help maintain blood flow. Underlying conditions associated with impaired renal blood flow and increased renal prostaglandin release include preexisting renal disease, renal artery stenosis, congestive heart failure, elderly patients, diabetics, and volume-depleted patients. Also, the use of NSAIDs to acutely treat musculoskeletal pain immediately after vigorous exercise should be discouraged until the patient has been adequately rehydrated.

NSAIDs may also cause a characteristic lesion manifesting as acute interstitial nephritis and nephrotic syndrome. The syndrome improves after stopping the offending agent, but immunosuppressive therapy may be necessary. A more detailed description of this lesion is beyond the scope of the current discussion.

Cisplatin

Cisplatin is concentrated in proximal tubular cells. Nephrotoxicity occurs because of cellular degeneration and tubular obstruction from cellular debris, resulting clinically in acute tubular necrosis. The severity of the lesion is dose- and duration-dependent and may be irreversible. Pre-dose hydration can attenuate renal toxicity. Normal saline with or without mannitol or furosemide before and after cisplastin therapy has been effective in providing renal protection.

Cyclosporine

CsA has become the cornerstone drug in the prevention of allograft rejection. It causes a dose-dependent decline in GFR and an associated rise in serum creatinine. CsA frequently leads to renal dysfunction, primarily as a result of renal vasoconstriction. This phenomenon may occur at any dose and at any serum level. BUN and serum creatinine should be monitored frequently and systemic hypertension treated aggressively

to reduce the risk of nephrotoxicity. CsA nephrotoxicity is increased by concomitant use of amphotericin B, aminoglycosides, NSAIDs, and ketoconazole. A number of agents have been used with varying degrees of success to decrease the risk of the nephrotoxicity caused by CsA, such as:

- Thromboxane A_2 synthetase inhibitors
- Pentoxifylline
- Misoprostol

Radiographic Contrast Media

The use of contrast media in high-risk patients (with conditions such as diabetes mellitus, preexisting renal failure, multiple myeloma, dehydration, hypertension) is associated with ARF. These agents can cause mild, nonoliguric ARF, with serum creatinine rising within 2 to 3 days and returning to baseline in 10 to 14 days. Oliguric ARF may develop and warrant dialysis. Available contrast agents include hyperosmolar (1500 mOsm/μg) or less hyperosmolar (750 mOsm/μg) forms, although the osmolarity seems to have little influence on the nephrotoxicity caused by these agents. The precise mechanism of nephrotoxicity from these agents is not known. Prevention of nephrotoxicity is more important. Hydration, especially in high-risk patients, seems to be effective in reducing nephrotoxicity. Intravenous saline with or without furosemide is generally effective if this therapy is given 12 hours before contrast study and for 24 hours following constrast study.

Drug-induced Crystal Formation and Nephrolithiasis

A number of drugs may cause tubular precipitation of drugs, giving rise to crystal formation or frank nephrolithiasis. As with any compound that may precipitate in the tubules, adequate hydration is important in preventing this process. Table 22.6 lists the drugs that can cause renal damage by crystallization or stone formation in the kidney.

SUMMARY

Patients with renal insufficiency can present with subtherapeutic or toxic responses to many medications. As discussed, a basic understanding of pharmacokinetic and pharmacodynamic principles will help the practitioner avoid such drug misadventures. The information in this chapter has been limited to the agents most commonly prescribed in general practice. The authors

TABLE 22.6   Drugs Causing Tubular Crystallization or Nephrolithiasis

Acyclovir[a]
Azathioprine
Bactrim (sulfas)
Ciprofloxacin
Indinavir[a]
Methotrexate[a]
Triamterene
Polyethylene glycol[a]
   (causes calcium oxalate stones)

[a]May result in diffuse tubular obstruction and acute renal failure.

KEY POINTS

- It is desirable to obtain a 24-hour C_{cr} measurement as a gauge of GFR for the purpose of drug dosing.

- If it is difficult to obtain a 24-hour C_{cr}, its value may be estimated using the Cockcroft-Gault equation.

- Gastrointestinal symptoms are common in renal patients and may prevent or delay oral absorption of drugs.

- Gastroparesis is especially common in diabetic renal patients and may cause a delay in absorption of many drugs.

- The increase in gastric pH in uremia hinders the conversion of ferrous iron to ferric iron, the form necessary for absorption. Thus, malabsorption of iron is common in uremic patients. For this reason, intravenous iron may be necessary to promote the effect of erythropoietin therapy.

- Increased gastric pH can delay the absorption of a common antiinfective drug, ciprofloxacin.

- In ESRD, free fraction of phenytoin is increased because of decreased protein binding. Although a total serum concentration of 5 to 10 mg/L appears subtherapeutic (as as result of increased volume of distribution), the free concentration remains within the therapeutic range.

- The most clinically significant example of the impact of altered volume of distribution is digoxin. As a result of decreased volume of distribution in renal failure, lower loading doses must be used to avoid toxicity.

- The metabolism of drugs can result in toxic or inactive metabolites. Because most metabolites are water soluble and excreted by the kidney, renal failure can result in accumulation of these metabolites. For example, oxypurinol, a metabolite of allopurinol, is retained in renal failure. Therefore, the daily dose of allopurinol should be reduced to one-third the regular dose in patients with renal failure.

- In dialysis patients, nephrotoxicity is no longer a concern, but ototoxicity remains a potential complication.

hope that the guidelines provided will be helpful in the medical management of all patients with renal failure.

SUGGESTED READINGS

Bennett WM. Mechanisms of aminoglycoside nephrotoxicity. Clin Exp Pharmacol Physiol 1989;16:1–6.

Bennett WM. Drug Prescribing in Renal Failure: Dosing Guidelines for Adults. 3rd ed. Philadelphia: American College of Physicians, 1994.

Carter BL. Dosing of antihypertensive medications in patients with renal insufficiency. J Clin Pharmacol 1995; 35:81–86.

Hoitsma AJ, Wetzels JFM, Koene RAP. Drug-induced nephrotoxicity. Drug Safety 1991;6:131–147.

Hoyer J, Karl-Ludwig S, Lenz T. Clinical pharmacokinetics of angiotensin-converting enzyme inhibitors in renal failure. Clin Pharmacokinet 1993;24:230–254.

Livornese LL, Benz RL, Ingerman MJ, et al. Antibacterial agents in renal failure. Infect Dis Clin North Am 1995;9: 591–614.

Talbert RL. Drug dosing in renal insufficiency. J Clin Pharmacol 1994;34:99–110.

Tozer TN, Winter ME. Phenytoin. In: Evans WE, Schentag JJ, Jusko WJ, eds. Applied Pharmacokinetics Principles of Therapeutic Drug Monitoring. 3rd ed. Vancouver: Applied Therapeutics Inc, 1992:523–524.

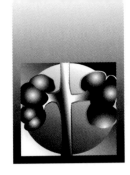

Counseling Patients with Hypertension and Diabetes Mellitus

Wanda G. Miller

BACKGROUND

The incidence of high blood pressure is greatest in African-Americans, in people older than age 60, and in those who lack education. High blood pressure is also more prevalent in lower socioeconomic groups. The incidence of high blood pressure is greater for men than for women until later middle age, when it reverses. High blood pressure, or hypertension, is diagnosed by three separate blood pressure recordings of a systolic reading of 140 or higher or combined with a diastolic reading of 90 and or higher.

Diabetes mellitus is caused by the lack of a pancreatic hormone, insulin, or by the body's incapability to use the insulin. The hormone insulin is essential in metabolism of carbohydrates, a process in which sugars and starches are changed into glucose (blood sugar), the body's principal fuel. Approximately fifty million Americans have what is considered high blood pressure, approximately eleven million have diabetes mellitus,

and roughly three million are diagnosed with both hypertension and diabetes mellitus.

Clients with both hypertension and diabetes mellitus have an increased incidence of renal disease, which accompanies other risk factors including dyslipidemia, increased fibrinogen, hyperuricemia, and left ventricular hypertrophy. Hypertension adds to the leading causes of morbidity and mortality in diabetics, which include organ diseases such as coronary heart disease and end-stage renal disease (ESRD). For these reasons, both hypertension and diabetes mellitus must be diagnosed early and treated aggressively through medications, proper counseling, and education by an informed health care provider.

MEDICATIONS IN COEXISTING CONDITIONS

When hypertension exists concomitantly with another condition, antihypertensive medications should be identified that will not worsen the coexisting condition but instead improve both hypertension and the coexisting condition. Diuretics and beta blockers are effective agents in alleviating hypertension. These drugs may be contraindicated in a diabetic patient; therefore, special precautions must be taken in the patient with coexisting diabetes mellitus (such as close monitoring of glucose levels). Other medications appear satisfactory in the prevention of diabetic nephropathy, such as ACE inhibitors for patients who have both hypertension and diabetes mellitus.

OVERCOMING BARRIERS AND IDENTIFYING PATIENTS' NEEDS

When counseling patients with hypertension or diabetes mellitus, certain barriers to self-care must be addressed. Patients may decide against caring for themselves if they have cultural beliefs or attitudes such as:

- There will be an early cure
- A self-care regimen is too difficult to follow
- My health condition will not improve by using a strict regimen

Additional psychological factors that can influence self-care include:

- Stressful events and the patient's prior coping mechanisms
- A patient's support system
- A patient's attitude and approach toward the medical care provided by the health care practitioner

When these factors have been assessed, the provider can proceed with counseling. Clearly, the first step in counseling is to determine the patient's needs. It is necessary to ascertain a patient's current knowledge of hypertension and/or diabetes mellitus so that an acceptable teaching plan can be developed to fit those needs.

DEVELOPING A TEACHING/COUNSELING PLAN

Hypertension

A teaching plan for hypertension should include:

- Definition of normal blood pressure versus high blood pressure
- Characteristics that facilitate primary or essential hypertension
- Causes of secondary hypertension
- Signs and symptoms of hypertension
- Algorithm of treatment
- Lifestyle modifications

- Dietary sodium restriction
- Alcohol limitations
- Exercise requirements
- Follow-up care as a lifelong process

Attempts to actively engage the patient in selecting and following a course of treatment can be challenging and rewarding for both patient and health care provider. The provider must ask the patient both specific and open-ended questions. Such conversations might identify the patient's individual strengths and the problem-solving strategies that enabled the patient to successfully meet past challenges.

Diabetes Mellitus

A teaching plan for diabetes mellitus requires:

- Definitions of diabetes mellitus, hypoglycemia, and hyperglycemia
- Characteristics of type I versus type II diabetes mellitus
- Complications caused by uncontrolled diabetes mellitus
- Signs and symptoms of hypoglycemia
- Treatment of hypoglycemia
- Signs and symptoms of hyperglycemia
- Treatment of hyperglycemia
- Algorithm of treatment
- Dietary requirements
- Exercise requirements
- Emphasis on blood sugar monitoring
- Foot care instruction
- Insulin therapy (type I) procedure and outcome
- Oral hypoglycemic agents (type II) outcome
- Emphasis on follow-up care as a lifelong process

If the provider believes that a patient knows little about diabetes mellitus or hypertension, the initial goal should be the patient's acknowledgment and acceptance of the condition(s). The next step is to have patients articulate to the health care provider how the disorder affects their daily life.

The next goal involves the patient's acceptance that lifestyle adaptations must be made. Explain to the patient that the treatment plan can be modified to minimize adverse reactions, such as those related to medication (i.e., impotence with certain hypertension medicines). This explanation may help to increase the patient's involvement in constructing a treatment plan, as well as ensure compliance. Additional issues that a diabetic patient must address include:

- Sick leave regulations of employer
- Travel rules

- Diet flexibility and exercise self-management
- Approaches for special occasions

It is advisable for diabetic patients to go beyond the basic rules and increase their knowledge and understanding of the disorder. Special educational sessions are offered by Certified Diabetes Educators (CDE). The primary health care provider can locate a CDE by contacting the American Association of Diabetes Educators, at 1-800-TEAM-UP-4.

Working with teaching plans, encouraging the client, and setting learning outcomes together (sometimes a signed agreement by both patient and provider is helpful) will add to the patient's ability to follow through with a treatment plan.

EVALUATING LEARNING OUTCOMES

Important learning outcomes in patients with diabetes mellitus and hypertension can be evaluated for effectiveness by the patient's ability to verbalize, describe, and demonstrate his or her understanding of the diseases. A list of tasks that the patient should be able to demonstrate to the health care practitioner is presented in Table 23.1.

CHOOSING TEACHING AND COUNSELING TOOLS AND TECHNIQUES

The health care provider uses explanation and discussion of the particular disorder's course and treatments to counsel patients about hypertension or diabetes mellitus. For example, beginning instruction for the patient with hypertension with dietary issues may be less threatening than describing adverse effects of medications. The provider should include demonstrations on the correct method of performing blood pressure monitoring and stress-reducing techniques for relaxation. Printed educational material about hypertension, examples of recipes of low-sodium meals, video materials on healthy diets and exercises, and counseling with a dietitian should be made available to hypertensive patients.

Further teaching and counseling strategies will be directed by how questions such as these are answered: Does the patient acknowledge having the disorder? Are the patient's eating habits changing? Is the patient exercising? Does the patient take all the medication required?

| **TABLE 23.1** | **Evaluating Patient Learning Outcomes** |

Patients with Hypertension Should Be Able To	Patients with Diabetes Mellitus Should Be Able To
Discuss perceptions and emotions about the disease	Discuss perceptions and emotions about disease
Describe how smoking, obesity, alcohol, and salt intake contribute to hypertension	Describe how smoking, obesity, alcohol, and salt intake contribute to diabetes mellitus
List their medications and possible adverse effects	List medications and check for possible adverse effects of drugs on diabetes
Explain how to take their medications	Explain how to take oral hypoglycemic agents
Identify foods with high sodium content	Describe sites suitable for subcutaneous injections of insulin
Develop a meal plan that is appropriate for hypertension	Demonstrate how to inject insulin
Verbalize willingness to perform home blood pressure monitoring	Demonstrate how to check glucose levels
Demonstrate ability to take blood pressure correctly	Explain what actions to take when experiencing hypoglycemia
Describe risks associated with uncontrolled hypertension	Verbalize willingness to perform glucose testing and take medications
Verbalize when regular follow-up care is needed	Describe risks associated with uncontrolled diabetes mellitus
	Verbalize when regular follow-up care is needed

The provider should include demonstrations on obtaining glucose readings and on stress-reducing techniques such as meditation or biofeedback. Printed educational material on diabetes mellitus, examples of meal plans, video materials on self-care related to diabetes, and counseling sessions to cover topics of eye care, nerve damage, and foot care should be made available.

Whichever disorder is being discussed, it is important to not overwhelm the patient with information. Offer only what information can be readily absorbed by a particular patient. Allow enough time for the patient to think about lifestyle adjustments and the impact of the disorder if the patient decides not to comply with treatment. It is equally important to allow time for the patient to express his or her feelings about a changing self-image and an altered lifestyle.

EVALUATING TEACHING AND COUNSELING TECHNIQUES

Research studies and clinical experiences produce compelling evidence that patients increase compliance with and adherence to planned regimens and self-care when a health care provider identifies a patient's particular needs and follows through by reinforcing that patient's progress with each visit. The provider must look at the ongoing evaluation and assessment. Observation indicates the patient's compliance with dietary recommendations; for example, a provider can ask the patient to share new recipes. If weight reduction is an issue, then weighing the patient at each visit is important. The provider can also use return demonstration evaluation: have the patient demonstrate how to take a blood pressure or glucose reading. This will assist the provider in assessing the patient's progress as well as the effectiveness of teaching tools and techniques.

Providers should be knowledgeable regarding the ethnic, regional, and religious issues of their patients. Long-term compliance to a carefully planned and maintained self-care therapeutic program, along with incorporating the use of home care, can prolong or prevent expensive inpatient hospital services. Health care providers should be aware of the economic issues present in providing optimal cost-effective care on a long-term basis.

The provider must recognize that a positive attitude on his or her part is vital in counseling the patient. Compliance with long-term therapy is enhanced when regimens are simplified, understandable, and reinforced.

KEY POINTS

- Hypertension adds to the morbidity and mortality in patients with diabetes, including organ damage caused by coronary artery disease and ESRD.

- Early detection of hypertension and diabetes mellitus and aggressive treatment through proper counseling and education are essential.

- When counseling clients with hypertension or diabetes mellitus, certain barriers to self-care should be addressed. These include a belief of early cure, and attitudes that a self-care regimen is too hard to follow or that a health condition will not improve by following a strict regimen.

- Additional psychological factors that can influence self-care include stressful events, a patient's support system, and a patient's attitude and approach toward his or her medical care.

- A teaching plan for both hypertension and diabetes mellitus is essential.

- Periodic evaluations of learning outcomes in patients with hypertension and diabetes mellitus are essential.

- Further teaching and counseling strategies will be directed by the response to questions that a patient asks.

- Avoid overwhelming patients with more information than they can currently assimilate.

- Allow a patient time to express emotions toward a changing self-image and an altered lifestyle.

- The health care provider must recognize that a positive attitude on his or her part is vital in counseling patients.

- Compliance with long-term therapy is enhanced when regimens are simple, understandable, and reinforced.

SUGGESTED READINGS

American Diabetes Association. Diabetes 1993 Vital Statistics. Chicago: American Diabetes Association, 1993.

Dawson KG, McKenzie JK, Ross SA, et al. Report of the Canadian Hypertension Consensus Conference, 5: hypertension and diabetes. Can Med Assoc J 1993;149:821–826.

Epstein M, Sowers JR. Diabetes mellitus and hypertension. Hypertension 1992;19:403–418.

Joint National Committee. The Fifth Report of the Joint National Committee on detection, evaluation, and treatment of high blood pressure. Arch Intern Med 1993;153:154–183.

Metropolitan New York Association of Diabetes Educators. Guide to Teaching Diabetes Survival Skills. Alexandria, VA: American Association of Diabetes Educators, 1995.

National High Blood Pressure Education Program Working Group. Working Group Report on hypertension and chronic renal failure. Arch Intern Med 1991;151:1280–1287.

U.S. Department of Health and Human Services. The Physician's Guide to Improving Adherence Among Hypertensive Patients. U.S. Department of Health and Human Services, 1987.

U.S. Department of Health and Human Services. The Prevention and Treatment of Complications of Diabetes. U.S. Department of Health and Human Services, 1982.

U.S. Department of Health and Human Services. Take Charge of Your Diabetes—A Guide For Care. U.S. Department of Health and Human Services, 1991.

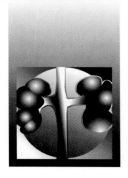

CHAPTER 24

Nutritional Treatment in the Management of Renal Disease

Beth A. Holthausen

BACKGROUND

Elliott Joslin is quoted as saying: "Heredity loads the cannon, but obesity and other stresses pull the trigger." Current epidemiologic and experimental research into the etiology and control of many of the chronic health problems in the United States substantiates Joslin's observation. What we eat and how it is prepared may indeed delay or encourage the pulling of that "trigger,"

affecting the potential development of hypertension, adult-onset diabetes, and cardiovascular disease. Changes in dietary habits, as with all lifestyle changes, are notoriously difficult to achieve, but the view that dietary modification is impractical, ineffective, or doomed to failure is not justified. The success demonstrated by a patient in changing any health habit depends in large part on the primary health care provider's attitude, knowledge, and skill in motivating patient change, as well as the provider's ability to organize a team approach.

No matter the medical problem being treated, nutritional health must be identified as a treatment goal. "Nutritional health," as defined by this author, is the capacity to access and assimilate essential nutrients and energy in a personally acceptable form in sufficient quantity to achieve and maintain medical and life-quality goals. Nutritional health demands a collaboration between the patient and primary care provider. The prevention and control of chronic conditions such as hypertension benefit from this interaction.

HYPERTENSION

Age, relative weight, and alcohol consumption are strong predictors for the development of hypertension and are strongly associated with other adult-onset chronic diseases. Hypertension, which is approximately twice as common in people with diabetes as in the rest of the population, is also closely linked to various manifestations of heart disease. Thirty to seventy-five percent of the complications that develop in diabetes can be attributed to elevated blood pressure. Not only does controlling blood pressure potentially reduce, or perhaps even prevent, those complications, but it may also slow the progress of renal failure and the development of heart disease. Hypertension is a major cause of morbidity and mortality in the United States and in other developed countries. The potential cost savings that could be derived by using low-risk, effective, non-pharmaceutical therapies have resulted in an increased medical interest in encouraging lifestyle modifications. Although there have been indications since the beginning of this century that dietary changes can influence blood pressure, cost-containment measures and an emphasis on prevention have given nutritional therapy a renewed and prominent role in hypertension management.

Nutritional Factors in the Development of Hypertension

The National Blood Pressure Education Program Working Group Report on primary prevention of hypertension summary states: "Weight loss, a reduction in sodium intake, increased physical activity, and avoidance of excessive alcohol consumption appear to be the most efficacious approaches to the prevention (and/or control) of hypertension." Those most likely to develop hypertension are individuals with high-normal blood pressure, a positive family history, and any one or more of the following:

- Caloric imbalance resulting in a body mass index (BMI) greater than 27
- High salt intake
- Lack of physical activity
- Relatively low potassium intake

One can conclude, then, that encouraging the public to adopt appropriate lifestyle changes offers a number of benefits with little cost and minimal risk.

Excessive Body Weight

Despite the development of sugar substitutes, fat substitutes, and calorie- and fat-reduced foods during the past decade, the incidence of overweight in this country continues to climb, reportedly reaching more than 33% of the adult sample evaluated during the 1988–1991 National Health and Nutrition Examination Survey (NHANES). The mean BMI has increased to 26.3 kilogram per square meter. Standards have developed establishing a BMI of 24 to 27 for women and 25 to 27 for men as indicative of overweight. All races and both genders demonstrated these dramatic increases. Those studies that examined the effect of weight on blood pressure show a stepwise increase in pressure with progressively higher levels of body weight. A nomogram has been developed and is readily available for use for determining BMI.

An individual who is 20% over the "ideal body weight" (IBW) has an increased risk of mortality 2.5 to 3 times that of the general population; a person 40% over the IBW increases this risk 5.2 to 7.9 times the average. Waist-to-hip ratios effectively provide a measure of central obesity. A waist-to-hip ratio greater than 0.85 in women and greater than 0.95 in men correlates to increases in hypertension, dyslipidemia, diabetes mellitus, and mortality from coronary heart disease. Indeed, 20 to 30% of cases of hypertension in the United States can be attributed to the prevalence of excess body weight: 53% of overweight women are hypertensive, as are 55% of overweight men. In the Framingham study, an increase in relative weight of just 10% was predictive of a 7 mm Hg rise in blood pressure.

Excessive Salt Intake

Salt intake is considered a key population-wide factor that can influence the frequency of hypertension. In societies where the average sodium intake is as low as 70 mEq/day, there is little hypertension. Hypertension is common and stroke a leading cause of death in those countries where the salt intake is very high (i.e., 9–12 g/day, or 120–150 mEq sodium/day). Although epidemiologic studies have shown this statistically significant relationship between individual habitual high salt intake and hypertension, this effect is by no means experienced by all individuals. Some segments of the population are more salt sensitive than others—particularly obese hypertensive people, the elderly, and African-Americans—although presently there is no reliable way to determine who those salt-sensitive individuals may be. Estimates indicate one of every three people is salt sensitive. The current average intake in the United States is 8 to 12 grams of salt per day (4000–6000 mg sodium), of which 65 to 85% comes from processed foods. The amount of sodium needed daily for health is approximately 500 mg. Despite some controversy over the advisability of a general recommendation to all Americans to reduce salt intake to moderate levels, it appears there is little to be lost and much to be gained from such a recommendation.

Alcohol Consumption

Alcohol contributes approximately 5% to the total calories in the American diet. Three ounces of alcohol, the amount in approximately three mixed drinks, can raise blood pressure in many people by approximately 2 mm Hg. To prevent high blood pressure, alcohol should be limited to no more than two drinks per day.

Exercise

The prevalence of hypertension in inactive adults is greater than in their more active counterparts in all weight categories. The value of an active lifestyle is well established, yet 35% of normal-weight men and 55% of obese men remain inactive. Physical activity not only aids in the maintenance of a healthier weight but also increases overall functional health status while decreasing the risk of cardiovascular disease. Sedentary and nonfit people increase their risk for the development of hypertension by 20 to 50%, compared with their peers who are more active and fit. The numerous health benefits of increased physical activity for all adults support its inclusion as a preventive and maintenance measure.

Other Nutritional Considerations

Potassium   In numerous population studies, potassium intake and blood pressure are inversely related. Potassium is also related to stroke mortality; this effect appears to be unrelated to any change in blood pressure. An increase in potassium intake of 10 mEq/day in one study was related to a 40% decrease in the incidence of stroke-related deaths. This increase in potassium can be easily achieved by increasing fruit and vegetable intake by

High Potassium-containing Foods[a]	TABLE 24.1
Fruits and Juices	**Amounts**
Apricots, dried	7 halves
Avocado	$\frac{1}{3}$
Banana	1 small
Cantaloupe	$\frac{2}{3}$ cup
Dates	7 dried
Grapefruit, fresh	1 whole
Grapefruit juice	1 cup
Honeydew melon	$\frac{1}{3}$ cup
Orange	$1\frac{1}{2}$
Orange juice	$\frac{2}{3}$ cup
Orange and grapefruit juice	1 cup
Pears, fresh	2 each
Pears, dried	4 halves
Prunes, dried	4–6
Prune juice	$\frac{1}{2}$ cup
Tomato juice	$\frac{2}{3}$ cup
Vegetables	**Amounts**
Dried beans and peas (all)	$\frac{1}{3}$ cup
Baked beans	$\frac{1}{3}$ cup
Lima beans	$\frac{1}{3}$ cup
Broccoli	1 cup
Brussels sprouts	$\frac{2}{3}$ cup
Kale	1 cup
Mustard greens	1 cup
Parsnips	$\frac{2}{3}$ cup
Potato, white or sweet	$\frac{2}{3}$ of potato
Spinach, cooked	$\frac{1}{3}$ cup
Swiss chard	$\frac{1}{3}$ cup
Stewed tomato	$\frac{1}{2}$ cup
Winter squash	$\frac{1}{3}$ cup
Succotash	$\frac{2}{3}$ cup

Data adapted from Pennington JAT. Bowes and Church's Food Values of Portions Commonly Used. 16th ed. Philadelphia: Lippincott, 1994.
[a]The following foods provide approximately 8 mEq of potassium per serving as listed.

one to two servings per day. A list of high potassium–containing foods is provided in Table 24.1.

Calcium   A low intake in dietary calcium has been associated with increased arterial pressure. It is worth noting that dietary calcium intake fails to meet recommended levels in virtually all categories in Americans, while sodium intake far exceeds needs. High dietary sodium leads to high urinary calcium levels; this calcium comes from bone. It would make sense that both normotensive and hypertensive individuals, whose intake of calcium is even lower, would benefit from an increase in calcium intake. Although increasing calcium intake is not a first-line treatment, nor perhaps a major preventive measure, studies show that adequate amounts of calcium may be associated with a decreased risk in developing hypertension. Studies are still needed to show if the inadequate calcium intake associated with elevated arterial blood pressure is correctable with calcium supplementation.

Magnesium   Although magnesium has come under considerable study, there is insufficient evidence at this time to support the routine use of magnesium supplementation for hypertension.

Fruits and vegetables   Recently, there has been added emphasis via the United States Department of Agriculture and the Department of Health and Human Services to lower the risk of developing chronic diseases by increased consumption of fruits and vegetables, such as the following:

- Dietary fiber
- Vitamins A and C
- Complex carbohydrates
- Other plant components that may contribute to a lower risk of developing chronic diseases

Approximately 50% of the population of the United States consumes, at most, one serving of vegetables on any given day; 75% of the population may have consumed as much as one fruit or fruit juice serving on any one day. Recommended daily intake is five to nine servings daily. Evidence continues to grow, showing that diets rich in foods of plant origin offer some protection against a number of chronic conditions, including obesity, heart disease, diabetes, and some forms of cancer. An inverse relationship is noted between the development of stroke and fruit and vegetable intake. For each three- to five-serving increment in intake each day, the risk of stroke falls 22%. However, the NHANES II study from which the preceding data originate indicates that this effect is independent of blood pressure, and a prospective study showed that intake of fruit and vegetables is inversely associated with systolic and diastolic pressure.

Nutritional Treatment of Hypertension

Weight reduction and salt restriction have been proven to be the most effective strategies in the nutritional management of high blood pressure. Weight loss can modify obesity and the associated distur-

bances of lipid and carbohydrate metabolism often seen in hypertension.

A reduction in blood pressure usually occurs early in a weight reduction program, often becoming apparent after a loss of only 4 to 5 kg. For overweight patients who require medication, the quantity of drug needed to achieve adequate therapeutic effect may be reduced almost 50% when a weight reduction diet is prescribed and followed in conjunction with such medical treatment.

Moderate salt restriction to 2400 mg of sodium per day, or approximately 6 grams of salt, is the current recommendation for all those with hypertension. A mild salt restriction may prove to be therapeutic in those segments of the population most at risk (i.e., African-Americans and the elderly). This degree of restriction remains a reasonable and achievable goal.

Nutritional management of hypertension relies on overall improvement of dietary habits. Primary focus should be on achievement and maintenance of healthy body weight through diet and exercise, moderating salt intake by reducing intake of high-sodium processed foods, and limiting alcohol intake to no more than two drinks per day. The intake of adequate dietary calcium and five or more servings of fruits and vegetables each day should be encouraged.

CONGESTIVE HEART FAILURE (CHF)

Hypertension that is left untreated or remains poorly controlled is the leading cause of CHF and is frequently associated with the development of left ventricular hypertrophy, cardiac dysrhythmias, and ischemic heart disease. In a recent study of individuals with moderate to severe hypertension, left ventricular mass had decreased after 12 months of sodium restriction, indicating that left ventricular hypertrophy could be decreased nonpharmacologically with moderate sodium restriction.

Undoubtedly, the best treatment for left ventricular hypertrophy is to prevent its development in the first place with early treatment of hypertension.

CHF may progress to cardiac cachexia, as characterized by protein-energy malnutrition, in 35 to 53% of patients with moderate to severe disease; however, cardiac cachexia can occur in any patient with severe malnutrition. These patients require intensive nutritional support and rehabilitation to improve their chances for survival.

Nutritional Treatment of CHF

Restriction of activity and a moderate sodium restriction are primary treatment for patients with CHF, with an overall goal to optimize nutritional status with minimal stress to the heart while minimizing or preventing edema.

The assessment of a patient's nutritional status may be compromised greatly by the presence of edema. Measured weight may appear to be within normal limits, but edema may mask a 10 to 15% weight loss. To monitor nutritional status over time, anthropometrics may be used. For cardiac patients retaining fluid, lean body mass (LBM) may be best estimated by using calf and thigh circumferences followed by measurement of midarm circumference. In those patients with severe CHF who are undernourished, energy needs may be increased 30 to 50% over the basal metabolic rate because of increased energy expenditure by the heart and lungs. This may be difficult to achieve in those experiencing anorexia, early satiety, or shortness of breath and will require creativity and commitment on the part of the caregiver if nutritional needs are to be achieved in the home setting.

General strategies for achieving optimal nutritional status include:

- Multiple small feedings of calorically dense foods offered at times preferred by the patient
- No supplements given with meals because they could result in meal replacement rather than supplement
- The patient being well rested to maximize the feeding opportunities
- Fluids offered at the end of the meal to minimize bloating
- Gas-forming foods limited to minimize bloating
- Referral to a registered dietitian to aid caregiver and patient in achieving improved nutritional health

If carefully planned oral feedings do not result in improvement of nutritional health, enteral feedings are indicated. No medical condition is improved by prolonged starvation.

CHF patients whose activities are limited by their illness yet remain overweight require weight reduction to reduce stress on the compromised heart muscle. Because of limitations on exercise, calories must be restricted to 1000 to 1200 kcal/day. These diets require careful planning to assure nutritional adequacy.

For patients with mild heart failure without symptoms or congestion, sodium restriction and sometimes fluid restriction is all that is required. Moderate to severe CHF is generally controlled with sodium restricted to 1 to 2 g/day. With improvement, sodium intake may be increased to 3 to 4 g/day. Although 1 mL of fluid per kcal of energy expended is generally needed by adults, a moderate restriction of 1000 mL/day may be an appropriate starting point when fluid restriction is required. Close monitoring of the patient's tolerance to restrictions and the effectiveness of those restrictions is indicated. Daily weighing before the first meal of the day is essential. An unexplained weight gain of 2 to 3 lbs in 24 hours must be evaluated. Extremely low sodium diets are rarely required and are not only nutritionally inadequate but also unpalatable. An increase in diuretic use and less severe sodium restriction improve compliance to the diet.

Very low sodium diets can result in hyponatremia, hypochloremia, and eventual azotemia with the fall in the glomerular filtration rate (GFR). Symptoms include weakness, lassitude, anorexia, vomiting, abdominal cramps, aching skeletal muscles, and mental confusion. Digitalis toxicity can cause these same symptoms, as well as the potential for hallucinations and depression and, more importantly, cardiac arrhythmias, especially in those patients who are treated with nonpotassium–sparing diuretics. Encouraging the patient to eat high potassium-containing foods may be adequate (Table 24.1), but some patients require potassium supplementation. Salt substitutes may contain 13 to 72 mEq potassium/teaspoon and can be highly effective in assuring adequate potassium intake in those patients with adequate renal function who are not taking potassium-sparing diuretics.

DIABETES MELLITUS

Of the complications that arise from diabetes, 30 to 75% can be attributed to hypertension. Thus, nutritional strategies used in the prevention and treatment of hypertension are equally, if not more, important for the diabetic patient.

The American Diabetes Association has established five goals for nutrition therapy to assist in preventing, delaying, or managing diabetes complications. These are summarized as follows:

- Maintain near-normal blood glucose levels by balancing food, insulin, and activity.
- Achieve optimal lipid levels.
- Provide adequate calories to achieve or maintain reasonable weight in adults. Reasonable weight is defined as "that level of weight individuals and health care providers acknowledge as achievable and maintainable both short- and long-term." Thus, this may be a weight that is considerably greater than the "ideal" weight based on height and frame size.
- Prevent, delay, or treat nutrition-related risk factors and complications.
- Improve overall health through optimal nutrition.

To assess individual progress toward attaining these goals, blood glucose, glycated hemoglobin, lipids, blood pressure, and weight must be monitored and management plans altered accordingly.

Nutritional Treatment of Diabetes Mellitus

For patients requiring insulin, it is important to implement dietary advice, which is based on usual eating and exercise patterns. An adult who has not eaten breakfast in 20 years is not likely to start now and continue with it. It is far better to achieve day-to-day consistency, synchronizing meal times with insulin peak actions. This action not only increases ease of adherence but also assists in achieving more nearly normal blood glucose levels. Analysis of the Diabetes Control and Complications Trial (DCCT) confirms that blood glucose control is the single most important factor in preventing or delaying the chronic complications of diabetes.

Ninety percent of people with diabetes have non–insulin-dependent diabetes mellitus (NIDDM), which is frequently complicated by obesity. For years, dietary advice has focused on achieving weight loss; however, currently used dietary strategies are often insufficient to achieve significant or long-term weight loss in the majority of people. Rather than concentrating on weight as a goal, the focus should be on improved metabolic control, requiring routine monitoring. Glucose monitoring can quickly give patients feedback on the degree of metabolic success they achieve when implementing a new dietary behavior, such as adjusting the spacing of meals throughout the day. Improved meal spacing helps to prevent exaggerated postmeal hyperglycemia, which occurs after large meals. Incorporating regular physical activity as a nutritional strategy not only facilitates weight control and improves metabolic control but also has the potential to prevent or delay the onset of type II diabetes in those individuals at risk.

A moderate daily caloric restriction of 250 to 500 kcal less than the average daily intake combined with an increase in physical activity may lead to gradual and perhaps more sustainable weight loss. A weight loss of 5 to 10 kg is often sufficient to improve glycemic control, increase insulin sensitivity and perhaps insulin secretion, and positively affect blood pressure and serum lipid levels. Those who are able to maintain this loss for 1 year continue to have significant improvement in fasting blood sugar, glycated hemoglobin, low-density lipoprotein cholesterol, and triglycerides.

Macronutrients

Protein   Currently, insufficient evidence exists to support protein intakes either higher or lower than the recommended intakes for the general population. The recommended dietary protein intake for adults is 0.8 g/kg/body weight. Recent surveys show that the average intake for all age groups of the United States population varies from 14 to 18% of total caloric intake, almost twice the recommended amount. A high protein intake may increase the workload on the kidney in the diabetic patient. Limiting protein intake may attenuate overt diabetic nephropathy and slow the progression of chronic renal failure (CRF). Protein intake corresponding to the recommended daily allowance of 0.8 g/kg body weight/day appears to be sufficiently restricted and is recommended for individuals with evidence of nephropathy.

Fat and carbohydrates   Individuals with type I diabetes exhibit an increase in triglycerides as a result of a lack of insulin. People with type II diabetes have twice the incidence of hypertriglyceridemia and elevated levels of low-density lipoproteins as those without diabetes; this incidence is thought to be related to insulin resistance and hyperinsulinism. The risk for heart disease as compared with those with normal carbohydrate tolerance and normal lipid levels is increased three- to fourfold. In view of this risk, saturated fat intake should be no more than 10% of total calories. The remaining total calories are then provided according to treatment goals, eating habits, and preferences of the individual being treated. Generally, total fat is restricted to 30% of calories or less, leaving the majority of calories to be supplied by carbohydrates. High carbohydrate diets, when followed by some patients with NIDDM, may result in elevated triglyceride and cholesterol levels, promote hyperinsulinemia, and cause a worsening of glycemic control. These patients may benefit from a diet high in monounsaturated fat. The so-called "Mediterranean diet," one component of which is large amounts of olive oil (monounsaturated fatty acids), reportedly improves not only glycemic control but also blood pressure control, while decreasing the risk of cardiovascular disease. The response to differing levels and types of fats varies, pointing to the need to individualize therapy.

Sucrose   Historically, sucrose (table sugar) has been the major food item forbidden for use by those with diabetes. All too frequently, it appears to be the only dietary concept with which those with diabetes seem to be concerned. However, studies examining the glycemic effects of sugar do not support this restriction, and recent recommendations allow for the use of sugar within the context of a healthful diet.

Within the general population, the average daily intake of sugar is approximately 41 grams (8 teaspoons), or 9% of total caloric intake. A prudent approach for the use of sugar is to:

- Recognize that sugar is a form of carbohydrate and must be substituted for other carbohydrates in the diet
- Incorporate sugar only if blood sugar is under control (i.e., serum glucose consistently under 200 mg/dL)
- Consider the presence of other nutrients frequently ingested in combination with sucrose, such as fat, which will affect not only total calories provided but also overall nutrient distribution

Sodium   As noted earlier, individuals with diabetes mellitus may be more sensitive to salt and its effect on blood pressure and have an increased incidence of hypertension than the general public. Because of this association, the American Diabetes Association affirms the position of the American Heart Association in recommending that total sodium intake not exceed 3000 mg/day. For those with moderate hypertension, sodium intake should be reduced to no more than 2400 mg/day.

Micronutrients

Vitamins and minerals   For those who follow a healthful diet, there is probably little need for vitamin or mineral supplementation. Some people may be at greater risk for suboptimal nutrition, indicating evaluation for possible supplementation. People on weight-reducing diets, strict vegetarians, the elderly, pregnant or lactating women, those in poor metabolic control, individuals taking medications known to alter micronutrient metabolism, and those in critical care environments are all at some risk for a less than optimal micronutrient status.

Despite many studies examining the theory that type II diabetes may be secondary to a micronutrient deficiency, particularly deficiencies of zinc or chromium, little data support these theories. A more important association has been identified with magnesium. Magnesium depletion has been associated with insulin insensitivity, which, in those with NIDDM, may improve with oral supplementation. Additionally, patients in poor glycemic control who receive diuretics may require magnesium supplementation.

NEPHROPATHY AND DIABETES

Diabetic nephropathy occurs approximately 15 years after the onset of diabetes in those with type I disease, but its onset is much more rapid in those with type II disease, frequently developing within 1 to 5 years. Nephropathy is an important cause of hypertension in this population. Adequate control of hypertension is probably the single most important determinant of renal outcome. Clinical evidence of nephropathy is first seen as proteinuria. Poor glycemic control increases the risk for developing this condition, while hypertension serves to hasten its progression. The progression of renal disease can be slowed by:

- Limiting protein intake to 0.8 g/kg/body weight
- Aggressively monitoring and treating high blood pressure
- Achieving and maintaining good glycemic control
- Addressing any cardiovascular risk factors present

These health measures can do much to reduce the incidence of end-stage renal disease (ESRD). Four of ten persons who have had insulin-dependent diabetes mellitus (IDDM) for more than 20 years develop ESRD. Approximately one-third of all new cases are attributable to diabetes, accounting for almost $1 billion per year in health care expense.

Nutritional Treatment of Diabetes

The complications of diabetes may be reduced with the following strategies:

- Decrease insulin resistance. Successful weight reduction together with increased activity improves glucose metabolism.
- Control hyperglycemia through diet.
- Reduce cardiovascular risk. Dietary strategies should be employed to assist in the management of hypertension and hyperlipidemia.
- Delay onset of nephropathy. Implement control of protein intake with the onset of proteinuria.

RENAL FAILURE

Nutritional Treatment of Renal Failure

Approximately 45% of all patients with ESRD experience mild to severe malnutrition. The causes are varied but may be categorized as follows:

- Reduced food intake as a result of anorexia or early satiety
- Intervening catabolic illnesses

- Nutrient loss to the dialysate
- Stimulation of protein catabolism by hemodialysis
- Acidemia

Because of the documented increase in morbidity and mortality rates associated with protein-calorie malnutrition, it is important to monitor nutritional status periodically using well-established criteria and alter treatment as indicated. A registered dietitian, preferably experienced in renal disease, should be consulted.

Protein

Protein restriction has been a mainstay in the treatment of renal failure for several decades, having first been shown to improve uremic symptoms in 1918. The Modification of Diet and Renal Disease (MDRD) multicenter trial has made recommendations of dietary protein intake of 0.8 g/kg/day for patients whose GFR is greater than 55 mL/min but reduced to 0.6 g/kg/day for those whose GFR is 25 to 55 mL/min, with 60% high biologic value in each case.

Protein needs for the patient undergoing peritoneal dialysis or hemodialysis are increased in part because of protein and amino acid loss during treatment and the catabolic stimulus of hemodialysis. Dietary intake should approximate 1.2 to 1.5 g/kg/day. This may be difficult to achieve in patients on peritoneal dialysis, who frequently have alterations in taste. In addition, the absorption of dialysate dextrose may suppress the appetite. Frequent evaluation of serum albumen levels and appropriate nutritional counseling are required.

Energy   Energy requirements for the patient with CRF do not differ from those for normal individuals. Most authorities recommend 35 kcal/kg/day for normal-weight individuals; those who are obese may be prescribed a lower caloric intake. The caloric contribution of the dextrose in dialysate must also be considered for those patients receiving peritoneal dialysis and may account for as much as 25 to 33% of daily caloric intake.

Lipids

Cardiovascular disease is the most frequently cited cause of death among hemodialysis patients. Some research also indicates that elevated levels of blood lipids can accelerate the decline in renal function. Elevated triglyceride levels may also respond to a dietary increase in polyunsaturated fats.

Calcium and Phosphorus

With a fall in GFR, phosphorus is retained in the plasma. This retention plays an important role in the development of secondary hyperparathyroidism and in an increase in parathyroid hormone (PTH). To protect against the development of renal osteodystrophy, calcium intake must be high while dietary phosphorus is restricted. Because phosphorus is closely tied to protein, a protein-restricted diet often is associated with adequate phosphorus restriction. However, high calcium foods are also high in phosphorus, necessitating calcium supplementation by nonfood sources. Calcium-containing phosphate binders in conjunction with a low phosphate diet, when taken as prescribed, effectively provide 1 to 2 grams of elemental calcium per day.

Many patients continue to have hypocalcemia despite calcium supplementation. Vitamin D in the form of calcitriol may be used to increase serum calcium levels, suppress PTH secretion, and promote normal bone architecture.

Magnesium

Patients with renal failure are at risk for developing hypermagnesemia, which can exacerbate already existing bone disease. Severe elevations of magnesium are rare unless the patient has received an excessive amount, commonly through medications such as Maalox, Gelusil, milk of magnesia, or cascara sagrada. Patients need to be cautioned that phosphate binders can be very constipating. The use of bran or other high-fiber foods in conjunction with light exercise should be encouraged, and the medications listed avoided.

Sodium and Fluid

The kidney's ability to adapt to large increases or reductions in sodium intake is impaired in advanced renal failure. A sudden increase in sodium intake may result in edema, worsening hypertension, and CHF. Renal concentrating and diluting mechanisms are usually impaired as well, affecting the patient's natural ability to regulate water balance. Usually, sodium is restricted to 70 mEq (3 g)/day, and fluid is restricted to 1000 mL/day, plus urinary output. Weight increases between hemodialysis treatments should be no more than 2 lb/day.

Potassium

Patients with advanced renal failure are at high risk for developing life-threatening hyperkalemia, particularly if they are ingesting a high potassium diet or inappropriately using potassium-containing salt substitutes. Insufficient caloric intake can also contribute to a rising serum potassium level because the body is forced to use protein stores for energy, releasing potassium into the extracellular space. When potassium levels slowly increase, patients may be asymptomatic; monitoring serum levels is essential. Restriction of 30 to 50 mEq/day is usually prescribed.

Vitamins

Diets that are restricted in protein, potassium, and phosphorus are deficient in water-soluble vitamins and should be replaced.

No supplements of fat-soluble vitamins are needed. Vitamin A supplements are not recommended because even a small excess may cause vitamin A toxicity, with increased bone resorption.

ACUTE RENAL FAILURE (ARF)

Nutritional Treatment of ARF

Early attention to adequate nutritional support, often in the form of total parenteral nutrition, improves patient survival rates. Close attention must be paid to protein and amino acid intake, energy needs, and fluid and electrolyte requirements.

NEPHROTIC SYNDROME

Nutritional Treatment of Nephrotic Syndrome

The recommended protein intake for patients remains controversial, although most authorities now caution against a high protein intake (> 1.5 g/kg/day), which increases glomerular pressure and accelerates the course of renal disease. A diet consisting of 0.7 g protein/kg/day plus 1 g protein/day for each gram/day urinary loss is usually employed. This diet may reduce urinary protein loss and minimize protein malnutrition.

CALCIUM NEPHROLITHIASIS

The development of kidney stones (calcium nephrolithiasis) may be prevented or reduced by increasing urinary volume. Many people, especially older men, habitually consume limited amounts of fluid; however, patients should be encouraged to consume enough fluid to produce at least 2 L/day of urine. One useful prescription is to consume two 8-ounce glasses of water every 4 hours while awake.

Nutritional Treatment of Calcium Nephrolithiasis

Hypercalciuria

Calcium oxalate stones comprise approximately 75% of all kidney stones; hypercalciuria may be the single most important condition underlying calcium stone formation. Idiopathic hypercalciuria is predominantly a disease of men in the third to fifth decade of life. Associated with obesity and hypertension, the condition is also familial. Hypercalciuria can be exacerbated by several dietary factors, the most important of which is dietary sodium, which increases renal calcium excretion. High intake of animal protein increases the excretion of urate and calcium. Calcium restriction should not be implemented because it may promote hyperoxaluria by enhancing intestinal oxalate absorption. Patients should be counseled to maintain a moderate calcium intake of two to three dairy servings per day to minimize bone loss and prevent increased urinary oxalate.

Hyperoxaluria

Enteric hyperoxaluria results from intestinal overabsorption commonly seen in diseases of the small intestine or with excessive intake of vitamin C (i.e., 2 g/day). Increased absorption can be caused by a diet high in oxalate, intestinal malabsorption, or calcium restriction in those with idiopathic hypercalciuria.

Although many foods may have high levels of oxalate, only the following nine foods have been shown to raise urinary oxalate excretion: rhubarb, spinach, strawberries, chocolate, wheat, bran, nuts, beets, and tea. Elimination of these foods may reduce urinary oxalate excretion.

NUTRITION COUNSELING

Nutritional factors to be considered in the management of hypertension, CHF, diabetes mellitus, renal failure, and renal stones have a great deal of commonality:

- Maintenance of desirable weight and activity levels
- Avoidance of excessive amounts of salt and alcohol
- A daily diet including a variety of fruits and vegetables

The food guide pyramid should be used as a basic counseling tool.

Poor adherence to lifestyle modifications and pharmacologic therapy has been identified as a major reason for inadequate control of blood pressure and blood sugar levels. Possible causes of poor adherence include:

- Low level of education on the part of the patient
- Unclear instructions
- Inadequate or no patient education
- Lack of patient involvement in the treatment plan

Printed materials are widely used in patient education programs but may be poorly understood by those for whom the information is intended. Promotion of a healthy lifestyle should begin in childhood and continue through adolescence, before dietary and activity habits that contribute to overweight are established. Adults benefit from repeated and continued interventions to assist them in making beneficial changes.

Although many health and professional organizations recommend that primary care physicians provide nutrition counseling as a routine part of preventive health care, surveys of both physicians and the public show that most physicians do not do so. Reasons include lack of nutrition knowledge and counseling skills, lack of reimbursement for time spent on nutrition counseling, and the physician's **expectations of patient noncompliance.**

The physician remains the most trusted source of diet and nutrition information for patients. The long-term relationships established with patients can be used to good advantage in educating the patient regarding diet and health. Many patients indicate that if they received such guidance from their physicians, they would be greatly helped in achieving a more healthful diet. Failure to receive this information causes many to turn to less reliable sources of information. Information and counseling, as well as other indications of personal interest, directly and positively influence patient satisfaction with the care provided.

PROGRAMS FOR NUTRITIONAL INTERVENTION

Several programs for incorporating brief nutritional interventions have been developed and successfully im-

KEY POINTS

- It is evident that blood pressure increases stepwise with progressively increasing body weight.

- A body weight that is 20% over the IBW increases the risk of mortality by a factor of 2.5 to 3.4; a body weight that is 40% over the IBW increases this risk 5.2 to 7.9 times the average.

- A waist-to-hip ratio greater than 0.85 in women and greater than 0.95 in men correlates with increases in hypertension, dyslipidemia, diabetes mellitus, and mortality from coronary heart disease.

- In societies with very high salt intake (9–12 g/day), hypertension is common and stroke a leading cause of death.

- Some segments of the population are more salt sensitive than others, particularly individuals who are obese, those who are hypertensive, and African-Americans.

- Increased physical activity has numerous health benefits and should be recommended as a preventive measure for hypertension.

- Although increasing calcium intake is not a first-line treatment, nor, perhaps, a major preventive measure, studies show

that it may be associated with a decreased risk in developing hypertension.

- Weight reduction and salt restriction have been proven to be the most effective strategies in the nutritional management of high blood pressure.

- For many people with mild hypertension, weight reduction alone may be all that is required to bring about adequate blood pressure control.

- There is little doubt that the best treatment for left ventricular hypertrophy is to prevent its development in the first place with early detection and treatment of hypertension.

- Individuals with CHF who are overweight and have limited activity should be restricted to 1000 to 1200 kcal/day.

- Approximately 45% of all patients with ESRD experience mild to severe malnutrition.

- Protein restriction has been recognized for decades as a mainstay in the treatment of renal failure.

- It is recommended that a registered dietitian, preferably experienced in renal disease, be involved in the treatment of patients with renal failure.

plemented. The Nutrition Screening Initiative, a project of the American Academy of Family Physicians, the American Dietetic Association, and the National Council on the Aging, strives to identify those patients who are most at risk for poor nutritional status. Specific interventions and suggestions for incorporating interventions into daily practice are provided.

The American Dietetic Association/Foundation, in cooperation with the American Academy of Family Physicians, the Society of General Internal Medicine, and the American Medical Association, has implemented an educational initiative designed to provide primary care practitioners with practical, efficient strategies for incorporating nutrition screening and intervention into daily patient care routines. Many registered dietitians have been trained to provide practitioners with the information and tools needed to use the information provided through this initiative.

One of the objectives of Healthy People 2000 is to "increase the proportion of primary care providers who provide nutrition assessment and counseling and/or referrals." Physicians and other primary care providers can play a limited but effective role in promoting healthy eating habits. Long-term dietary change is more likely to occur after high-contact intervention through multiple channels; a team approach is recommended.

The American Dietetic Association recommends that all patients with NIDDM be referred to a registered dietitian within the first month of diagnosis, with follow-up scheduled within 1 to 2 weeks. For this referral to be effective, the physician needs to communicate appropriate treatment goals to the dietitian, which include glycemic, lipid, and blood pressure control, as well as weight management. Treatment also needs to consider educational and behavioral objectives; quality of life issues; possible reduction or change in medications; and strategies to delay long-term complications.

Nutritional treatment provided by registered dietitians can have significant and positive impact on the patient's ability to understand and adhere to prescribed dietary changes. Dietitians available to do individual counseling can be found through the American Dietetic Association's Nationwide Nutrition Network.

SUGGESTED READINGS

American Diabetes Association. Maximizing the Role of Nutrition in Diabetes Management. Alexandria, VA: American Diabetes Association, 1994b.

Dietary Guidelines Advisory Committee. Report of the Advisory Committee on the Dietary Guidelines for Americans. Hyattsville, MD: USDA, USDHHS, 1995.

Fishman P. Healthy People 2000: what progress toward better nutrition? Geriatrics 1996;51:38–42.

Healthy People 2000: National Promotion and Disease Prevention Objectives. Washington, DC: USDHHS, US Government Printing Office, 1990.

Herman W , ed. The Prevention and Treatment of Complications of Diabetes: A Guide for Primary Care Practitioners. Atlanta, GA: Division of Diabetes Translation, DHHS, PHS, CDC, National Center for Chronic Disease Prevention and Health Promotion, 1991.

Joint National Committee on Detection, Evaluation, and Treatment of High Blood Pressure. The Fifth Report of the Joint National Committee on detection, evaluation, and treatment of high blood pressure (JNC V). Arch Intern Med 1993;153:154.

Kumanyika SK. Feasibility and efficacy of sodium reduction. Trials of hypertension prevention, phase I. Hypertension 1993;22:502–512.

National Heart, Lung, and Blood Institute. Workshop on salt and blood pressure. Hypertension 1991;17 (suppl I):1–222.

National High Blood Pressure Education Working Group. Report on primary prevention of hypertension. Arch Intern Med 1993;153:186.

Patterson BH, Block G, Rosenberger WP, et al. Fruit and vegetables in the American diet: data from NHANES II survey. Am J Pub Health 1990;80:1443.

Registered Dietitians Association Subcommittee on the Tenth Edition of the RDA. Recommended Dietary Allowances. 10th ed. Washington, DC: National Academy Press, 1989.

Index

Page numbers in *italics* denote figures; those followed by "t" denote tables.